Color Atlas and Text of

BONE MARROW TRANSPLANTATION

Edited by

Jennifer Treleaven
MD FRCP FRCPath
Consultant Haematologist and Honorary Senior Lecturer
The Royal Marsden Hospital
London, England

and

Peter Wiernik
MD
Department of Oncology
Montefiore Medical Center
Bronx, New York
USA

Foreword by

A John Barrett
MD, MRCP, FRCPath
Hematology Unit
National Institute of Health
Bethesda, MD
USA

Mosby-Wolfe

London Baltimore Bogotá Boston Buenos Aires Caracas Carlsbad, CA Chicago Madrid Mexico City Milan Naples, FL New York Philadelphia St. Louis Sydney Tokyo Toronto Wiesbaden

Copyright © 1995 Times Mirror International Publishers Limited

Published in 1995 by Mosby-Wolfe, an imprint of Times Mirror International Publishers Limited

Printed by Grafos, S.A. ARTE SOBRE PAPEL

ISBN 0 7234 1798 9

All rights reserved. No part of this publication may be reproduced, stored in a retrieval system, copied or transmitted, in any form or by any means, electronic, mechanical, photocopying, recording or otherwise without written permission from the Publisher or in accordance with the provisions of the Copyright Act 1956 (as amended), or under the terms of any licence permitting limited copying issued by the Copyright Licensing Agency, 33–34 Alfred Place, London, WC1E 7DP.

Any person who does any unauthorised act in relation to this publication may be liable to criminal prosecution and civil claims for damages.

Permission to photocopy or reproduce solely for internal or personal use is permitted for libraries or other users registered with the Copyright Clearance Center, provided that the base fee of $4.00 per chapter plus $.10 per page is paid directly to the Copyright Clearance Center, 21 Congress Street, Salem, MA 01970. This consent does not extend to other kinds of copying, such as copying for general distribution, for advertising or promotional purposes, for creating new collected works, or for resale.

For full details of all Times Mirror International Publishers Limited titles, please write to Times Mirror International Publishers Limited, Lynton House, 7–12 Tavistock Square, London WC1H 9LB, England.

A CIP catalogue record for this book is available from the British Library.

Library of Congress Cataloging-in-Publication Data Applied For

Project Manager:	Roderick Craig
Developmental Editor:	Jennifer Prast
Cover Design:	Lara Last
Illustration:	Lee Smith & Linda Payne
Production:	Jane Tozer
Index:	Jill Halliday
Publisher:	Richard Furn

CONTENTS

List of Contributors		6
Foreword and Preface		7
Acknowledgements		8
I	**INTRODUCTION**	9
	Sylvia Benjamin	
	Early history of bone marrow transplantation	9
	Recent history of allogeneic bone marrow transplantation	10
	Tissue typing	11
	Types of bone marrow transplantation	13
	Goals of bone marrow transplantation	15
	Indications for bone marrow transplantation	15
	The course of bone marrow transplantation	16
	Results of bone marrow transplantation	17
II	**CONDITIONS CORRECTABLE BY BONE MARROW TRANSPLANTATION**	**19**
	1. Inborn Errors of Metabolism	19
	Peter Hoogerbrugge, Ashok Vellodi and Roberto Pasquini	
	Introduction	19
	Bone marrow transplantation in animal models of lysosomal enzyme deficiency	20
	Results of bone marrow transplantation in patients suffering from lysosomal storage diseases	21
	Hurler's disease (MPS-IH) and San Filippo's disease (MPS-III)	22
	Gaucher's disease	28
	Conclusions	29
	Fanconi's anaemia	30
	2. Inherited Defects in Red Cell Production	37
	Caterina Borgna-Pignatti	
	Thalassaemia	37
	Sickle cell anaemia	43
	3. Severe Aplastic Anaemia	49
	Roberto Pasquini	
	4. Primary Immunodeficiency Diseases	55
	Jayesh Mehta	
	The nature of stem cell engraftment required for correction	56
	Conditioning regimens	56
	Graft rejection	57
	Graft-versus-host disease	57
	Use of alternative sources of normal stem cells	58
	Recovery of immune function post–transplant	58
	B-lymphocyte proliferative disease	59
	Results	59
	Alternative therapy	59
	Gene therapy	60

	5. Leukaemias, Lymphomas and Myeloma *John Luckit and Jennifer Treleaven*	63
	Leukaemias	63
	Lymphomas	69
	Multiple myeloma	72
	6. Solid Tumours *Joseph A Sparano, Nicolae Ciobanu and Rasim Gucalp*	77
	Preclinical evidence supporting a dose–response effect	77
	Drugs amenable to dose escalation	79
	Clinical evidence supporting a dose–response effect	80
	High-dose chemotherapy plus autologous bone marrow transplantation for the treatment of solid tumours	82
	Conclusions	97
III	**BONE MARROW HARVESTING** *Keith Patterson*	**101**
	Donor preparation	101
	Harvest procedure	102
	Bone marrow reinfusion	106
IV	**BONE MARROW PROCESSING** *Keith Patterson*	**109**
	Red cell, plasma and T-cell depletion	109
	Stem cell cryopreservation	110
	Cryopreservation without a programmable freezer	114
	Quality control of stem cell cryopreservation	114
	Marrow purging	115
V	**BONE MARROW PURGING** *John Kemshead and Adrian Gee*	**117**
	Detection	117
	Physical techniques	121
	Chemical techniques	122
	Immunological techniques	123
VI	**VENOUS ACCESS** *Richard Stacey and Jacqueline Filshie*	**129**
	Central venous catheters	130
	Implantable devices	138
VII	**GRAFT-VERSUS-HOST DISEASE** *Edward Kanfer*	**143**
	Acute and chronic Graft-versus-host disease	143
	Aetiology	144
	Options for prophylaxis	145
	Conclusion	150

VIII	**PATIENT CONDITIONING**	**155**
	1. Total Body Irradiation *Peter Barrett-Lee*	155
	2. Chemotherapy Conditioning Agents *Edward Kanfer*	161
	Complications of conditioning therapy	162
	Individual agents	162
	Combinations of cytotoxic agents	165
	Conclusions	165
IX	**PROBLEMS FOLLOWING BONE MARROW TRANSPLANTATION**	**169**
	1. Pulmonary Complications *Susan Height*	169
	Pneumothorax	169
	Pulmonary oedema	170
	Pulmonary haemorrhage	170
	Pulmonary embolus	170
	Infections	170
	Idiopathic pneumonitis	177
	Long-term pulmonary complications	178
	2. Cerebral Infections *Rosemary Barnes*	181
	3. Graft-Versus-Host Disease *Jane Norton*	185
	Clinical features	185
	Histological features	188
X	**LATE EFFECTS OF BONE MARROW TRANSPLANTATION** *Jennifer Treleaven*	**193**
	Chronic graft-versus-host disease	194
	Growth and development	195
	Fertility	196
	Ophthalmic complications	196
	Respiratory function	196
	Infection	197
	Second malignancies	197
	Autoimmune disorders and thyroid disfunction	198
	Bone problems and musculoskeletal dysfunction	198
	Neurological problems	198
	Renal function	198
	Hepatic function	199
INDEX		**201**

CONTRIBUTORS

Peter Barrett-Lee MD MRCP
Senior Registrar in Radiotherapy
The Middlesex Hospital
London, UK

Sylvia Benjamin MRCP
Senior Registrar in Haematology
The Radcliffe Hospitals
Oxford, UK

Rosemary Barnes MD MRCP MRCPath
Consultant in Medical Microbiology
University of Wales College of Medicine
Cardiff, Wales, UK

Caterina Borgna-Pignatti MD
Clinica Pediatrica, Policlinico Roma
Verona, Italy

Nicolae Ciobanu MD
Albert Einstein Cancer Center
New York, USA

Jacqueline Filshie FFARCS
Consultant Anaesthetist,
The Royal Marsden Hospital,
Sutton, Surrey, UK

Adrian P Gee PhD
Division of Transplant Medicine
University of South Carolina
Columbia, South Carolina, USA

Rasim Gucalp MD
Assistant Professor of Medicine
Montefiore Medical Center
New York, USA

Susan Height MRCP
Research Fellow and Honorary Senior Registrar
in Haematology
The Royal Marsden Hospital
Sutton, Surrey, UK

Peter M Hoogerbrugge MD PhD
Department of Paediatrics
University Hospital
Leiden, The Netherlands

Edward Kanfer MRCP MRCPath
Consultant in Haematology
Charing Cross Hospital
London, UK

John Kemshead PhD
ICRF Laboratories
Franchay Hospital
Bristol, UK

John Luckit MRCP MRCPath
Consultant Haematologist
The North Middlesex Hospital
London, UK

Jayesh Mehta MD
Leukaemia Unit
Royal Marsden Hospital
Surrey, UK

Jane Norton MB BS
Senior Registrar in Histopathology
St. Mary's Hospital
London, UK

Roberto Pasquini MD
University Hospital
Federal University of Paran
Curitiba, Brazi

Keith Patterson MRCP MRCPath
Senior Lecturer in Haematology
and Honorary Consultant
The Middlesex Hospital
London, UK

Joseph A Sparano MD FACP
Assistant Professor of Medicine,
Montefiore Medical Center,
New York,
USA

Richard Stacey FFARCP
Consultant Anaesthetist
The West Middlesex Hospital
London, UK

Jennifer Treleaven MD FRCP FRCPath
Consultant Haematologist and
Honorary Senior Lecturer
The Royal Marsden Hospital
Surrey, UK

Ashok Vellodi MRCP
Department of Paediatrics
Institute of Child Health
London, UK

FOREWORD

Bone marrow transplantation is being used increasingly worldwide in the treatment of a wide spectrum of malignant and non-malignant disorders. It requires complicated procedures and a high quality of patient care, involving a wide range of health-care staff from the laboratory to the operating room and bedside. The high level of expertise required from the transplant team cannot be achieved without training.

In the last decade there has been a deluge of publications on marrow transplantation, including scientific papers, articles and reviews, two dedicated journals and a number of textbooks. For the newcomer wishing to obtain a grasp of the practical aspects of the subject, this profusion of information can be daunting. There is, therefore, a need for an introductory overview. The *Color Atlas and Text of Bone Marrow Transplantation* amply fills this requirement. The editors, Jennifer Treleaven and Peter Wiernik, both experts in the field of bone marrow transplantation, have assembled a unique collection of pictures, text and diagrams that speak louder than many words. Bone marrow transplantation is a vast discipline. We use our eyes to diagnose and monitor our patients, and diagrams to understand complicated procedures and biological interactions. An atlas is an excellent way to accomplish this, combining text and images that help to demystify the subject. The book is full of clinical photographs, photomicrographs and photographs of x-rays, amply covering such subjects as graft-versus-host disease and infective complications. Readily accessible to a wide readership it compliments the larger textbooks that have recently been produced on the subject. The *Color Atlas and Text of Bone Marrow Transplantation* should find a home in all marrow transplant units. It will be an invaluable review for all the staff involved in this multidisciplinary field.

A John Barrett MD, MRCP, FRCPath

PREFACE

This little book is designed to provide an overview of the vast discipline of bone marrow transplantation and to highlight its more pictorial aspects. We have aimed to briefly discuss the disorders for which the procedure is used and to provide an historical perspective of the discipline. The problems encountered during and after bone marrow transplantation are numerous, and encompass among other things, infective complications, graft-versus-host disease and the various late effects of bone marrow transplantation. The latter are particularly relevant now as many treated patients may be expected to live a normal life span. We have also introduced some material concerning preparation of patients for the procedure, including harvesting bone marrow or peripheral blood stem cells, bone marrow purging, and an outline of some of the preparative chemoradiotherapy regimens.

Some aspects of bone marrow transplantation are, naturally, more pictorial than others, and this book is not in any way designed to be all-embracing in what it covers of the subject. However, we hope that it will provide a starting block for further in-depth reading for all health-care staff working in the field, especially medical and nursing staff. The book should also be of use to those studying for medical and nursing examinations, particularly as some of the subjects discussed, such as infections in the immune compromised host, are relevant to other branches of medicine.

Jennie Treleaven
Peter Wiernik

ACKNOWLEDGEMENTS

We should like to thank all our contributors for the time they have taken to find suitable photographs to illustrate their subjects, and for preparing their texts.

Our thanks are also due to Ben Hilditch for his invaluble desk-top publishing skills and the time he spent checking references and the script.

I Introduction

Sylvia Benjamin

The techniques of bone marrow transplantation (BMT) have been developing over the past few decades and now permit opportunities to treat diseases which were previously invariably fatal. However, problems may arise as a result of the following:
- The underlying disease for which transplantation is being used.
- The conditioning therapy administered to create space within the bone marrow cavity, eradicate the underlying disease and render the patient able to accept the incoming graft.
- The clinical consequences of mixing material of differing immunological types in the allogeneic situation.

The purpose of this book is to outline some of these problems, and to illustrate them where appropriate.

Early history of bone marrow transplantation

The importance of clinical research in the field of bone marrow transplantation was recognised with the award of the 1990 Nobel Prize in Physiology and Medicine to E. Donnall Thomas, one of the pioneers of BMT in humans. Bone marrow was first used to treat human disease in 1891 by Brown-Sequard, and this was reported by Quine in 1896. One dram of an aromatic glyceride of red marrow was given orally after meals for the treatment of leukaemia. Subsequently, attempts were made to treat pernicious anaemia using a glycerol extract of animal bone marrow administered orally, and in 1899 intramedullary injections of marrow were used to treat aplastic anaemia with some success. However, any positive effects seen after such therapy were refuted by Billings (1894) and Hamilton (1895), who, probably correctly, attributed them to the mineral and iron content of the material. Saline extracts of red bone marrow and spleen were also tried as haemopoietic stimulants and some successes were observed where other treatments had failed, and in 1937 Schretzenmayr administered intramuscular injections of freshly aspirated autologous or allogeneic bone marrow to patients suffering from parasitic infections, again with some success.

The first intravenous infusion of bone marrow was carried out by Osgood in 1939, although this route of administration was subsequently discarded for many years. Bernard, in 1944, injected allogeneic bone marrow directly into the medullary cavity and attributed the ensuing poor results to the possibility that the injected material had largely entered the general circulation of the recipient, a situation subsequently shown to be true.

Jacobson *et al.* (1951) showed that mice could recover from lethal irradiation if the haemopoietic areas in their femurs were shielded, having previously observed that marrow aplasia in irradiated mice could be reversed by shielding the spleen (Jacobson *et al.*, 1949). Subsequently, mice given potentially lethal doses of radiation were protected by marrow infusion, and in 1952 Lorenz showed that recovery was due to the cells in transplanted marrow.

Immediately after the Second World War, the haematological effects observed following irradiation in atom bomb survivors of Hiroshima and Nagasaki stimulated research into the potential of bone marrow to confer radioprotection in experimental animals. The idea of marrow transplantation was rapidly taken up by experimental clinicians who saw its potential for correcting bone marrow failure syndromes, and as a means of protecting patients against the myeloablative effects of radiation and chemotherapy.

The problems confronting clinicians in the early years of bone marrow transplantation were numerous. Autologous marrow transplantation necessitated the development of reliable systems for cryopreserving marrow (see review by Pegg, 1966), and allogeneic BMT was beset by the immunological problems of graft rejection, and the poorly understood phenomenon of 'secondary disease' (Barnes *et al.*, 1962). Until the human leukocyte antigen (HLA) system was recognised and HLA typing developed, the only compatibility test available was the mixed lymphocyte culture (MLC), characterized by Friedman in 1961. Without proper matching, donor selection was a random affair, and because of the high risk of serious incompatibility, only occasional transplants were successful. There were, however, seven reported cases of correction of aplastic anaemia by syngeneic transplant, and at least four of these may well have represented successful correction of haematopoiesis by BMT (Giraud and Desmontis, 1959, 1960). However, the novelty of BMT as a therapeutic modality in the minds of most clinicians was such that these reports were treated with scepticism.

Recent history of allogeneic bone marrow transplantation

Until the mid-1960s, allogeneic haemopoietic stem cell infusions were not established as a practical procedure in clinical medicine. Out of 417 reported cases, only three prolonged allografts were documented, and no more than 10% of the patients experienced clinical improvement attributable to the marrow infusion (Pegg, 1966).

George Mathé was a pioneer in the early development of clinical BMT. He was the first to propose the need for a large radiation dose to eliminate recipient malignancy, the use of substantial amounts of donor marrow to ensure engraftment, and the application of sterile nursing techniques. In 1958, six physicists were accidentally exposed to large doses of mixed χ and neutron irradiation at Vinca in Yugoslavia (Mathé, 1959). The most severely irradiated died, but of the remaining five, four were judged to have received a radiation dose of 600–1000 rads. They were treated with allogeneic bone marrow infusions, and red cell antigen studies demonstrated that successful but temporary engraftment ensued (**1**). It is also of interest that donor red cell output paralleled the amount of marrow initially infused. Presumably, autologous haemopoietic recovery occurred eventually, but the allogeneic bone marrow served to protect the patients until recovery occurred (**1**).

Mathé *et al.* (1963) were the first to describe graft-versus-host disease in man. A leukaemic patient, conditioned with methyl-nitro-imidazole, mercaptopurine, and total body irradiation followed by allogeneic bone marrow infusion from six donors, developed desquamating dermatitis, diarrhoea and weight loss. The patient was treated with steroids and antibiotics, and recovered. Mathé suggested at this time that the occurrence of secondary disease might favour elimination of leukaemia cells, and may have helped towards achieving remission in this case (Mathé and Amiel, 1964). These early proposals have now been substantiated, and are termed the graft-versus-leukaemia effect (Gale and Champlin, 1984): there is a smaller incidence of leukaemia relapse in patients surviving graft-versus-host disease than is the case in patients experiencing no graft-versus-host disease.

McFarland, in 1961, treated 20 cases of aplastic anaemia with no marrow ablation. He used a cell dose of between 0.7 and 40×10^9 nucleated cells, and seven patients showed improvement, with five recovering completely. Prior to this, very small quantities of bone marrow had been used, which almost certainly contained insufficient stem cells to effect engraftment. In general, however, successful 'take' of the infused marrow did not parallel an ultimately successful clinical outcome. In many cases there was graft failure after initial documented take, and it was rare for true chimerism to result. It was therefore realised that some form of 'conditioning' prior to allogeneic bone marrow infusion was necessary, in order to suppress host reaction to infused bone marrow, and, in the cases of malignant disease, to irradicate evidence of the disease prior to BMT.

Much of the subsequent work concerning the development of BMT was carried out by E. Donall Thomas (Thomas *et al.*, 1957). He initially concerned himself with autologous BMT and

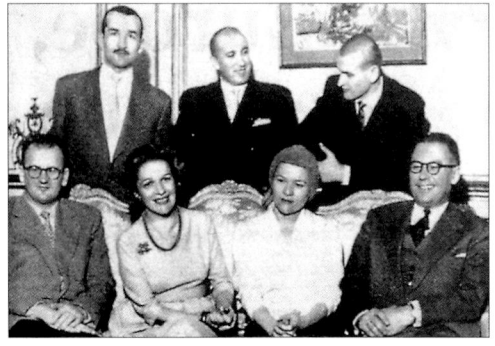

1 Some of the physicists irradiated in the Yugoslavian accident and treated by George Mathé, during their convalescence.

systematically examined the various components of the BMT procedure. He used the dog as an experimental model to develop effective total body irradiation schedules and introduced methotrexate as a means of preventing graft-versus-host disease. These technical advances, the characterization of the HLA system by Dausset *et al.* (1965), Payne (1964) and Van Rood (1958), and the miniaturization of the HLA assay by Terasaki and McLelland in 1964, prepared the way for a new era in BMT where transplants were carried out between HLA-matched sibling donor–recipient pairs. Pioneering work in severe combined immunodeficiency disease (SCID) by the Leiden group demonstrated the ability of BMT to cure this otherwise fatal disorder (De Koning *et al.*, 1969). In Seattle, led by Donall Thomas, BMT was carried out with increasing success in aplastic anaemia and leukaemia. The Seattle group maintained a lead in the clinical application of BMT which persists to this day.

Tissue typing

The human leukocyte antigen (HLA) system

HLA expression is not confined to leukocytes. Most tissues, including erythrocytes, express Class I antigens. However, Class II molecules are expressed by only a limited range of cells including activated T lymphocytes, B cells, macrophages, dendritic cells and Kuppfer cells. The primary function of the HLA system is to react with foreign antigens in the context of HLA identity rather than disparity, although the ability to recognise allogeneic HLA molecules even if never previously exposed to them, is well preserved.

The original studies were carried out using mice, when the major histocompatibility complex (MHC) was recognised. This is now known to be present in all mammalian species. The genes of the human MHC are arranged on chromosome 6 (**2, 3**), and the human genome bears at least 17 HLA Class I genes. To date, six functional Class I genes have been recognised, and 11 pseudogenes (Shimizu *et*

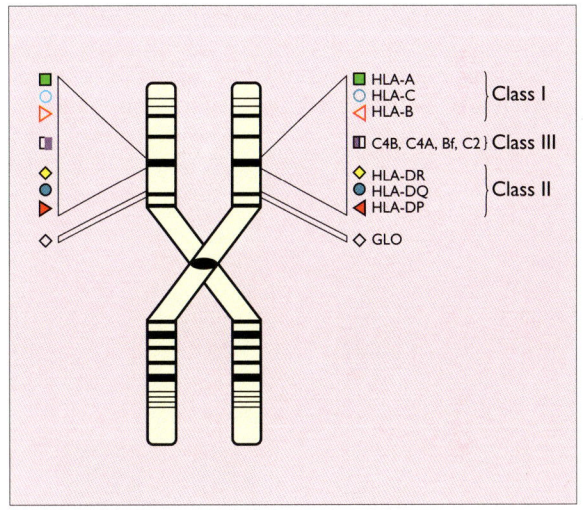

2 The HLA system and other genetic loci on chromosome 6.

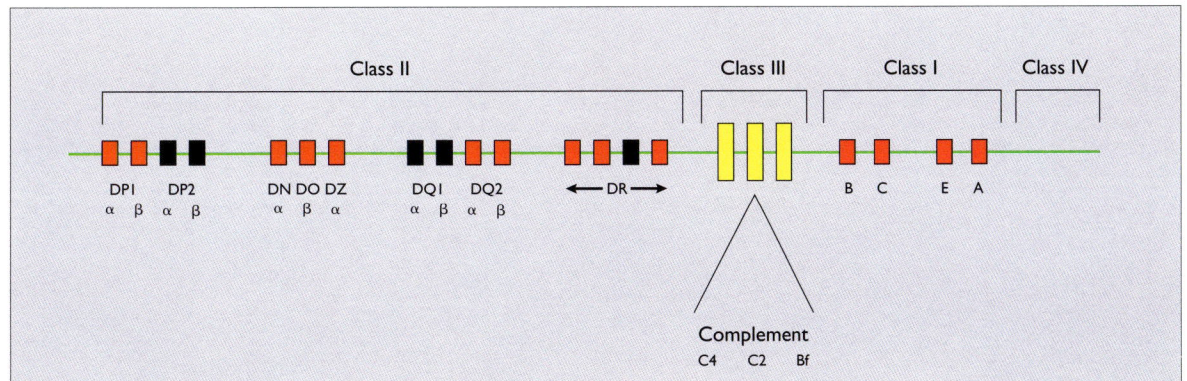

3 The HLA locus on chromosome 6.

al., 1988). The Class I MHC interacts closely with the CD8 antigen on T cells.

Class II molecules consist of an α- and a β-chain. They are transmembrane molecules and interact closely with the CD4 antigen of the T-helper cells. In transplantation, HLA-DR is the most important of the Class II molecules.

There are also several 'minor' loci outside the MHC region that encode molecules thought to be important and are strongly implicated in the pathogenesis of graft-versus-host desease and in histocompatibility recognition

The three loci of major importance in BMT are the HLA-A, B and DR, loci. Their closely linked, multiple alleles lead to four possible haplotype combinations within a family (**4**). There is, therefore, a 1 in 4 chance of a sibling donor being a match for a patient. Tissue typing identifies the phenotype of patients and potential donors. Serological tests are used for A, B and DR typing and a mixed lympho-cyte reaction (MLR) is used to confirm DR identity. More recently, molecular biology technology has been used to give accurate DR typing. However, even with matched sibling bone marrow transplants, some 10–20% of recipients experience severe graft-versus-host disease due to minor histocompatibility mismatches. *Ex vivo* T-lymphocyte depletion of the graft results in a significant decrease in graft-versus-host disease, but also in loss of graft-versus-host disease effect and consequent high relapse rates, and the incidence of graft rejection is also increased.

The demonstration that the HLA system is the human MHC, analogous to that found in mice, led to matching of transplants. This led to a more logical selection of the donor, but did not eliminate graft-versus-host disease. Post-transplant immunosuppression allowed modification of graft-versus-host disease and survival. The first patients treated had end-stage leukaemia and many died of infection or disease, but as the procedure has become safer, it is now applied earlier in disease to effect cures impossible with any other therapy. BMT may offer a prolonged survival and may even be repeated. The last 20 years have seen BMT move from being a scientific curiosity to the established treatment for many conditions.

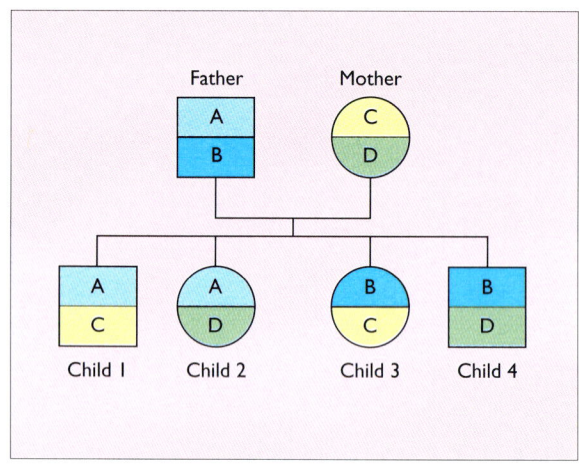

4 Schematic representation of the inheritance haplotypes for HLA.

Types of bone marrow transplantation

The pluripotent stem cells from which all committed blood cells arise (**5**) are located within the bone marrow space, and, to a lesser extent, are found in the peripheral blood. Both of these sites can therefore be exploited as a source of bone marrow stem cells, whether for autologous or allogeneic marrow transplantation.

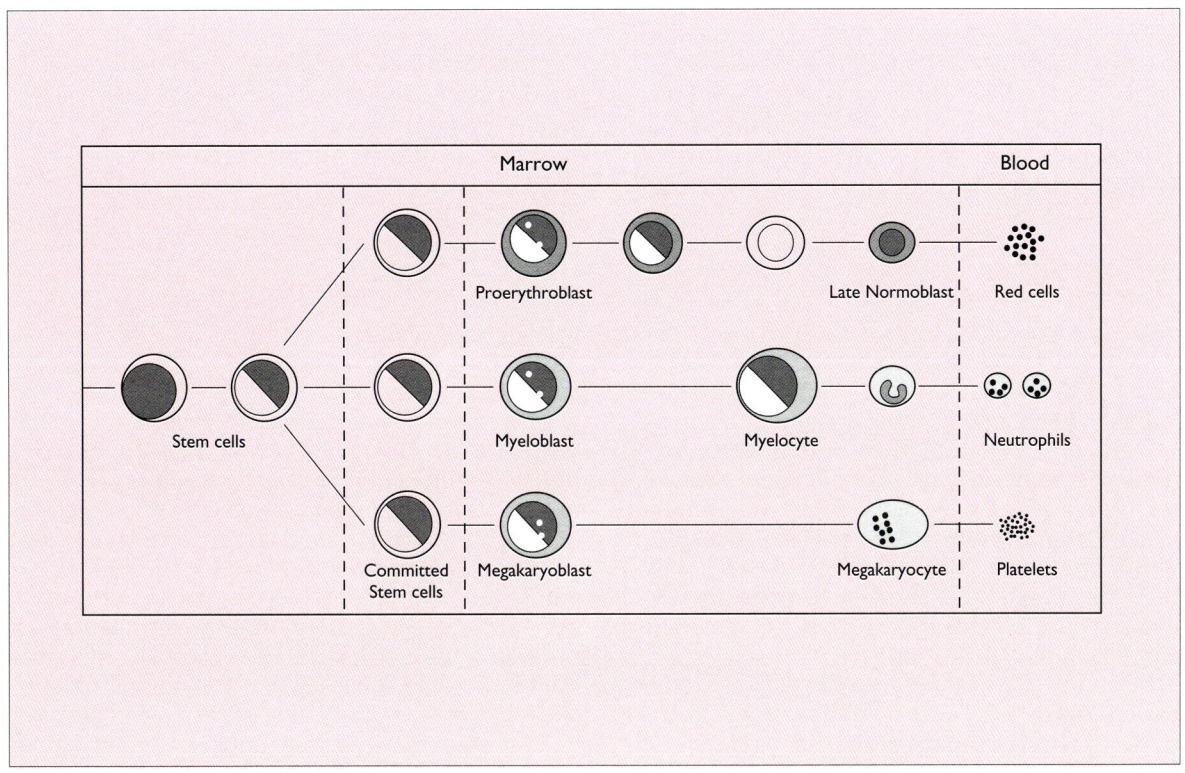

5 Simplified representation of the stages of blood cell development from stem cell stage through to maturation.

Allografting

Allografting involves transplanting marrow or peripheral blood stem cells to a recipient of the same species who is genetically different, except where monozygotic twins are concerned, in which case the transplant is termed syngeneic. In the syngeneic situation there is no graft-versus-host disease, and thus no antileukaemic effect is derived from the transplanted marrow because the host does not recognise the donated marrow as extraneous. The more common situation is for marrow to be donated by a fully HLA-matched sibling, in which case some degree of graft-versus-host disease is to be anticipated and the recipient should receive immunosuppressive therapy in the form of cyclosporin with or without methotrexate (see Section VII).

Partially matched family members, or matched but unrelated donors from a volunteer panel may also be used as donors, but in these situations the incidence of severe graft-versus-host disease increases, as does the incidence of graft rejection.

Matched but unrelated donor transplants (MUDs)

In the average family with 2.7 children, about 35% of patients may expect to find a sibling donor. The lack of an HLA identical sibling for the majority of patients who might benefit from BMT has led to the setting up of panels of potential donors, which can be searched to look for a MUD. Potential donors are either volunteers on a donor panel, for example, the Anthony Nolan Research Centre, or recruited from the National Blood Transfusion Service via the British Bone Marrow and Platelet Donor Panel (Bristol, UK). The chances of finding a match depend on several factors including the size of the panel, the frequency of a specific HLA type in the population and the ethnic background of donor and recipient. Usually, several months are necessary for a search to be completed. In a panel of 100 000 potential donors, 42% of patients may ultimately find a matched donor and 75% may find a donor with a one-antigen mismatch. The chance of finding a match varies with each individual patient. The occurrence of a few relatively common haplotypes together with linkage disequilibrium leads to a high expectancy of finding a donor for Caucasians, but a relatively low chance when attempting to find a match for patients of ethnic minorities.

Autografting

Since only approximately 1 in 4 patients who needs a bone marrow transplant has an HLA identical sibling available to act as a source of stem cells, autologous bone marrow or peripheral blood stem cell transplantation is also used as a method of treating a number of malignant disorders including leukaemias, lymphomas and some solid tumours. Clearly, such approaches are not feasible as treatments for patients who have a deficiency of their functional bone marrow, as is the case with aplastic anaemia, the inborn errors of metabolism and the immunodeficiency states.

Since the transplanted material derives from the patient, no graft-versus-host disease occurs, and hence there is no graft-versus-leukaemia effect. Relapse rates are higher than is the case in parallel situations where allogeneic marrow is used, a fact which also pertains when syngeneic marrow is used, again because of the lack of an antileukaemic effect from the transplanted material. In the autologous situation, it has been questioned whether a low level of tumour cells persisting in the material to be autografted may promote relapse, and this has led to a number of workers using various tumour cell purging techniques in an effort to rid material destined for autologous transplantation of contaminating tumour cells (see Section V). In the autologous situation it has proven extremely difficult to separate the potential of transplanted tumour cells to effect relapse from the lack of a graft-versus-leukaemia effect. Randomized trials are desirable, but variations in prior treatment, different disease stages, varying patient ages, small patient numbers and many other factors make these difficult to conduct in a manner which will yield unambiguous results.

Stem cell transplants

Stem cells recovered from the peripheral blood either of patients to be used in the autologous setting, or from donors for allogeneic use engraft rapidly provided that sufficient are harvested in relation to the body weight of the patient. Such an approach avoids the problems associated with general anaesthesia, especially desirable where normal donors are being used, since stem cells can be obtained by placing the donor on a cell separator. It also renders autologous transplantation possible in situations where the bone marrow itself cannot be harvested, as is the case with extensive marrow fibrosis.

Administration of growth factors such as granulocyte colony-stimulating factor (G-CSF) or granulocyte–macrophage colony-stimulating factor (GM-CSF) prior to procedures, or priming of patients with chemotherapy result in an increased number of circulating stem cells and consequent reduction in the amount of time that donors need to spend attached to the cell separator (see Section IV).

Goals of bone marrow transplantation

Although the procedure of BMT is similar in all cases, the goals vary depending upon the disease being treated. Where inborn diseases of the marrow are concerned (enzyme deficiencies, disorders of cellular immunity or abnormalities of haemoglobin synthesis), the defect may be corrected after the original marrow has been destroyed by high-dose chemoradiotherapy and replaced by normal donor marrow. Examples of such situations include SCID where a normal immune system may be established without prior conditioning therapy (Kenny and Hitzig, 1979). In β-thalassaemia major, where abnormal haemoglobin synthesis occurs, normal synthesis can be restored with the transplanted marrow. In Hurler's disease, the deficient enzyme, $α_1$-iduronidase, may be replaced by transplanted allogeneic bone marrow.

Severe aplastic anaemia of any cause has a very poor prognosis and in situations where pharmaceutical preparations have failed to restore haemopoiesis, allogeneic BMT is the only option.

The bone marrow is usually the major site of disease in haematological malignancies, where the aim of BMT is to eradicate the diseased marrow cell population, together with the normal cells, and then replace it with allogeneic marrow which, as well as reconstituting the haemopoietic system, has an antileukaemic effect.

Some solid tumours are sensitive to chemotherapy and show a dose–response in that higher doses of drugs or radiotherapy result in more cures. However, dose intensification is limited by marrow toxicity, and this can be overcome by autologous transplantation of the patient's own haemopoietic cells which are removed prior to therapy either by bone marrow or peripheral blood stem cell harvesting, and which are therefore protected from the effects of treatment. Autograft procedures are also performed for marrow diseases where no allogeneic donor is available or if patients are too old to withstand the problems associated with allografting, and, in some situations, results in terms of disease-free survival have been improved over those seen with chemotherapy alone. However, in the autologous setting, a graft-versus-leukaemia effect is not present since the haemopoietic cells with which patients are 'rescued' after high-dose therapy are not recognised as foreign.

Indications for bone marrow transplantation

Table 1 shows the conditions for which bone marrow transplantation has been used. It is indicated for some congenital abnormalities of the bone marrow function, or where there is disease involving the marrow not amenable to cure with standard chemoradiotherapy treatment. These approaches are being tried out as potentially curative therapy for an increasing number of tumours, but, because of the continuing high morbidity and mortality associated with BMT procedures, patients must be carefully selected for transplantation so that only those with a prognosis known to be poor with conventional therapy, and those who are likely to survive the procedure in terms of age and other risk factors are selected. Results of previous studies are used to define low- and high-risk groups with alternative treatments. For example, childhood common acute lymphoblastic leukaemia has a very good prognosis with chemotherapy, and therefore BMT is not indicated in first remission unless specific factors are present including some chromosome abnormalities known to be associated with poor outcome. In other diseases, such as chronic myeloid leukaemia, BMT offers the only chance of a cure (see Section II.5).

Transplants have been carried out on patients aged less than 1 year up to 60 years. The best results are seen in those who are less than 30 years of age at transplant, particularly in allografts where graft-versus-host disease tends to be more severe. Because of the universally poor outcome in the older age groups, allografts are now usually reserved for patients under 50 years of age.

Table 1. Indications for bone marrow transplantation.

Malignant disorders	Non-malignant disorders
Leukaemias	Bone marrow failure syndromes
Acute myeloblastic leukaemia	Aquired severe aplastic anaemia
Acute lymphoblastic leukaemia	Fanconi's aplasia
Chronic myelogenous leukaemia	Reticular dysgenesis
Myelodysplastic syndromes	
Acute myelofibrosis	
Lymphoproliferative disorders	Immunodeficiency states
Hodgkin's lymphoma	Severe combined immunodeficiency disease
Non-Hodgkin's lymphoma	Some less severe combined immunodeficiency disorders
Multiple myeloma	Wiskott–Aldrich syndrome
Chronic lymphocytic leukaemia	
Solid tumours	Haematological disorders
Neuroblastoma	Thalassaemia syndromes
Bronchial carcinoma	Some sickle-cell anaemias
Breast carcinoma	Congenital neutropenia
Melanoma	Severe congenital platelet disorders
Cerebral tumours	Osteopetrosis
Osteosarcoma	
Ewing's sarcoma	Non-haematological genetic disorders
Teratomas	Mucopolysaccharidoses
Others	Leukodystrophies
	Other rare metabolic disorders

The course of bone marrow transplantation

Patients are prepared for transplant by high-dose chemotherapy with or without radiotherapy (see Section VIII) This creates space within the marrow cavity, causes immunosuppression, treats any residual disease and allows acceptance of infused marrow. Conditioning therapy ablates residual haemopoiesis which is reconstituted by the pluripotent stem cells present in the infused marrow or peripheral blood. Evidence of engraftment is usually present 2–3 weeks after infusion, and the period of aplasia can usually be shortened by administering haemopoietic growth factors such as G-CSF or GM-CSF (Powles et al., 1990).

Prior to engraftment there may be significant clinical problems including anaemia, bleeding and sepsis. Patients are nursed in isolation by highly trained staff, thus reducing the risk of exogenous infection. Blood product support and antibiotics are administered until the graft is functional. In order to facilitate these treatments, continuous intravenous access is provided with a Hickman line (see Section VI). The marrow for transplant is infused through this line into a central vein and the pluripotent stem cells find their own way into the marrow, where they settle and divide to eventually re-populate the entire haemopoietic, immune and supporting tissues.

There are few immediate side effects of BMT, except for those associated with volume load or anticoagulant therapy. Subsequent complications involve the toxic effects of chemoradiotherapy, pancytopenia, veno-occlusive disease, graft rejection and acute graft-versus-host disease. Later complications may include chronic graft-versus-host disease, interstitial pneumonitis, viral infections, radiotherapy effects and disease relapse. Children may have additional problems related to chemo-radiotherapy, including learning difficulties and hormonal and growth retardation (see Section X).

Results of bone marrow transplantation

Disease free survival after BMT varies widely depending upon the disease being treated. Mortality is due to underlying disease or complications of the procedure. The best results are in children treated for inherited abnormalities of the marrow. Unacceptably high death rates result from transplants in older patients (over 50 years for allograft and over 60 years for autograft). However, there is still a procedure-related mortality of about 20%. The overall survival for all transplants in adults is 30–60%, the causes of death being different for allografts (graft failure and graft-versus-host disease) and autografts (disease relapse). Survival is better if the patient is younger and in good clinical condition prior to BMT. As new advances lead to improved results, indications for the procedure may become more widespread.

References

Barnes DW, Loutit JF, Micklem HS. 'Secondary disease' of radiation chimeras: a syndrome due to lymphoid aplasia. *Ann New York Acad Sci* 1962; **99**: 374–385.

Bernard J. Discussion. *Sang* 1944; **16**: 434.

Billings JS. Therapeutic use of extract of bone marrow. *Bull Johns Hopkins Hosp* 1894; **5**: 115.

Daussett J, Rapaport FT, Ivanyi P, Colombani J. Tissue alloantigens and transplantation. In: *Histocompatibility Testing*, 1965. Eds: Balner H, Cleton FJ, Eernisse JG. Munksgaard, Copenhagen, pp.63–78.

De Koning J, Van Bekkum DW, Dicke KA et al. Transplantation of bone marrow cells and foetal thymus in an infant with lymphopenic immunological deficiency. *Lancet* 1969; **1**: 1223–1227.

Friedman EA, Retan JW, Marshall DC, Henry L, Merrill JP. Accelerated skin graft rejection in humans preimmunised with homologous peripheral leucocytes. *J Clin Invest* 1961; **40**: 2162–2170.

Gale RP, Champlin RE. How does bone marrow transplantation cure leukemia? *Lancet* 1984; **2**: 28–29.

Giraud G, Desmontis T. Bone marrow transplantation in bone marrow aplasias of toxic, infectious and post-haemolysin aetiology. *7th European Congress of Haematology, London, 7–12 September 1959*.

Giraud G, Desmontis T. Medullary transfusion in toxic, infectious and post-haemolysin medullary aplasias. *Montpellier Med* 1960; **57**: 503.

Hamilton AM. The use of medullary glyceride in conditions attended by paucity of red blood corpuscles and haemoglobin. *New York Med J* 1895; **61**: 44.

Jacobson LO, Marks EK, Robson MJ et al. The effect of spleen protection on mortality following X-irradiation. *J Lab Clin Med* 1949; **34**: 1638.

Jacobson LO, Simmons EL, Marks EK, Eldredge JH. Recovery from radiation injury. *Science* 1951; **113**: 510.

Kenny AB, Hitzig WH. Bone marrow transplantation for severe combined immunodeficiency disease. *Eur J Pediatr* 1979; **131**: 155–177.

Lorenz E, Congdon CC, Uphoff D. Modification of acute irradiation injury in mice and guinea pigs by bone marrow injections. *Radiology* 1952; 58: 863–877.

Mathé G, Jammet H, Pendic B et al. Transfusions and grafts of homologous bone marrow in humans accidentally irradiated to high doses. *Rev Fr Etudes Clin Biologiques* 1959; **4**: 226–229.

Mathé G, Amiel JL, Schwarzenberg L et al. Haematopoietic chimera in man after allogeneic (homologous) bone marrow transplantation (control of secondary symptoms, specific tolerance due to chimerism). *B Med J* 1963; **2**: 1633–1635.

Mathé G, Amiel JL. Immunotherapy: new method of treating leukaemias. *Nouv Rev Fr Hématologique* 1964; **4**: 211–216.

Osgood EE, Riddle MC, Mathews TJ. Aplastic anaemia treated with daily transfusions and intravenous marrow. *Ann Intern Med* 1939; **13**: 357.

McFarland W, Granville NB, Schwarz R et al. Therapy of hypoplastic anaemia with bone marrow transplantation. *Arch Intern Med* 1961; **108**: 23-33.

Payne R, Tripp M, Weigle J et al. A new leucocyte isoantigen system in man. *Cold Spring Harb Symp Quant Biol* 1964; **29**: 285–295.

Pegg DE. Allogeneic bone marrow transplantation in man. In: *Bone Marrow Transplantation*, 1966. Lloyd-Luke Medical Books, London, pp.77–101.

Powles R, Smith C, Milan S et al. Human recombinant GM-CSF in allogeneic bone marrow transplantation for leukaemia: double-blind, placebo-controlled trial. *Lancet* 1990; **336**: 1417–1420.

Quine WE. The remedial application of bone marrow. *J Am Med Assoc* 1896; **26**: 1012.

Schretzenmayr A. Treatment of anaemia by bone marrow injection. *Klin Wissenschaftschreiben* 1937; **16**: 1010–1012.

Shimizu Y, Geraghty DE, Koller BM et al. Transfer and expression of three cloned human non-HLA-A,B,C Class I major histocompatibility genes in mutant lymphoblastoid cells. *Proc Natl Acad Sci USA* 1988; **85**: 227–331.

Terasaki PI, McLelland JD. Microdroplet assay of human serum cytotoxins. *Nature (London)* 1964; **204**: 998–1000.

Thomas ED, Lochte HL, Wan Ching Lu, Ferrebee JW. Intravenous infusion of bone marrow in patients receiving radiation and chemotherapy. *N Engl J Med* 1957; **257**: 491.

Van Rood JJ, Eernisse JG, Van Leeuwen A. Leucocyte antibodies in serum from pregnant women. *Nature (London)* 1958; **181**: 1735–1736.

II Conditions Correctable by Bone Marrow Transplantation

1. Inborn Errors of Metabolism

Peter Hoogerbrugge, Ashok Vellodi and Roberto Pasquini*

Since 1980, bone marrow transplantation (BMT) has been used in the treatment of children and young adults suffering from lysosomal enzyme deficiencies (Hobbs et al., 1981). Different animal models of lysosomal storage diseases have also been investigated. This chapter describes the possible contribution of marrow transplantation in the treatment of subjects with such diseases.

Introduction

Allogeneic BMT has been used successfully for the treatment of patients suffering from haematological malignancies and other diseases of cells of the haemopoietic system such as aplastic anaemia and severe combined immunodeficiency disease. Following appropriate recipient conditioning, the haemopoietic system is replaced by that of the bone marrow donor and a chimaeric state is achieved. Engraftment of haemopoietic stem cells from an allogeneic donor requires intensive cytoreduction and immunosuppression of the immunologically competent recipient, with three principal aims:
1. To create space.
2. To achieve engraftment.
3. To prevent rejection of the graft.

Pretransplant conditioning of children with lysosomal storage disorders has consisted predominantly of cyclophosphamide (4×50mg/kg/day) and busulfan (4mg/kg/day $\times$ 4). Alternatively, total body irradiation or total lymph node irradiation have been used. Following allogeneic BMT in a conditioned recipient, the engrafted haemopoietic stem cells give rise to progeny of all haemopoietic lineages, including the monocyte lineage as precursors of tissue macrophages found in the skin, lung and liver tissue (Wagemaker, 1985). Based on this knowledge, Hobbs et al.(1981) proposed that a bone marrow graft may serve as a permanent source of the missing enzyme α-iduronidase in the treatment of patients with Hurler's disease.

At least four different mechanisms may contribute to a beneficial effect of allogeneic BMT in the treatment of lysosomal storage disorders. Replacement of the enzymatically deficient cells by enzymatically normal cells may be important, particularly in those diseases in which the mononuclear phagocytic cell system is primarily affected. The prototype of such a disease is Gaucher's disease Type I, in which the storage product is present predominantly in the macrophages of liver and spleen (Barranger and Ginns, 1989).

A second mechanism by which BMT may be effective is the transfer of enzyme from the enzymatically normal, bone-marrow derived cells to deficient cells by direct cell–cell contact. *In vitro* studies have shown that macrophages and lymphocytes can transfer lysosomal enzymes into deficient cells (Olsen et al., 1983). It can be anticipated that the effect of BMT due to enzyme transfer by cell–cell interaction will be limited to tissues rich in bone-marrow-derived cells, e.g. spleen, liver, lung and skin.

Thirdly, BMT may be effective through the release of enzyme into plasma, as may occur, for

---

* Contribution on Fanconi anaemia

example, with disintegration of donor-derived white blood cells. Subsequently, the circulating enzyme may be taken up by enzymatically deficient cells, analogous to the *in vitro* correction of lysosomal enzyme defects as initially reported in many enzyme deficiencies (Olsen *et al.*, 1983).

Finally, the presence of a concentration gradient of storage product between the tissues and the plasma compartment may result from the breakdown of circulating substrate by the lysosomal enzymes present in white blood cells and tissue macrophages of donor origin, and give rise to clearance of the storage product.

Bone marrow transplantation in animal models of lysosomal enzyme deficiency

In inbred strains of animals, the biochemical abnormalities, histological findings and the course of the disease are identical in all affected animals, which makes animal models very suitable for precise evaluation of the possible effect of bone marrow transplantation (Taylor *et al.*, 1986; Wenger *et al.*, 1986; Hoogerbrugge *et al.*, 1987, 1988a; Shull *et al.*, 1987, 1988; Birkenmeyer *et al.*, 1991). For example, the distribution of donor enzyme as well as its quantity in the various tissues or even cell types of the recipient can be determined.

In all animal models studied, the enzyme activity in white blood cells following successful BMT increased to donor levels concurrently with the development of haemopoietic chimaerism. In the visceral organs (spleen, liver and lung), enzyme activity attained a level between that of donor and recipient within a few weeks (Taylor *et al.*, 1986; Hoggerbrugge *et al.*, 1987, 1988a; Shull *et al.*, 1987, 1988). The rising enzyme activity in these tissues can be partly explained by replacement of host macrophages such as Kupffer cells and alveolar macrophages by those of the donor. In addition, transfer of enzyme from grafted macrophages into liver parenchymal cells of the host (Hoggerbrugge *et al.*, 1988b) and decrease of storage products in liver tissue (Shull *et al.*, 1987) have been reported in twitcher mice and mucopolysaccharidosis I (MPS-I; Hurler's disease) dogs, respectively.

The effect of BMT on the enzyme levels in the central nervous system (CNS) is less uniform: a rise of enzyme activity above background level was absent in the CNS of MPS-VI cats at one year (Wenger *et al.*, 1986) and in β-glucuronidase-deficient mice at six months after BMT (Hoggerbrugge *et al.*, 1987), which for mice is a long period of follow-up. In the CNS of MPS-I dogs, only enzyme activity in small amounts, i.e. 1–3% of donor value, was reported, together with a decrease of glycosaminoglycans (GAG) storage in cerebrospinal fluid and meninges at more than one year follow-up (Shull *et al.*, 1987). In transplanted twitcher mice and fucosidosis dogs, the enzyme activity in the CNS gradually increased to 15–25% of that found in control animals. In twitcher mice, this was explained by infiltration into the brain tissue of enzymatically competent donor-derived cells (**6**). Data in twitcher mice and fucosidosis dogs show clearly the contribution of the time-point of transplantation to the final outcome: mice transplanted early, before the onset of symptoms, showed prolonged survival after BMT, in contrast to mice transplanted at disease progression (**7**).

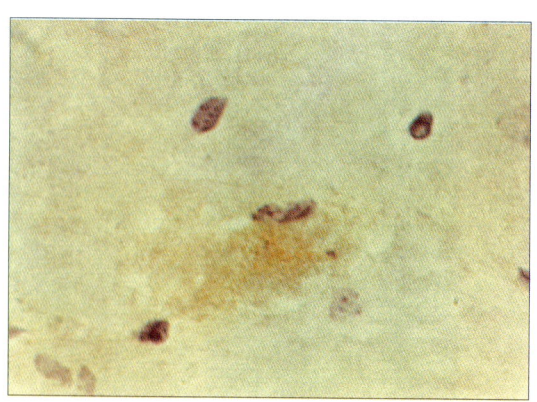

6 Light micrograph of frozen section of brain tissue of a twitcher mouse 100 days after allogeneic BMT. This shows the presence of donor antigens stained with biotinylated antibody recognising donor tissue, followed by immune-peroxidase (brown staining; magnification × 800).

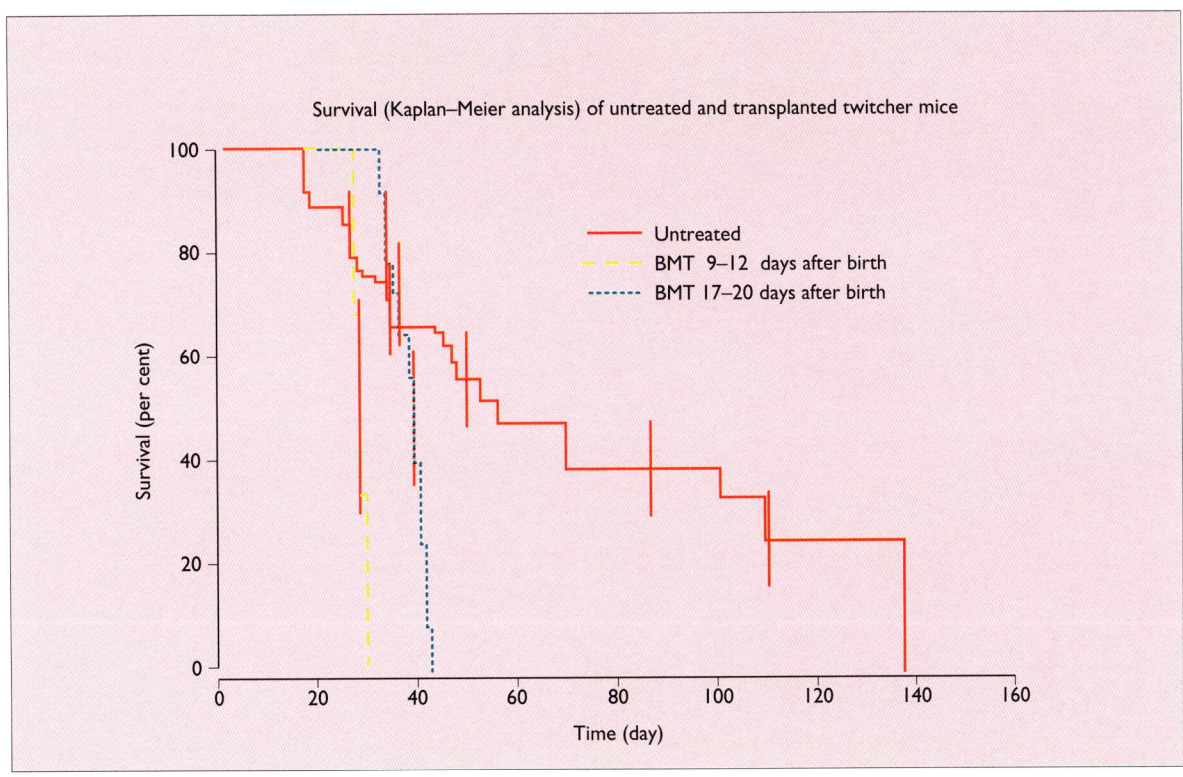

7 Effect of age at BMT on survival of twitcher mice: prolonged survival was seen if BMT was performed before the onset of symptoms (days 9–12) but not if performed after the onset of symptoms (days 17–20).

Results of bone marrow transplantation in patients suffering from lysosomal storage diseases

Since the first report on BMT in a patient suffering from Hurler's disease (MPS-I) by Hobbs *et al.* (1981), many patients with lysosomal storage diseases have undergone BMT (**Table 2**). The majority of such transplants have been performed at the BMT units of the Westminster Hospital (London, UK) and the University of Minnesota (Minneapolis, USA). These patients have recently been reviewed in detail elsewhere (Krivit *et al.*, 1992). By the end of 1992, approximately 70 patients had been reported to the registry of the European Bone Marrow Transplantation (EBMT) group, most of whom suffered from mucopolysaccharidoses.

As would be expected, the results of BMT were closely correlated with the type of disease involved and disease progression at the time of BMT. Here, we discuss three typical examples of diseases involved, namely mucopolysaccharidoses I and III (with skeletal and neurological symptoms), metachromatic leukodystrophy (with severe neurological involvement) and Gaucher's disease TYPE-I, in which storage occurs predominantly in macrophages.

Table 2. Conditions for which bone marrow transplantation has so far been attempted.

Lysosomal storage disorders		Non-lysosomal disorders
Mucopolysaccharidoses	Sphingolipidoses	Lesch–Nyhan syndrome
Hurler's disease (MPS-I H)	GM1 gangliosidosis	Adrenoleukodystrophy
Scheie's disease (MPS-I S)	Niemann–Pick disease	
Wolman's disease		
Hunter's disease (MPS-II)	Other lipidoses	
San Filippo A (MPS-III A)	Gaucher's disease	
San Filippo B (MPS-III B)	Pompe's disease	
Morquio's disease (MPS-IV)		
Maroteaux–Lamy disease (MPS-VI)	Others	
Leukodystrophies	Farber's disease	
Metachromatic leukodystrophy	Mucolipidosis Type II	
Globoid leukodystrophy (Krabbe's disease)	Alpha-mannosidosis	
	Fucosidosis	

Hurler's disease (MPS-IH) and San Filippo's disease (MPS-III)

Hurler's disease

Most patients transplanted for MPS suffered from MPS-IH (Hurler's disease **8, 9**). Skeletal deformities, neurological impairment and organomegaly are striking features of this disease. Following successful bone marrow engraftment in MPS patients, the enzyme levels in white blood cells rose rapidly to donor levels, indicating stable haemopoietic engraftment. Another common phenomenon in all successfully grafted MPS patients has been rapid reduction of urinary excretion of GAGs. Clinically, marked regression of hepatosplenomegaly has been noted. The main problems in these patients are commonly incapacitating skeletal symptoms (**10–13**) and neurological defects. The effects of BMT on these symptoms are unclear.

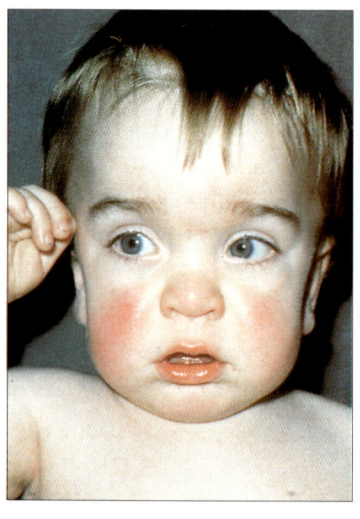
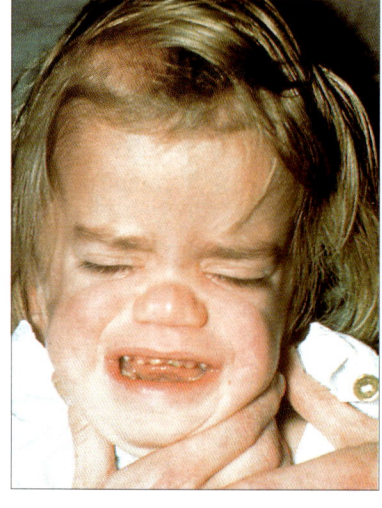

8, 9 Hurler's disease (MPS-IH). Typical features include the large head, coarse facial features, depressed nasal bridge, large tongue and widely spaced teeth (McKusick and Neufeld, 1983).

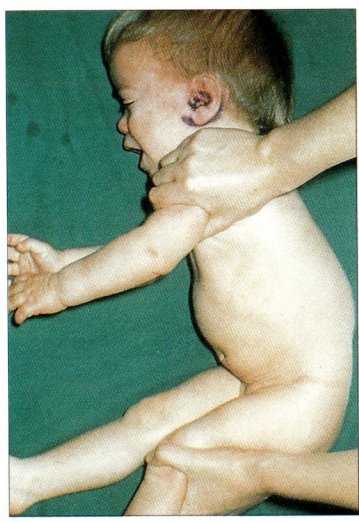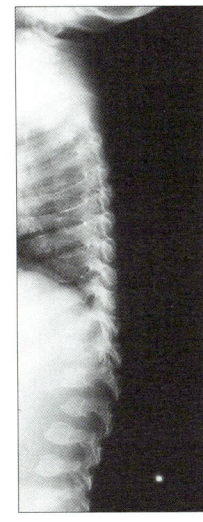

10, 11 The lumbar gibbus is one of the hallmarks of MPS-IH. It is present early in life and in its absence the diagnosis should be suspect. It results from anterior 'beaking' of the first lumbar vertebra. It is seen on X-rays taken soon after birth, and is clearly, therefore, not stress-related. The results of at least one post-mortem study show that the vertebral growth plate appears to be intact. Its aetiology is, therefore, unclear.

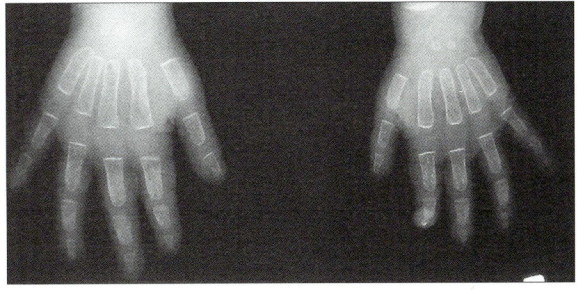

12 X-ray of hands in MPS-I showing the broad phalanges.

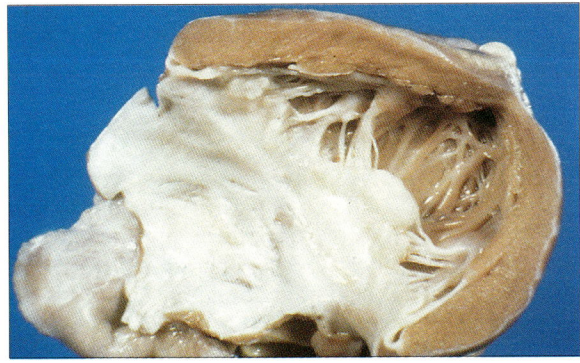

13 Cardiomyopathy is a frequent complication of MPS-I. It can present in various ways including congestive cardiac failure in the first year of life, sudden death resulting from coronary occlusion, or the clinical finding of a cardiac murmur. Frequently, however, there are no cardiac signs or symptoms. This figure shows endocardial fibroelastosis. The patient died 18 months post-BMT from pneumococcal septicaemia.

Recently, the Westminster group (Downie *et al.*, 1992) reported long-term follow up (7–11 years) of BMT in seven children with MPS-IH (**14–20**). In these seven surviving patients, the lumbar vertebrae have remained deformed and spinal growth is impaired. Psychomotor development has been

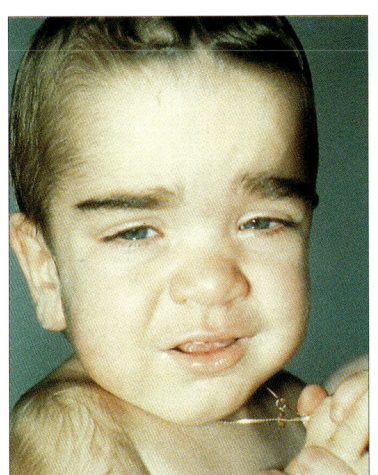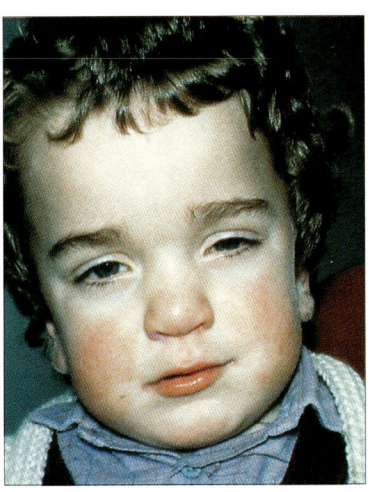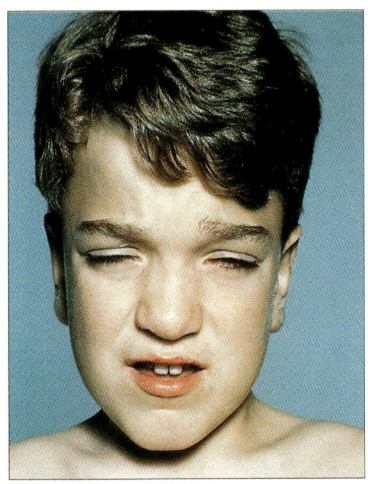

14–16 Facial features of MPS-I before, three years post-BMT and eight years after BMT. There is striking remodelling, resulting in a near-normal appearance. It is clear, however, that (a) not all the manifestations of the disorder respond to the same degree, and (b) there is a marked variation between patients in the observed response.

Bone Marrow Transplantation

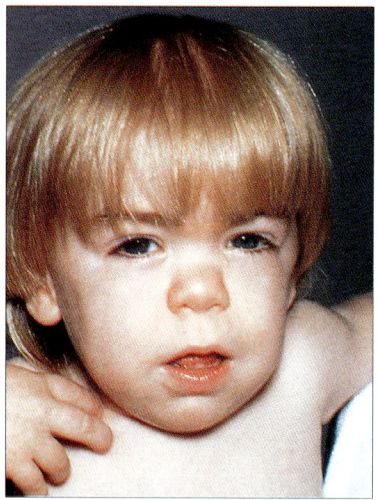
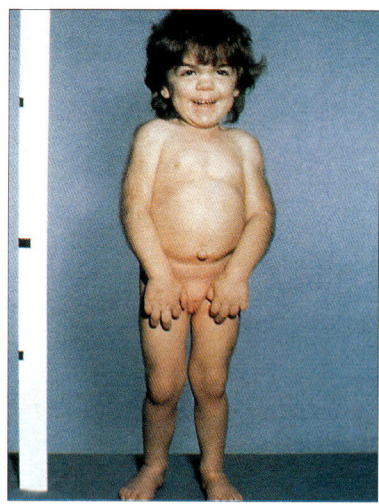
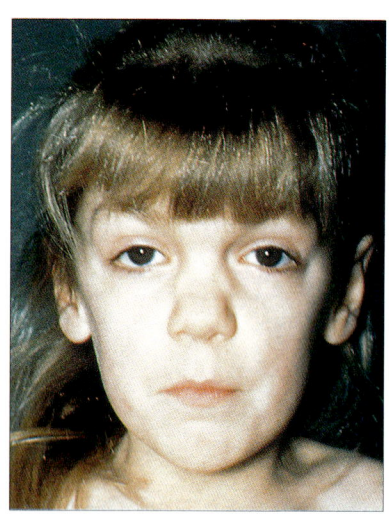

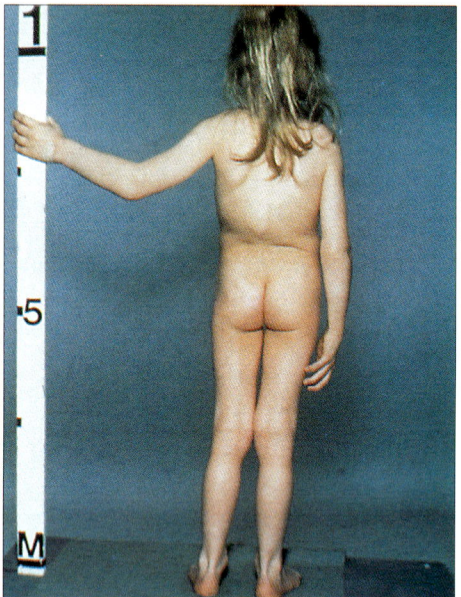

17–20 Points (a) and (b) from the previous set of pictures are illustrated here. They show progression of kyphoscoliosis in spite of obvious resolution of the facial features (Downie *et al.*, 1992).

studied in long survivors by serial assessment. These showed deterioration in two patients, stabilization in four and marked improvement in another patient (Downie *et al.*, 1992). Corneal clouding (**21, 22**), although reduced, had not completely cleared in all patients after several years of follow-up. Although follow-up is necessarily long to determine the effect of BMT in MPS-I (**23, 24**), a similar pattern has been seen by others (Krivit *et al.*, 1989). Data from the EBMT indicate that BMT seldom results in improvement of skeletal or neurological symptoms that are already present at BMT (**25, 26**). It remains to be clarified whether BMT, if performed before the onset of clinical symptoms, can prevent the occurrence of these symptoms (**27, 28**).

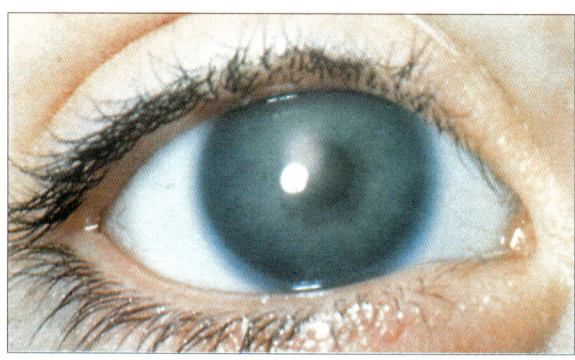
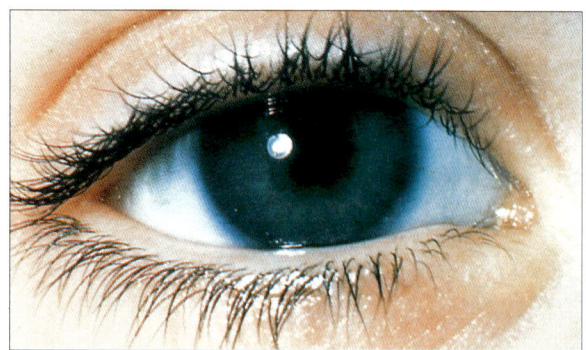

21, 22 Corneal clouding in MPS-I before and after BMT. There is obvious improvement. However, complete resolution never occurs. The reason for this is probably that the clouding is due not only to the deposition of mucopolysaccharide, which may be reversible, but also to mechanical disruption, which may not be. Residual photophobia and impairment of visual acuity have been seen in a number of children.

Inborn Errors of Metabolism

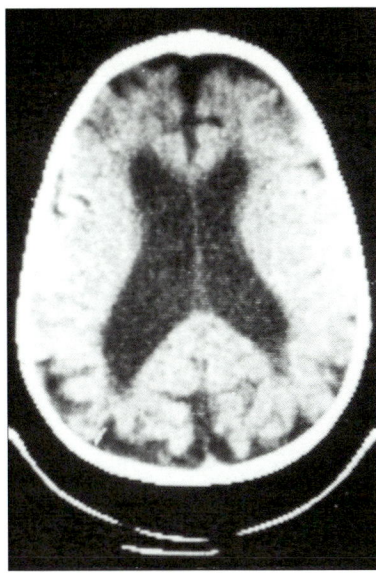
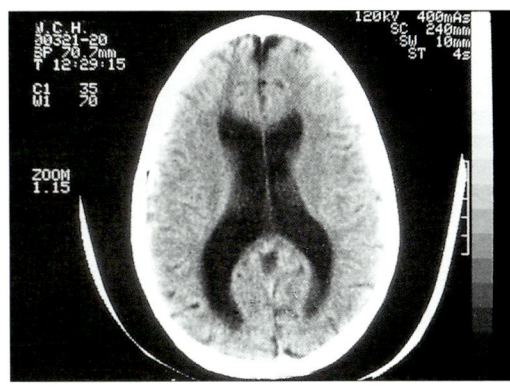

23, 24 CT scan of brain in MPS-I before BMT and 10 years after BMT. The pretransplant scan shows ventricular dilatation and prominence of the cerebral sulchi. These appearances appear to have resolved to some extent in the post-transplant scan. These findings lend some weight to the suggestion that the sulcal prominence is due to a communicating hydrocephalus, and not to cerebral atrophy, as has been suggested. Cerebral atrophy would be irreversible.

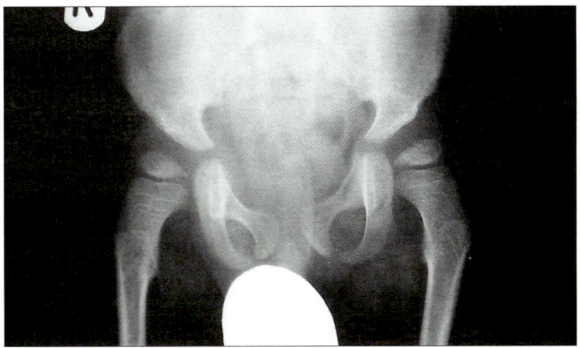
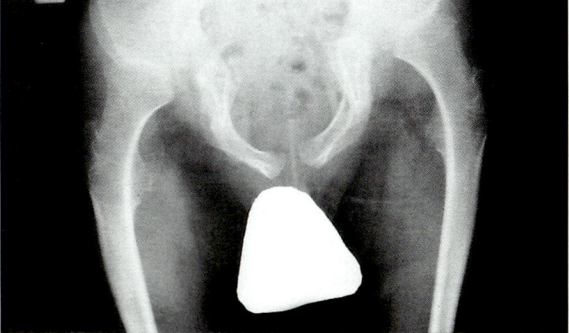

25, 26 X-rays of the hips in MPS-I before and eight years after BMT. The shallow, flat acetabula predispose to hip dislocation. Later, degenerative changes set in. It is, therefore, clear that BMT, while correcting the underlying biochemical defect, has failed to prevent the onset of degenerative joint changes. What is less clear is whether BMT has slowed down the degenerative process. There is insufficient information regarding the natural history of the disease.

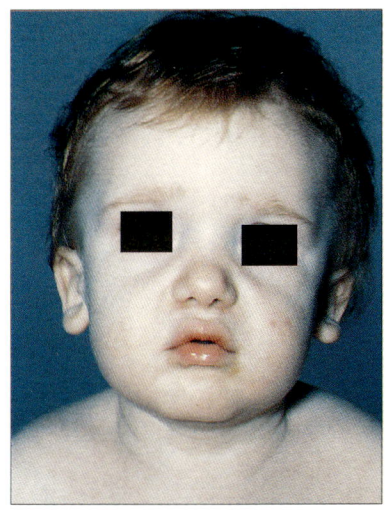
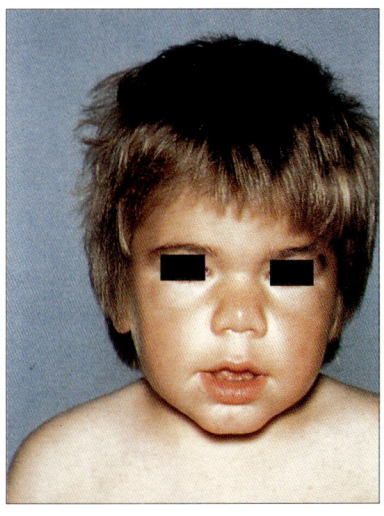

27, 28 Hunter's disease (MPS-II). This condition, unlike the other MPS disorders, is an X-linked recessive disorder. In younger children (left) the clinical features are not obvious. Hence, the diagnosis is easily missed. The right picture shows an older child, in whom the coarse facial features, similar to those found in Hurler's disease, have developed. The absence of corneal clouding is an important clinical distinction. It appears that, as in MPS-I, there is marked heterogeneous variation (Wilson *et al.*, 1991).

San Filippo's disease

San Filippo's syndrome (MPS-III) (**29, 30**), severe progressive mental deterioration and mild somatic manifestations are prominent. More than 25 BMTs have been performed for MPS-III. In all patients followed for more than 18 months, severe neurological deterioration was present (Krivit *et al.*, 1992). Even in two patients transplanted before onset of symptoms, severe deterioration occurred after BMT (Vellodi *et al.*, 1992).

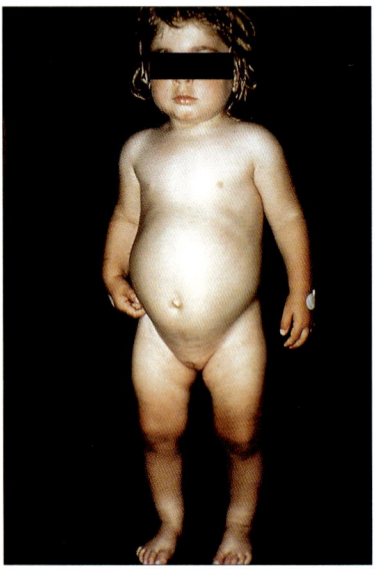
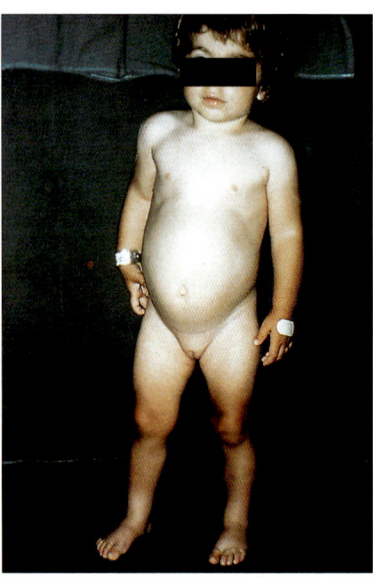

29, 30 Twin girls with San Filippo disease type B (MPS Type III), aged 2 years. They were asymptomatic. The diagnosis was made when an older sibling was found to be affected. As in Hunter's disease, therefore, the diagnosis is often not made until the child is older (Vellodi *et al.*, 1992).

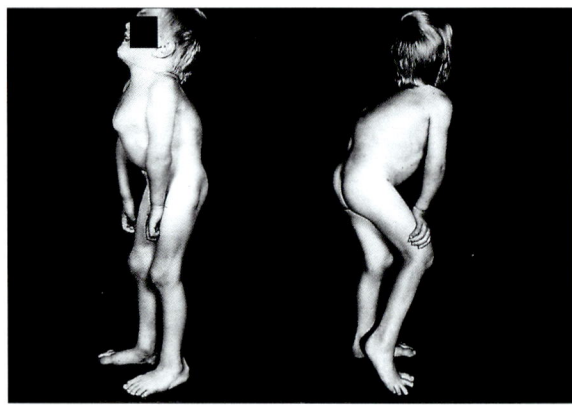
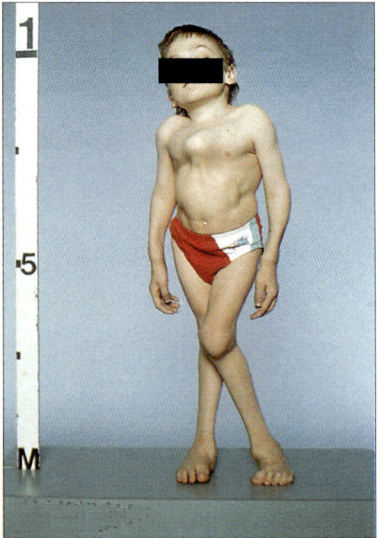

31, 32 Morquio disease (MPS Type IV), pre- (**31**) and two (**32**) years post-BMT. Note the severe skeletal deformities (dysostosis multiplex). There has been little, if any, response to treatment (Kato *et al.*, 1989).

Inborn Errors of Metabolism

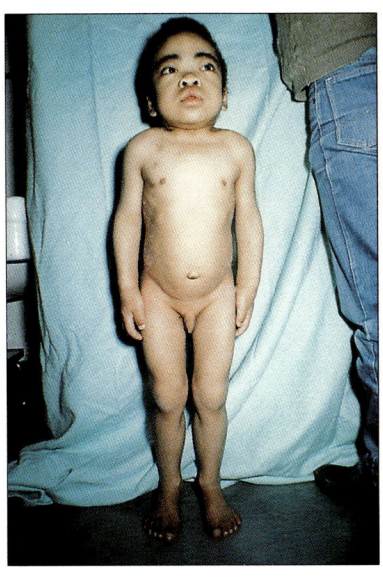

33 Maroteaux–Lamy syndrome (MPS Type VI). Note the obvious skeletal deformities (dysostosis multiplex) and coarse facies. Intellectual function is relatively well maintained. Complications include cervical instability, upper airway obstruction and cardiomyopathy, all of which may be life-threatening (McKusick and Neufeld, 1983). Upper airway obstruction and cardiomyopathy are indications for BMT. The presence of skeletal abnormalities is not an indication in itself as these do not respond to treatment (Krivit *et al.*, 1990b).

Metachromatic leukodystrophy

Two long-term surviving patients treated for metachromatic leukodystrophy have been reported by Krivit *et al.* (1990a) and by Ladisch (Bayever *et al.*, 1985; Ladisch *et al.*, 1986). In the first patient, (**34**) transplanted at four years of age, the brain-stem-evoked potentials and nerve conduction velocity have stabilized since BMT from levels that were slightly abnormal. The child's condition has not deteriorated. In the other long-term survivor (**35**), no detailed follow-up is available after BMT. EBMT data include 11 patients who under- went BMT. Clinical follow-up is lacking in five patients due to BMT-related complications (n = 1), graft rejection (n = 3), short follow-up (n = 1). All six patients with clinical follow-up were affected to a greater or lesser extent at BMT. In the patients already severely affected at BMT, no resolution of symptoms or signs occurred. It is not known whether occurrence of symptoms can be prevented by BMT if this takes place before their onset.

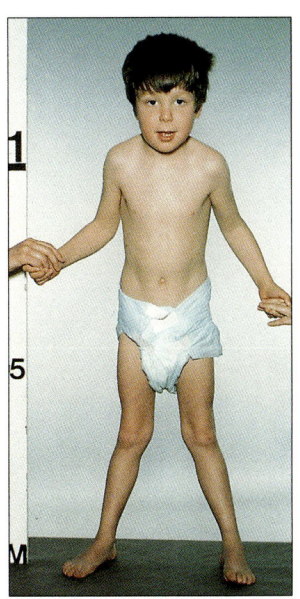

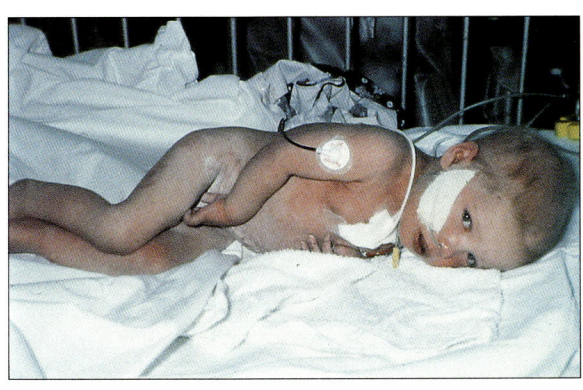

34, 35 Metachromatic leukodystrophy. The child in **34**, aged 8 years, has the juvenile form. Note the obvious pyramidal signs and urinary incontinence. Although the transplant was successful in correcting the enzyme defect, it had no effect on the clinical progression of the disease in this particular patient. However, if the diagnosis is made earlier, then disease progression can be prevented by transplantation. The same does not apply in the infantile form (**35**) which is perhaps illustrative of those conditions characterized by rapidly progressive disease (Moser *et al.*, 1992).

27

Bone Marrow Transplantation

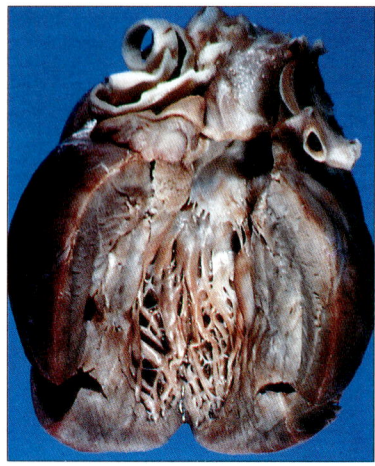

36 Pompe's disease (glycogen storage disease Type II) is characterized by severe hypertrophic cardiomyopathy. The onset is early (within the first few weeks of life) and a rapidly progressive downhill course is the rule. It is not surprising, therefore, that BMT has a uniformly disappointing outcome (Harris *et al.*, 1986).

Gaucher's disease

As glucocerebroside is stored predominantly in the macrophages of patients with Gaucher's disease, it may be anticipated that replacement of macrophages would result in amelioration of symptoms. Bone marrow aspirates and liver biopsies have shown that clearance of glucocerebroside-laden macrophages is a slow process, although it occurs more rapidly from bone marrow. It has been clearly demonstrated that clinical problems, including hepatosplenomegaly and growth retardation, diminish following successful BMT (Ringden *et al.*, 1988; Erikson *et al.*, 1990). In a follow-up period of more than nine years, growth rate improved and Gaucher cells disappeared from the bone marrow at

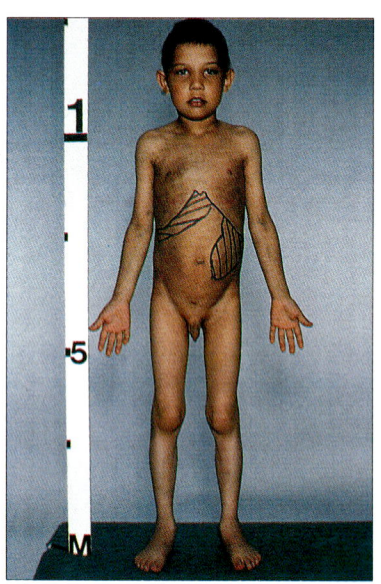
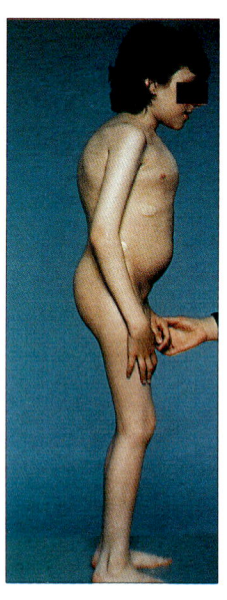
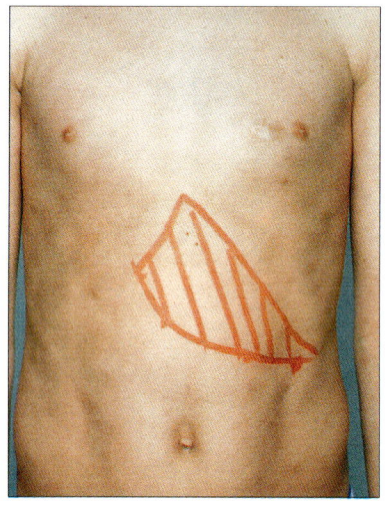

37–39 Gaucher's disease. The condition is caused by deficiency of leukocyte glucocerebrosidase. It is clinically heterogeneous. There are three major phenotypes. Type 1 (**37**, above left) presents in late childhood or early adult life with visceromegaly due to accumulation of glucocerebroside in macrophages, and is a slowly progressive condition. Type 2 causes death in infancy with severe central nervous system damage. Type 3 disease is characterized predominantly by visceral involvement. However, some neurological involvement also occurs and survival is longer than in Type 2. Bone involvement, resulting in pathological fractures and skeletal deformities (**38**, above centre) is common. Splenomegaly may be gross, resulting in severe physical discomfort and pancytopenia, and occasionally necessitating splenectomy (Brady *et al.*, 1983). Bone marrow transplantation results in a marked feeling of well-being, disappearance of bone pains and resolution of splenomegaly (**39**, above right). However, it is advisable to carry out splenectomy prior to BMT as otherwise prolonged pancytopenia may result and haematological support may be very difficult. The patient shown in **37**, **38** required over 300 units of platelets.

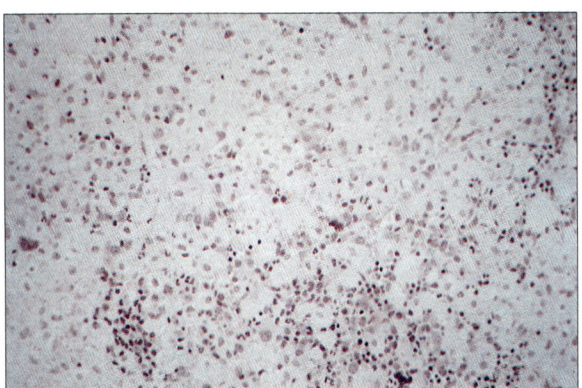 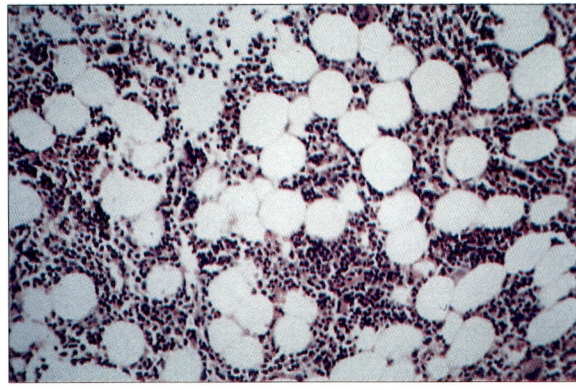

40, 41 The clinical events evident in **37–39** are paralleled by disappearance of Gaucher cells from the bone marrow (Hobbs *et al.*, 1987). Enzyme replacement therapy is now available, and BMT should therefore now only be considered in selected cases (Barton *et al.*, 1992).

three years after BMT. The issue of splenectomy prior to BMT is not yet resolved. Improved BMT results have been reported in patients following splenectomy as compared to patients with spleens (Hobbs *et al.*, 1987). However, Ceredase®, a modified, macrophage-targeted form of glucocerebrosidase, results in reduction of hepatosplenomegaly and improvement of haematological parameters (Barton *et al.*, 1990, 1992). This drug may be used to decrease the spleen size prior to HLA-identical BMT, but this point requires clarification in clinical trials. If no HLA-identical related donor is present, Ceredase® may be less toxic than BMT. So far, beneficial effects have only been reported in non-neurological forms of Gaucher's disease. No data concerning neurological forms are available.

Conclusions

Despite the number of BMT performed in patients with lysosomal storage diseases, it is still unclear for many diseases whether this experimental form of treatment is of any benefit. In contrast to inbred animal models, the natural course of the disease in humans suffering from lysosomal storage diseases can be variable, even within one family. Caution is therefore required in evaluating the possible effects of BMT in individual patients.

However, various common patterns are emerging from data so far reported. Enzyme activity determined in white blood cells and liver tissue after BMT merely reflects stable engraftment and replacement of tissue macrophages in most patients. A reduction of storage material in liver and spleen suggests replacement of storage-product laden host macrophages by enzymatically competent donor-derived cells. These cells may also induce clearing of stored material from neighbouring cells including hepatocytes. This may improve the well-being of patients with non-neurological forms of Gaucher's disease, but is insufficient to improve the quality of life of some patients with musculoskeletal or neurological involvement.

Most authors agree that improvement of skeletal deformities in lysosomal storage diseases is absent following BMT. Detailed studies in β-glucuronidase-deficient mice (Birkenmeyer *et al.*, 1991) have shown that transplantation very early in life, preferably before the onset of GAG accumulation, can prevent skeletal deformities. Whether this can also be achieved in human MPS patients is not yet known.

Neurological involvement is another major problem for the majority of patients with lysosomal storage diseases. Due to the blood–brain barrier, neuronal cells cannot be reached by circulating enzyme. In twitcher mice, infiltration of the brain by enzymatically competent, donor-derived cells played a role in diminishing the neurological symptoms (Hoogerbrugge *et al.*, 1988b). A similar phenomenon may have contributed to the neurological stabilization reported in one metachromatic leukodystrophy patient (Krivit *et al.*, 1990b). However, in a recent report of a patient who died of septicaemia two years after BMT for non-neurological Gaucher's disease, no enzyme was found in the brain tissue (Tsai *et al.*, 1992). However, animal work has shown that circulating enzyme can reach the leptomeninges, resulting in decreased storage in these structures (Shull *et al.*, 1987). Should this be the case in humans, a diminution of hydrocephalus may result. This, and the possible amelioration of airway obstruction following reduction of storage products in structures including the tonsils, may account for neurological improvement or prevention of symptoms.

So far, the metabolic corrections seen after BMT for lysosomal storage diseases exceed those previously seen after other forms of treatment such as intravenous infusion of purified human enzyme or fibroblast implantation. However, definite clinical improvement has been documented in only a few long-term survivors. Longer follow-up in transplanted patients and vigilant follow-up in patients grafted early in the course of their disease may reveal whether metabolic correction is paralleled by long-term clinical improvement.

Fanconi's anaemia

Fanconi's anaemia (FA) is an autosomal recessive disorder characterized by bone marrow hypoplasia, usually beginning with thrombocytopenia and later developing into severe pancytopenia. Abnormalities of the skeleton, heart and kidneys, microcephaly, strabismus, genital hypoplasia, skin pigmentation, growth and mental retardation are findings seen in more than half of the patients suffering from Fanconi's anaemia (Fanconi, 1967) (**42–50**). The typical physical stigmata are lacking in 30% of patients

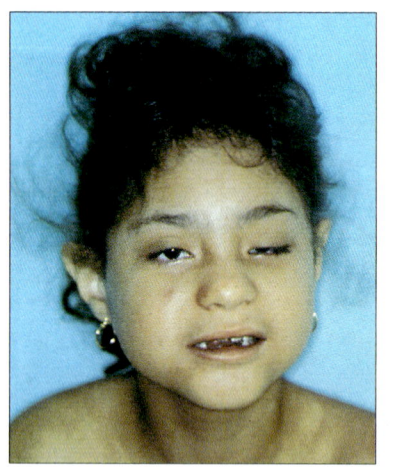
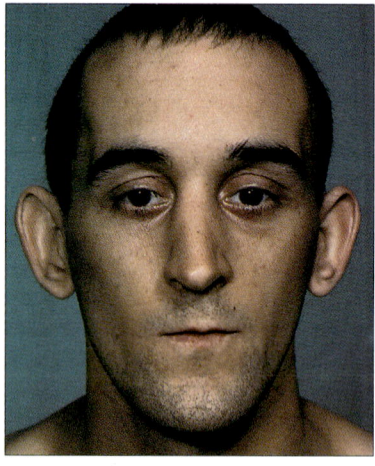

42 Fanconi's anaemia patient: an 8-year-old girl who presented with abnormal tooth implantation, strabismus and palpebral ptosis.

43, **44** Fanconi's anaemia patient, aged 24 years, with typical facies including close-set eyes and small chin.

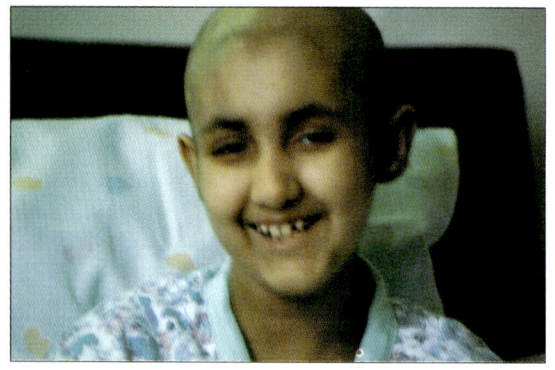

45 Fanconi's anaemia patient, an 11-year-old girl with typical Fanconi facies.

Inborn Errors of Metabolism

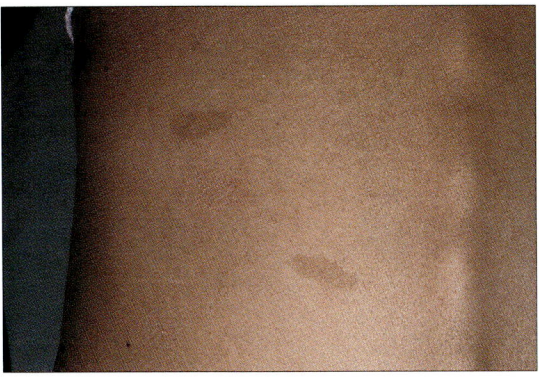

46 Characteristic hyperpigmented areas of skin seen in Fanconi's anaemia.

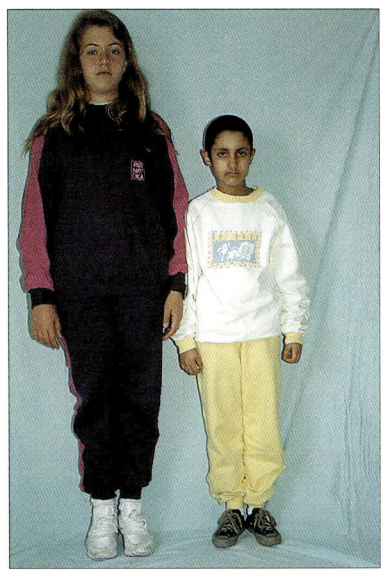

47 Comparison of height and appearance in an 11-year-old girl with Fanconi's anaemia (right) and her 13-year-old sister (left) who was the marrow donor.

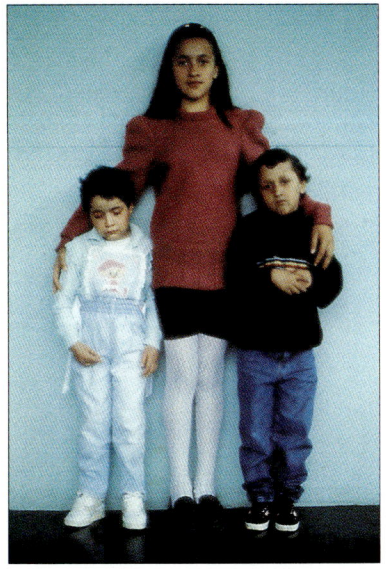

48 Two Fanconi's anaemia patients transplanted using marrow from their sister (middle), an 11-year-old girl. On the left is a 6-year-old girl transplanted two years previously, and on the right her 8-year-old brother three years' post-transplant.

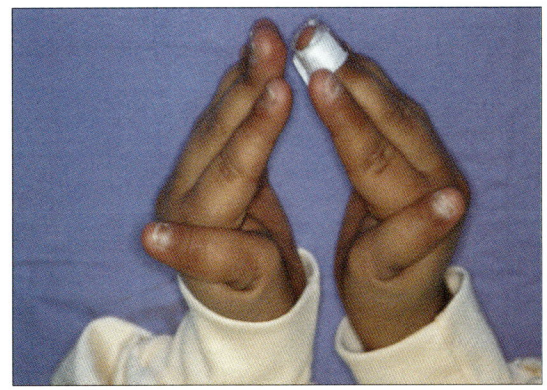

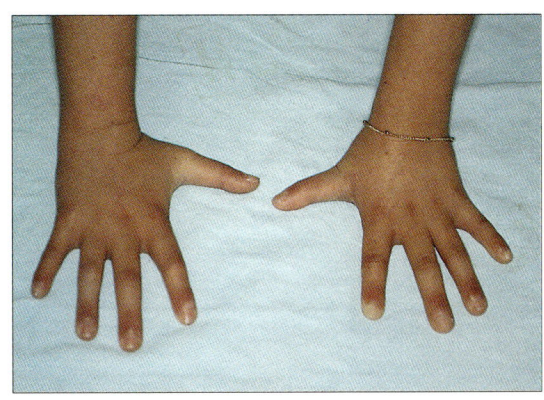

49, **50** Abnormal thumb implantation (**49**, top) and atypical thumb adduction (**50**, bottom) in two Fanconi's anaemia patients.

and the diagnosis is only confirmed by cytogenetic analysis, best carried out on peripheral blood (Auerbach *et al.*, 1989). Bone marrow cells, lymphocytes and fibroblasts cultured from homozygous FA patients show a high breakage rate and rearrangements with gaps, rings and triradial and quadriradial configurations (Schuler, 1969; Auerbach, 1978, 1983). The last is pathognomonic of FA (Auerbach *et al.*, 1981) (**51**). These abnormalities appear to be the result of failure of DNA repair, through mechanisms that remain incompletely explained (Digweed *et al.*, 1989). The cytogenetic abnormalities become more obvious when cells are incubated with alkylating agents (diepoxybutane, cisplatin, etc.), also called clastogenic agents, which cause further chromosome damage (Auerbach *et al.*, 1981). The International Fanconi Anaemia Registry has proposed the criteria for diagnosis of FA based on clinical features and cytogenetics findings (Auerbach, 1989).

FA patients may not show evidence of bone marrow failure until adulthood (Glanz and Fraser, 1982). The wide variations of phenotypic expression, even within kindreds, the long delay in the appearance of pancytopenia in some individuals and the apparent link between drug or chemical exposure and clinical manifestations suggest that genetic factors predispose to rather than predetermine aplasia.

The evolution of FA is always fatal with progression of pancytopenia and marrow aplasia resulting in the death of most patients due to haemorrhage or infection. Myelodysplasia, acute leukaemia and solid tumours develop in some patients and also contribute to the mortality of this disease (Alter, 1990).

Although FA may respond transiently to therapy with such agents as oxymethalone, BMT remains the only available means of permanently correcting the pancytopenia. The optimal timing of BMT is a matter for discussion, and is appropriate when progressive cytopenia develops, associated with transfusion dependency or infectious complications (Gluckman, 1990).

Allogeneic BMT in FA is associated with a high incidence of severe mucositis and skin toxicity (**52, 53**) due to the extreme sensitivity of FA patients to alkylating drugs and radiotherapy. Graft-versus-host disease and haemorrhagic cystitis are also

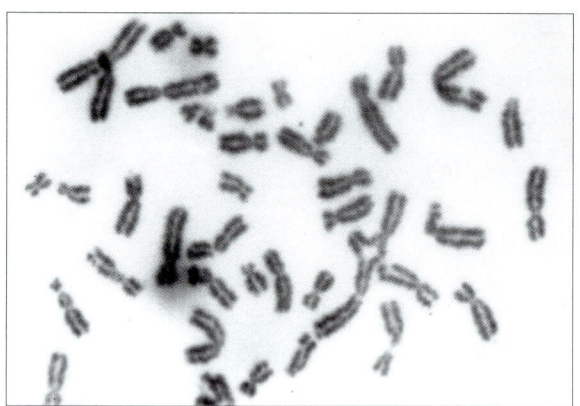

51 Typical chromosomal abnormalities in Fanconi's anaemia. Note chromosomal breaks, gaps, rearrangements and chromatid interchange. Preparation after exposure to cisplatin.

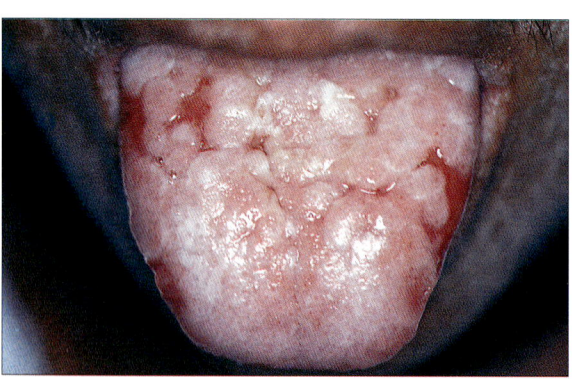

52 Irregular superficial hypertrophy of the tongue, a common complication of marrow transplantation in Fanconi's anaemia patients.

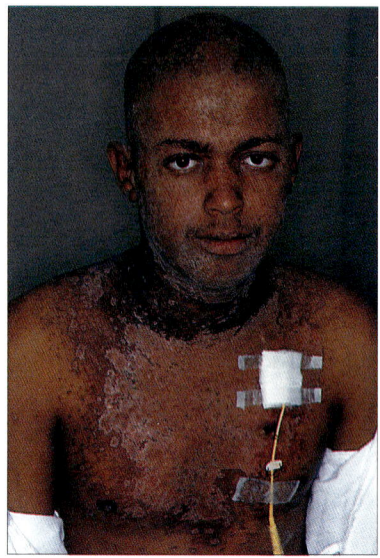

53 Skin toxicity in a Fanconi's anaemia patient after cyclophosphamide, 200 mg/kg was used in the preparative regimen for BMT.

commonly severe. The doses of alkylating agents and radiation usually used in transplant preparative regimens may therefore induce unacceptable morbidity and mortality in patients with FA (Gluckman, 1980), and should be reduced before BMT is undertaken in this patient group.

Gluckman (1990) has recently reported a long-term survival rate of 75% after allogeneic BMT for FA with a conditioning regimen in which low doses of cyclophosphamide (20 mg/kg) were given with 6 Gy thoracoabdominal irradiation. In Seattle (Flowers, 1992), and at our centre, results are similar using cyclophosphamide in doses higher than 100 mg/kg with or without antithymocyte globulin and without irradiation. Improved results have been seen in both centres following inclusion of cyclosporin A in the immunoprophylactic regimen. If these results are confirmed in a larger study population, radiation could be eliminated from the preparative regimen, and its side effects thus avoided (**Table 3**). Mucositis during BMT may be so severe that sloughing of large mucosal fragments occurs (**54**). Haemorrhagic cystitis can be very troublesome, and acute and chronic graft-versus-host disease occur at a higher rate in FA patients than in aplastic anaemia transplant recipients.

Acute graft-versus-host disease grades II–IV occurred in 60% of the FA patients conditioned with Gluckman's protocol, while those patients receiving only cyclophosphamide and cyclosporin A as immunoprophylaxis had less than a 25% incidence of this complication (**Table 3**). Graft failure is unusual.

Oesophageal stricture may be a late complication probably related to the use of alkylating agents during conditioning for BMT (**55**).

Transplants utilising non-identical family donors or unrelated donors have been performed in a few FA patients, but experience in this patient group is limited to date.

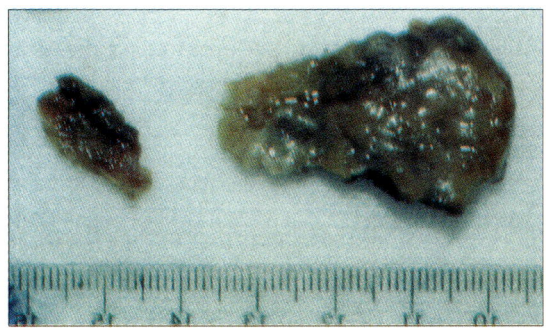

54 Oesophageal fragment expelled three weeks after marrow transplantation in a Fanconi's anaemia patient.

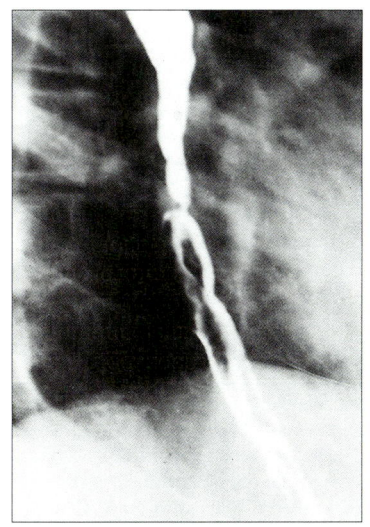

55 Oesophagram showing severe stricture three months after BMT.

Table 3. Results of BMT for Fanconi's anaemia from several different centres.

Study	Age (years) Range	(Median)	Conditioning regimen*	Immunosuppressive*	Acute GvHD	Survival
Gluckman (1990), France	5–20	(11)	CPAl + TAI	CSA	11/19	14/19
Hows (1989), UK	5–23	(9)	CPAl + TBI	CSA	9/15	8/19
Di Bartolomeo (1992), Italy	7–14	(13)	CPAl + TBI	CSA + MTX	2/5	5/5
Flowers (1992), USA	5–8	(6)	CPAh	CSA + MTX	1/4	4/4
Pasquini, Brazil	4–30	(14)	CPAh±ATG	CSA + MTX	4/14	10/14

*CPAl = low-dose cyclophosphamide (Gluckman); CPAh = high-dose cyclophosphamide (>100mg/kg); TAI = thoracoabdominal irradiation; TBI = total body irradiation; ATG = antithymocyte globulin; CSA = cyclosporin; MTX = methotrexate.

References

Alter BP. Constitutional aplastic anaemia. In: *Aplastic Anaemia and Other Bone Marrow Failure Syndromes*, 1990. Ed: Shahidi NT. Springer-Verlag, New York, pp. 38–50.

Auerbach AD, Wolman SR. Carcinogen-induced chromosome breakage in Fanconi's anaemia heterozygous cells. *Nature (London)* 1978; **271**: 69–70.

Auerbach AD, Adler B, Chaganti RS. Prenatal and postnatal and carrier election of Fanconi anaemia by cytogenetic method. *Pediatrics* 1981; **67**: 128–135.

Auerbach AD, Adler B, O'Reilly RJ *et al*. Effects of procarbazine and cyclophosphamide on chromosome breakage in Fanconi anaemia cells — relevance to bone marrow transplantation. *Cancer Genet Cytogenet* 1983; **9**: 25–36.

Auerbach AD, Rogatko A, Schroeder-Kurt TM. International Fanconi Anaemia Registry: relation of clinical symptoms to diepoxybutane sensitivity. *Blood* 1989; **73**: 391–396.

Barranger JA, Ginns EI. Glucocsylceramide lipidoses: Gaucher disease. In: *The Metabolic Basis of Inherited Diseases*, 1989. Eds: Scriver CR *et al*. McGraw Hill, New York, pp. 1677–1698.

Barton NW, Furbish FS, Murray GJ *et al*. Therapeutic response to intravenous infusions of glucocerebrosidase in a patient with Gaucher disease. *Proc Natl Acad Sci USA* 1990; **87**: 1913–1916.

Barton NW, Brady RO, Dambrosia JM *et al*. Dose dependent responses to macrophage targetted glucocerebrosidase in a child with Gaucher disease. *J Pediatr* 1992; **120**: 277–280.

Bayever E, Ladisch S, Phillipart M *et al*. Bone marrow transplantation for metachromatic leukodystrophy. *Lancet* 1985; **2**: 471–473.

Birkenmeyer EH, Barker JE, Vogler CA *et al*. Increased life span and correction of metabolic defect in murine mucopolysaccharidosis VII after syngeneic bone marrow transplantation. *Blood* 1991; **78**: 3081–3092.

Brady RO, Barranger JA. Glucosylceramide lipidoses: Gaucher's disease. In: *The Metabolic Basis of Inherited Disease*, 1983. Eds: Stanbury JB, Wyngaarden JB, Friedrickson DS, Goldstein JL, Brown MB. McGraw-Hill, New York, pp. 842–856.

Di Bartolomeo PD, Girolamo GD, Olioso P *et al*. Allogeneic bone marrow transplantation for Fanconi anaemia. *Bone Marrow Transplant* 1992; **10**: 53–56.

Digweed M, Sperling K. Identification of a Hela mRNA fraction which can correct the DNA-repair defect in Fanconi anaemia fibroblasts. *Mutat Res* 1989; **218**: 171–177.

Downie C, Hancock MR, Hobbs JR. Long term outcome after BMT for Hurler's syndrome. In: *Correction of Certain Genetic Diseases by Transplantation*, 1992. Eds: Hobbs JR, Riches PG. Cogent Trust, Middlesex, pp. 1–13.

Erikson A, Groth CG, Mansson JE *et al*. Clinical and biochemical outcome of marrow transplantation for Gaucher disease of the Norrbottnian type. *Acta Ped Scand* 1990; **79**: 680–685.

Fanconi G. Familial constitutional panmyelocytopathy. Fanconi's anaemia (FA). I. Clinical aspects. *Semin Hematol* 1967; **4**: 233–249.

Flowers ME, Doney KC, Storb R Marrow transplantation for Fanconi anaemia with or without leukemic transformation: an update of the Seattle experience. *Bone Marrow Transplant* 1992; **9**:167–173.

Glanz A, Fraser FC. Spectrum of anomalies in Fanconi anaemia. *J Med Genet* 1982; **19**: 412–416.

Gluckman E. Bone marrow transplantation for Fanconi's anaemia. In: *Aplastic Anaemia and Other Bone Marrow Failure Syndromes*, 1990. Ed: Shahidi NT. Springer-Verlag, New York, pp. 134–144.

Gluckman E, Devergie A, Schaison G *et al*. Bone marrow transplantation in Fanconi's anaemia. *Br J Haematol* 1980; **45**: 557–564.

Harris RE, Harron D, Vogler C, Hug G. Bone marrow transplantation in Type IIa glycogen storage disease. *Birth Defects* 1986; **22**: 119–132.

Hobbs JR, Hugh-Jones K, Byrom N *et al*. Reversal of clinical features of Hurler's disease and biochemical improvement after treatment by bone marrow transplantation. *Lancet* 1981; **2**: 709–712.

Hobbs JR, Hugh-Jones K, Shaw P *et al*. Beneficial effect of pre-transplant splenectomy on displacement bone marrow transplantation for Gaucher's disease. *Lancet* 1987; **1**: 1111–1115.

Hoogerbrugge PM, Poorthuis BJ, Mulder AH *et al*. Correction of lysosomal enzyme deficiency in various organs of beta-glucuronidase deficient mice by allogeneic bone marrow transplantation. *Transplantation* 1987; **43**: 609–614.

Hoogerbrugge PM, Poorthuis BJ, Romme AE *et al*. Effect of bone marrow transplantation on enzyme levels and clinical course in the neurologically affected twitcher mouse. *J Clin Invest* 1988a; **81**: 1790–1794.

Hoogerbrugge PM, Suzuki K, Suzuki K *et al*. Donor-derived cells in the central nervous system of twitcher mice after bone marrow transplantation. *Science* 1988b; **239**: 1035–1038.

Hows J, Chapple M, Marsh JC *et al*. Bone marrow transplantation for Fanconi's anaemia: the Hammersmith experience 1977–1989. *Bone Marrow Transplant* 1989; **4**: 629–634.

Kato S, Kubota C, Yabe H *et al*. Bone marrow transplantation in Morquio's disease. In: *Correction of Certain Genetic Diseases by Transplantation*, 1989. Ed: Hobbs JR. Cogent Trust London, pp. 120–126.

Krivit W, Whitley CB, Chang P *et al*. Lysosomal storage diseases treated by bone marrow transplantation. In: *Bone Marrow Transplantation: Current Controversies*, 1989 Eds: Gale RP, Champlin R. Alan R. Liss, New York, pp. 367–378.

Krivit W, Shapiro E, Kennedy E *et al*. Treatment of late infantile metachromatic leukodystrophy by bone marrow transplantation. *N Engl J Med* 1990a; **322**: 28–32.

Krivit W, Witley CB, Change PN *et al.* Lysosomal storage disease treated by bone marrow transplantation: review of 21 patients. In: *Bone Marrow Transplantation in Children*, 1990b. Eds: Johnson FL, Pochedly P. Raven Press, New York, pp. 261–287.

Krivit W, Shapiro E, Hoogerbrugge PM, Moser HW. State of the art review: Bone marrow transplantation treatment for storage diseases. *Bone Marrow Transplant* 1992; **10** (suppl): 87–96.

Ladisch S, Bayever E, Phillipart M, Feig SA. Biochemical findings after bone marrow transplantation for metachromatic leukodystrophy: A preliminary report. In: *Bone Marrow Transplantation for Treatment of Lysosomal Storage Diseases*, 1986. Eds: Krivit W, Paul NW. March of Dimes Birth Defects Foundation, Original Article Series, **22**, 1: 69–76, Alan R. Liss, New York.

McKusick VA, Neufeld EF. The mucopolysaccharide storage disorders. In: *The Metabolic Basis of Inherited Disease*, 1983. Eds: Stanbury JB, Wyngaarden JB, Fredrickson DS, Goldstein JL, Brown MS. McGraw-Hill, New York, pp. 750–777.

Moser HW, Moser AB, Smith KD *et al.* Adrenoleukodystrophy: phenotypic variability and implications for therapy. *J Inherited Metab Dis* 1992; **15**: 645–664.

Olsen I, Muir H, Smith R *et al.* Direct enzyme transfer from lymphocytes is specific. *Nature* 1983; **306**: 75–77.

Pasquini, R. Unpublished data.

Ringden O, Groth CG, Erikson A *et al.* Long term follow up of the first successful bone marrow transplantation in Gaucher disease. *Transplantation* 1988; **46**: 66–70.

Schuler D, Kiss A, Fabian F. Chromosomal peculiarities and *in vitro* examinations in Fanconi's anaemia. *Humangenetik* 1969; **7**: 314–322.

Shull RM, Hastings E, Selcer RR *et al.* Bone marrow transplantation in canine mucopolysaccharidosis. I: Effects within the central nervous system. *J Clin Invest* 1987; **79**: 435–443.

Shull RM, Breider MA, Constantopoulos G. Long-term effects of bone marrow transplantation in canine lysosomal storage disease. *Pediatr Res* 1988; **24**: 347–352.

Taylor RM, Farrow, BR, Stewart GJ, Healy PJ. Enzyme replacement in nervous tissue after allogeneic bone marrow transplantation for fucosidosis in dogs. *Lancet* 1986; **2**: 772–774.

Tsai P, Lipton JM, Sahdev I *et al.* Allogeneic bone marrow transplantation in severe Gaucher disease. *Pediatr Res* 1992; **31**: 503–507.

Vellodi A, Young E, New M *et al.* Bone marrow transplantation for San Filippo disease type B. *J Inherited Metab Dis* 1992; **15**: 911–918.

Wagemaker G. Hemopoietic cell differentiation. In: *Bone Marrow Transplantation: Biological Mechanisms and Clinical Practice*, 1985. Eds: van Bekkum DW, Loewenberg B. Dekker, New York, pp. 1–72.

Wenger DA, Gasper PW, Thrall MA *et al.* Bone marrow transplantation in the feline model of arylsufatase-B deficiency. In: *Bone Marrow Transplantation for Treatment of Lysosomal Storage Diseases*, 1986. Eds: Krivit W, Paul NW. March of Dimes Birth Defects Foundation, Original Article Series, Alan R. Liss, New York **22**:177–186.

Wilson PJ, Suthers GK, Callen DF *et al.* Frequent deletions at Xq28 indicate genetic heterogeneity in Hunter syndrome. *Hum Genet* 1991; **86**: 505–508.

2. Inherited Defects in Red Cell Production

Caterina Borgna-Pignatti

Over the last decade, improvements in bone marrow grafting have permitted application of this kind of therapy, once limited to life-threatening conditions, to diseases that are not rapidly fatal but that profoundly affect patient quality of life. Among these are the haemoglobinopathies that can be defined as defects of structure (the haemoglobin variants) or defects of synthesis of the haemoglobin chains (the thalassaemias). It has been calculated that some 250 000 children with major haemoglobinopathies are born each year worldwide. Allogeneic bone marrow transplantation has been used in the treatment both of homozygous β-thalassaemia and related severe structural haemoglobinopathies, and sickle cell anaemia.

Thalassaemia

The thalassaemias are a heterogeneous group of genetic disorders characterized by abnormal synthesis of one or more globin chains, with autosomal recessive inheritance. In its homozygous form, the absent or reduced synthesis of the beta-chain (β° and β^+, respectively), is responsible for a serious clinical condition known under the names of Cooley's anaemia, Mediterranean anaemia or thalassaemia major, in which ineffective erythropoiesis and haemolysis give rise to severe anaemia. A skull X-ray with 'hair-on-end' appearance secondary to ineffective erythropoiesis and subsequent marrow hyperplasia and widening of the marrow space is shown in **56**.

More than 30 000 patients are affected by thalassaemia major worldwide, one third of whom are in Europe (Weatherall and Clegg, 1981). The prognosis of the disease, once invariably fatal within the first decade of life, has improved in recent years. Survival at 15 years for patients born between 1970 and 1974 has been reported to be 94.4% (Zurlo *et al.*, 1989) (**57**), and well-treated patients have a normal

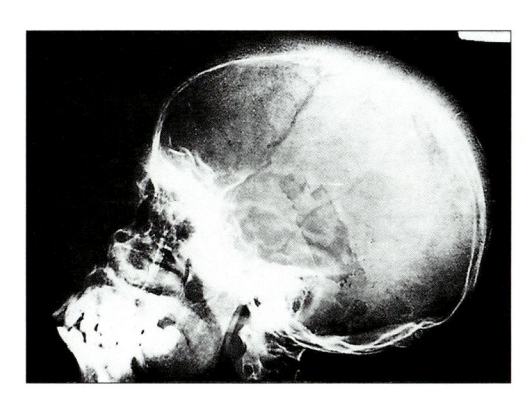

56 Skull X-ray with 'hair-on-end' appearance in untreated thalassaemia major. This is due to widening of the bony plates of the skull secondary to erythroid hyperplasia and ineffective erythropoiesis

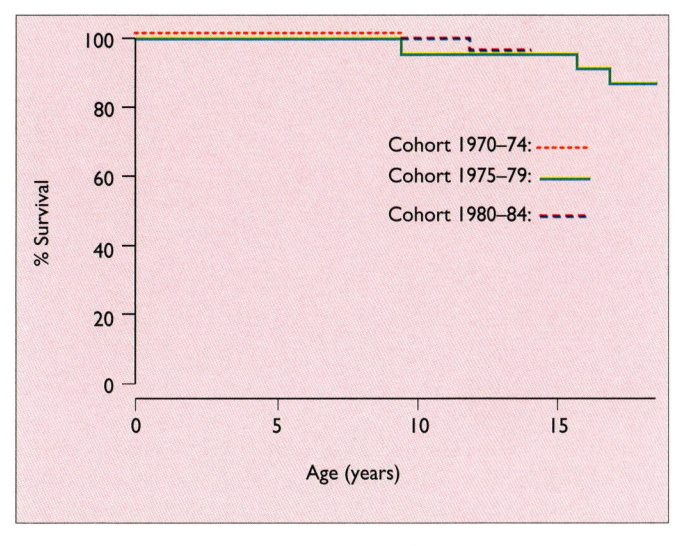

57 Survival of patients with thalassaemia major, born since 1970 and receiving conventional treatment.

appearance (**58**). The most recent therapeutic protocols include transfusions of filtered red cells every 2–3 weeks designed to maintain a mean haemoglobin of 11–12 g/dl, and iron chelation therapy. The only drug now available to prevent, or at least reduce, transfused iron accumulation is desferrioxamine. This requires administration subcutaneously every night, for 8–10 h. Nevertheless, iron overload continues to be a frequent complication of thalassaemia (**59, 60**). Heart disease is the primary cause of death, followed by infection in patients under the age of 15 years. Liver disease occurs, and diabetes mellitus affects 6% of patients over the age of 10 years (De Sanctis *et al.*, 1988). Puberty fails to occur in 40% of boys and 25% of girls over 12 years of age (Borgna-Pignatti *et al.*, 1985).

Bone marrow transplantation (BMT) has been introduced as an alternative approach to the treatment of thalassaemia after animal studies (Weiden *et al.*, 1981) had shown the feasibility of curing genetically determined haemolytic anaemias by marrow grafting, and good results had been obtained in patients with leukaemia and aplastic anaemia.

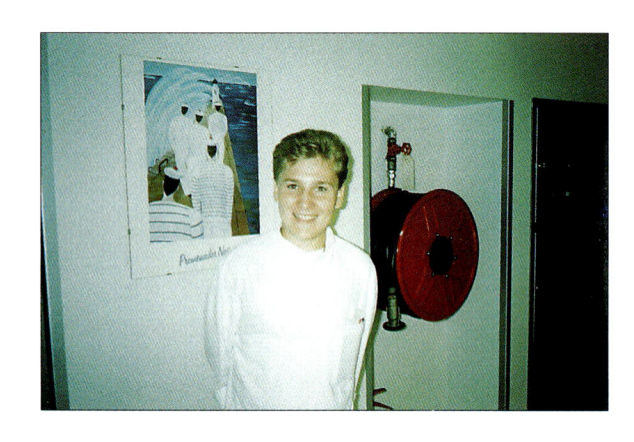

58 The appearance of a well-transfused and iron chelated patient with thalassaemia is normal.

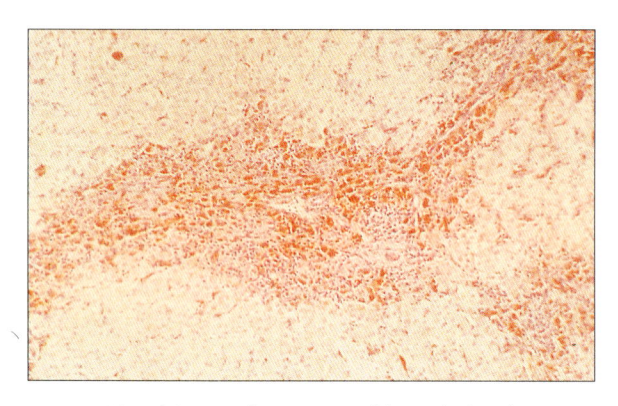

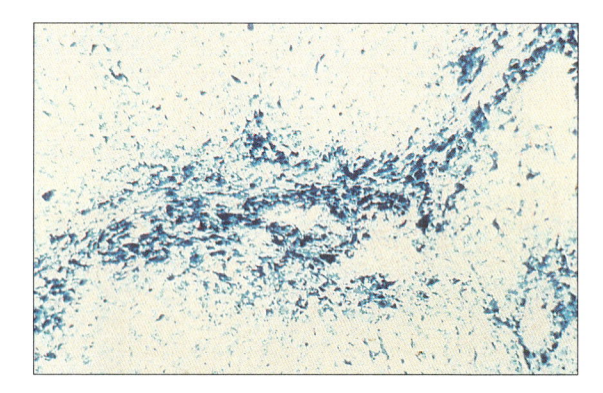

59, 60 Liver biopsy of a 14-year-old, unchelated patient with thalassaemia major: **59** Portal space with inflammatory infiltrates and iron pigment in the macrophages (EE × 100). **60** The Perl's staining demonstrates intense iron deposition.

Bone marrow transplantation

The first patient with thalassaemia was transplanted in Seattle in 1981 (Thomas *et al.*, 1982) (**61**). He is now 12 years old and in excellent general condition (**62**). Since then, several hundred transplants have been performed worldwide, the majority of these in Italy. The world experience has recently been reviewed (Borgna-Pignatti, 1992). Patient ages at BMT have been between 6 months and 24 years, and the number of transfusions received has ranged from none to several hundred. A few patients underwent BMT for thalassaemia intermedia and a few others were affected by HbE/β-thalassaemia or HbS/β-thalassaemia. Overall survival among patients with a follow-up of at least three months was 80%, ranging in the four largest series from 82 to 95%. Disease-free survival was 67% (67–90%). Most patients were chelated, but compliance had often been poor. In the hope of avoiding transfusion-

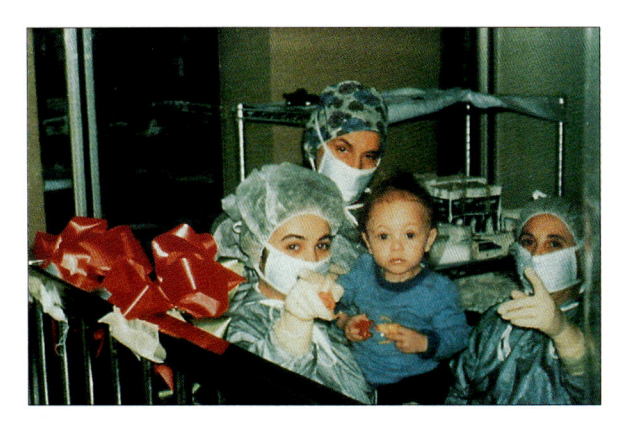

61, 62 The first thalassaemia patient to undergo bone marrow transplantation in 1981, and at the age of 12 years.

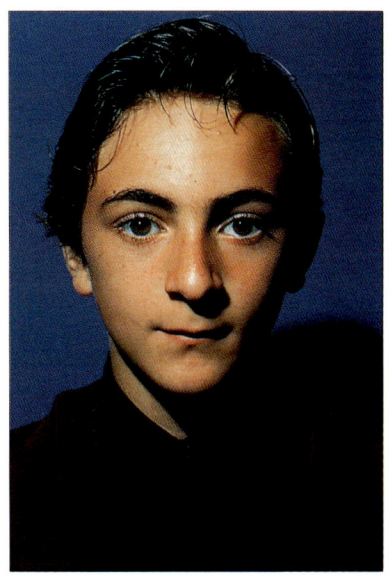

induced sensitization and the risks posed by haemosiderosis, the majority of transplants were performed in young patients, the median age being 4–8 years in the largest series reported. Age, however, does not seem to significantly influence results, as long as the general condition of the patient at the time of grafting is good. However, according to Lucarelli *et al.* (1990, 1991), outcome seems to be significantly affected by the presence of liver disease and by compliance with chelation. These investigators reported a disease-free survival at three years of 53% in poorly chelated patients without liver disease.

Because thalassaemia patients receive multiple blood transfusions, they are exposed to numerous blood-borne viral infections, especially those affecting the liver. However, infection with hepatitis B virus, once almost universal in transfused patients from the Mediterranean area, has now almost disappeared as a consequence of testing donor blood, and of the immunization programme introduced in the early 1980s. Antibodies to hepatitis C virus are present in 72% of thalassaemia patients in Italy (Rebulla *et al.*, 1992). Chronic persistent or chronic active hepatitis is therefore a frequent finding, especially in the older age group (Jean *et al.*, 1984). The combined effects of infections and of iron overload, with its fibrogenic effect, contribute to liver damage.

Before donated blood was systematically screened, 57 out of 3633 (1.5%) European patients had become HIV-positive (Lefrère and Girot, 1987). With screening, the risk of receiving an infected unit of blood appears to remain in the order of 1:50 000 (Mozzi *et al.*, 1992). Two HIV-positive patients have undergone BMT to date, but in both, the procedure was soon followed by death.

The prevalence of cytomegalovirus (CMV) seropositivity in thalassaemia patients before transplantation has been found to be 69%, increasing with age. This is similar to that of a control group made up of healthy bone marrow donors (Baronciani *et al.*, 1989). To limit the impact of CMV infection in the post-transplant period, i.v. human immunoglobulin, acyclovir or ganciclovir, blood filters and CMV-negative blood products have been included in the routine management of thalassaemia patients.

Donors

In order to minimize the risk of rejection and of graft-versus-host disease the ideal donor should be an HLA-identical sibling, which restricts the possibility of transplantation to approximately 34% of patients. Consanguinous marriage, which is frequent in many ethnic groups among whom the gene of thalassaemia is also common, increases the pool of potential donors. It has been observed, in fact, that 8.5% of the patients have phenotypically identical parental donors (Delfini *et al.*, 1985). The experience accumulated so far with imperfectly matched relative donors has been disappointing, with a high percentage of rejection and death. Unrelated volunteer donors are not considered a viable option in thalassaemia, because of the increased risk of severe graft-versus-host disease.

Because thalassaemia trait is transmitted in an autosomal recessive manner, two-thirds of donors will be carriers of β-thalassaemia, and one-third will be normal. It has been shown that there is no difference in the two groups as far as engraftment is concerned and that the initial post-transplant phase of medullary expansion is characterized by smaller erythrocytes (mean corpuscular volume, MCV = 72 ± 3fl), when the donor is heterozygous, as compared with the absolute macrocytosis (MCV = 94 ± 7fl) observed when the donor is haematologically normal (Cao et al., 1989). After two years, haemoglobin, MCV and MCH (mean cell haemoglobin) reach values similar to those of the respective donors, while levels of HbA_2 and globin chain synthesis reach the donor values within two months of BMT. Interestingly, in recipients of marrow from heterozygous donors, there is a more marked and protracted activation of HbF synthesis, as compared to those patients transplanted from normal donors (Galanello et al., 1989) This is most likely to be a result of the more marked erythropoietic stress on erythroid progenitors heterozygous for β-thalassaemia.

Preparative Regimen

In thalassaemia, the bone marrow is hypercellular, and requires complete ablation by the preparative therapy to permit engraftment of the donor marrow. In addition to pretransplant immunosuppression, which can effectively be achieved with cyclophosphamide, total body irradiation, busulphan dimethylbusuphan, melphalan, antithymocyte globulin (ATG) or total lymph node irradiation (TLI) have been used to effect myelo-ablation. The preparative regimens most often used include cyclophosphamide (30–50 mg/kg × 4 days) and busulphan (3.5–4 mg/kg × 4 days). A dose of busulphan lower than 14 mg/kg has resulted in an increased risk of rejection, whereas a higher dose, or the addition of irradiation, carries an increased risk of death from transplant-related causes. Moreover, irradiation of young children should be avoided, as it affects growth and thyroid and gonadal function, and can induce secondary malignancies.

For patients with liver problems, Lucarelli and his group (1991) have adopted a modified protocol, in which the dose of cyclophosphamide is reduced, and ALG (anti-lymphocyte globulin) is added from –5 to day +5. The results seem to be promising, with a reduction in the death rate, counterbalanced, however, by an increased risk of rejection. Graft-versus-host disease prophylaxis, in the past effected almost exclusively with methotrexate, is now usually with cyclosporin, alone or in combination with methotrexate. The use of cyclophosphamide and T-cell depletion of the marrow graft has also been reported.

Complications

Graft 'take' is usually documented by globin chain synthesis (**63–65**), isoelectrofocusing of globins (**66, 67**), study of DNA hypervariable loci or, when appropriate, by chromosomal analysis. Risk of rejection is highest when the recipient has been sensitized to minor donor transplantation antigens by previous blood transfusions. Rejection, or failure of engraftment, has complicated 13% of the transplants performed in thalassaemic children. Of these, two-thirds underwent autologous reconstitution, while one-third remained aplastic. Rejection is usually an early event, but in two cases the graft failed more than one year after the procedure. A second transplant can be done, and may be successful in one-half of cases. As an alternative, autologous bone marrow can be cryopreserved prior to the procedure and infused as a 'rescue' in those patients developing aplasia. The primary causes of death are bacterial and fungal infections, followed by acute graft-versus-host disease, which complicates the post-transplant course in one-quarter of the patients.

Chronic graft-versus-host disease, of moderate or severe degree, has been reported in approximately 6% of the patients surviving with a functioning graft for at least 150 days. This complication, characterized by disabling and disfiguring symptoms, is particularly feared by patients who undergo transplantation more to rid themselves of a chronic disease than to avoid impending death.

The occurrence of non-Hodgkin's lymphoma between 40 and 210 days after grafting, has been reported in four patients (Polchi et al., 1989; Slavin S, personal communication). Only one survives, after surgery and radiotherapy. An excess of malignancies has been reported in patients receiving conventional treatment (Zurlo et al., 1989), and whether bone marrow transplantation will increase or decrease this risk remains to be seen.

As mentioned above, iron overload now represents the main problem for patients receiving conventional treatment. When patients are transplanted before a large load of iron has accumulated, normal growth

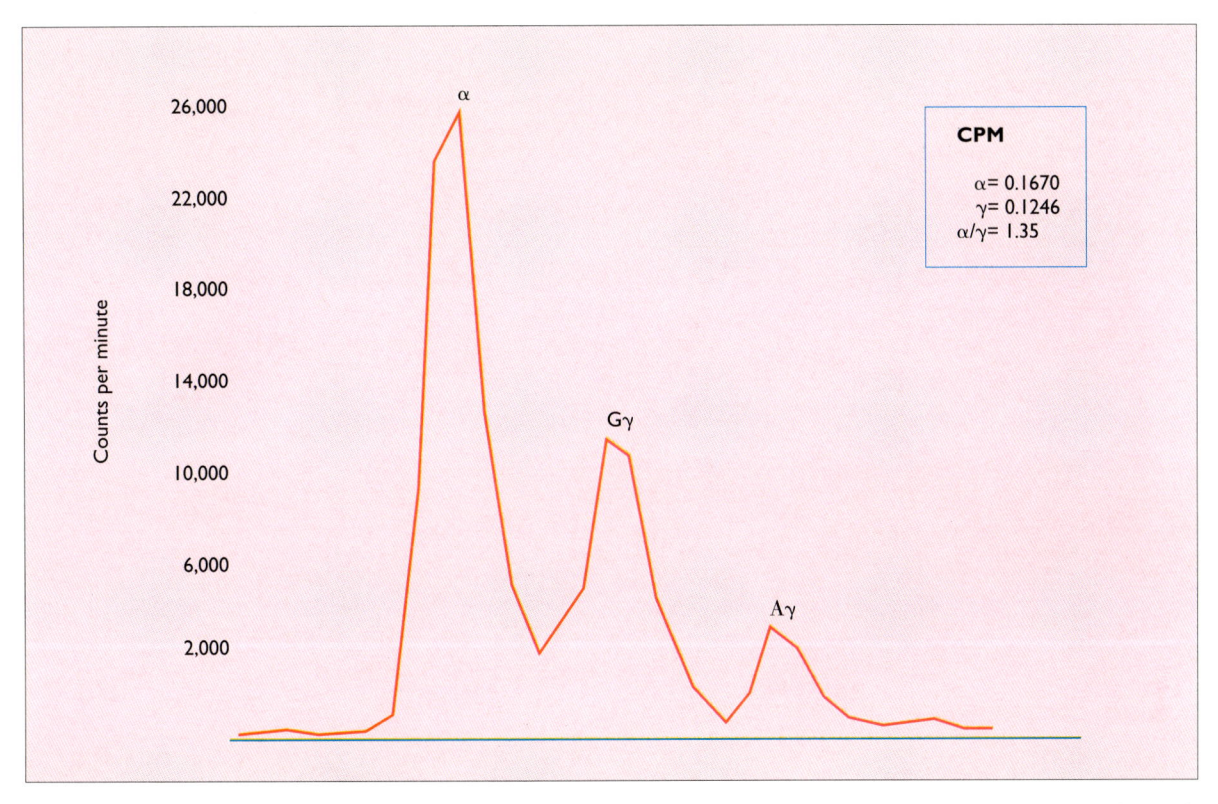

63 Globin chain synthesis (high-performance liquid chromatography) of a patient with β° thalassaemia (the peak corresponding to the β chain is absent).

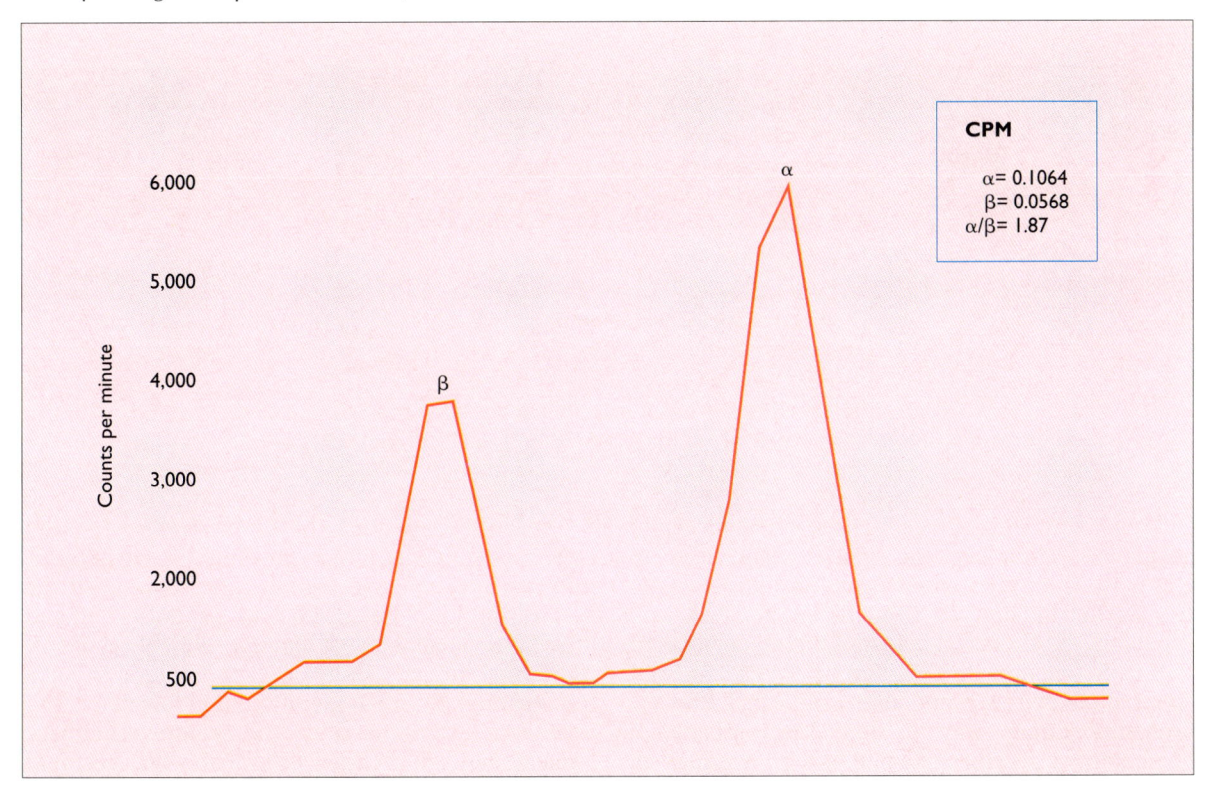

64 Globin chain synthesis (high-performance liquid chromatography) of the patient in **63**'s donor, carrier of thalassaemia trait.

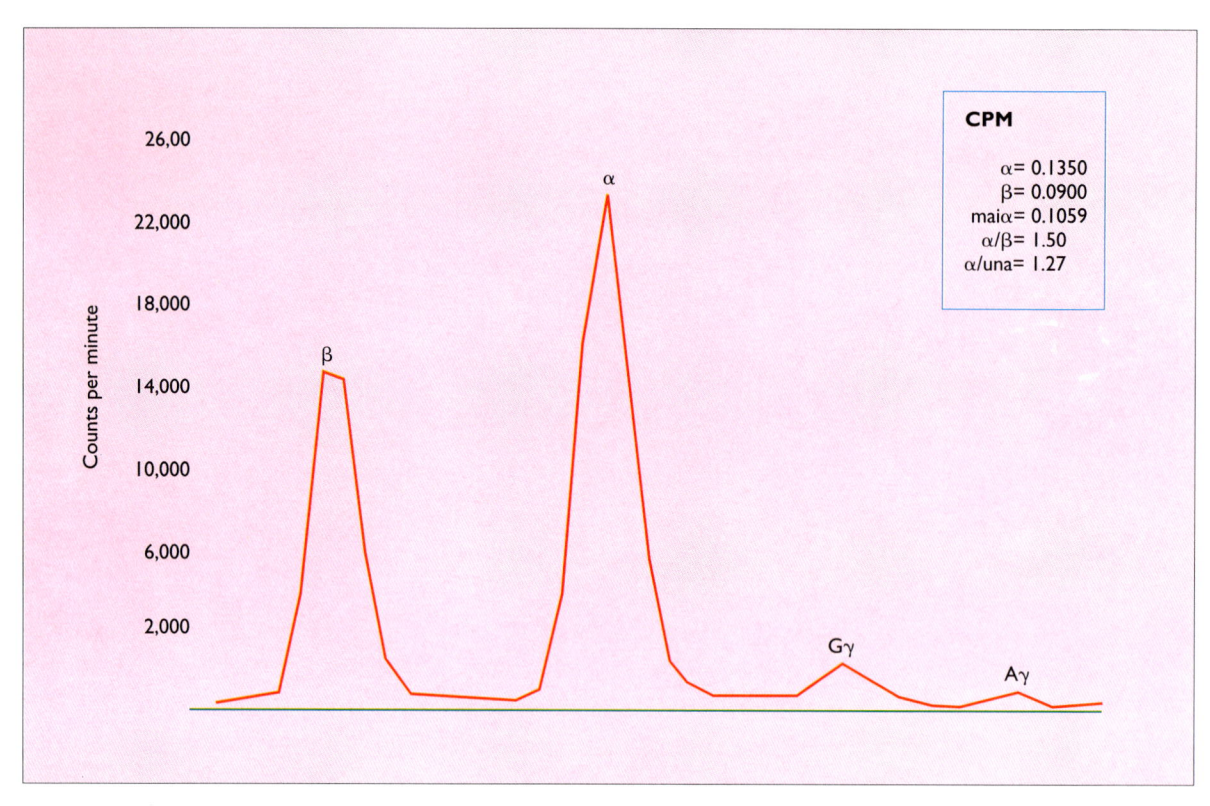

65 Globin chain synthesis (high-performance liquid chromatography) of the patient in **63**, 60 days after bone marrow transplantation. (Courtesy of Dr Galanello.)

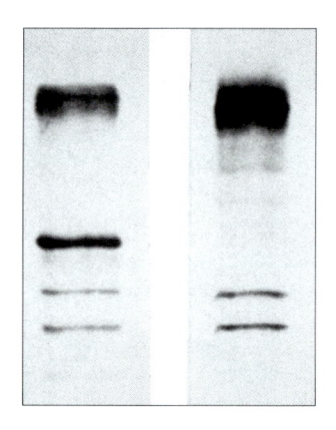

66 (left) Isoelectrofocusing of globins, before and 1 month after bone marrow transplantation of a child with β^0 thalassaemia from a normal donor. The presence of γ-chains after transplant can be considered an expression of stress erythropoiesis. (Courtesy of Dr Papayannopoulou.)

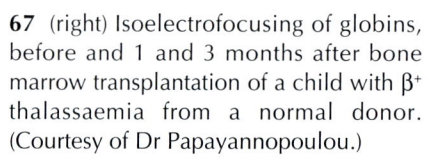

67 (right) Isoelectrofocusing of globins, before and 1 and 3 months after bone marrow transplantation of a child with β^+ thalassaemia from a normal donor. (Courtesy of Dr Papayannopoulou.)

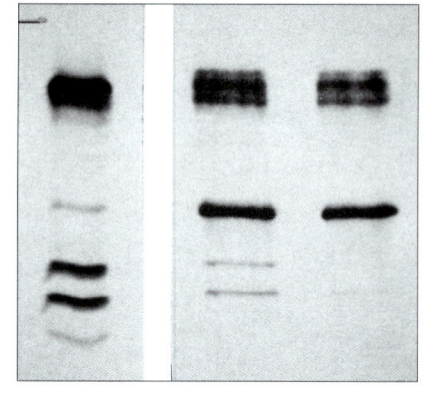

and renewed haematopoietic activity, are sufficient to normalize ferritin level and even, in some cases, to eliminate the excess liver iron (Angelucci *et al.*, 1989). After the first few years of life, however, and especially if chelation has not been performed regularly, haemosiderosis can be severe and not spontaneously reversible after grafting. Trials are presently under way to test the efficacy of phlebotomy or erythrocyte pheresis on overloaded, in successfully transplanted patients.

The consequences of iron overload upon endocrine function may be prevented by early BMT. It is possible, however, that the drugs administered as conditioning for BMT may provoke delayed growth, gonadal damage and infertility in their own right. A preliminary study on 30 prepubertal patients transplanted for thalassaemia, and followed for 0.7–5 years (De Sanctis *et al.*, 1991) showed severe gonadal damage in the girls, probably as a result of chemotherapy. There was, however, no obvious damage in boys. A longer follow-up will be necessary to define the severity of sexual dysfunction, if any, in these patients, and the relative roles of iron overload and conditioning therapy in its aetiology. In the meantime, it is encouraging that several transplanted patients have undergone spontaneous pubertal maturation (**68**).

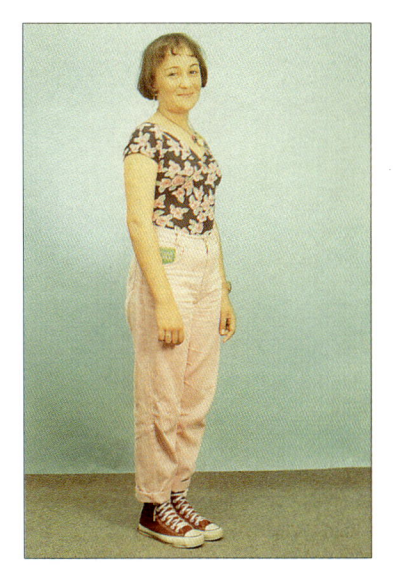

68 An 11-year-old girl transplanted for thalassaemia major at the age of 2 years. She had a completely normal puberty, including menarche, but still suffers from chronic skin graft-versus-host disease. This severly limits her social life as it affects her eyes.

Sickle cell anaemia

Haemoglobin S is characterized by the substitution of valine for glutamic acid, at the sixth position of the β-globin chain. This derives, in turn, from the substitution of thymine for adenine in the glutamic acid DNA codon on chromosome 11. The inheritance is autosomal recessive. The distribution of the gene corresponds closely to that of falciparum malaria, and is common in West Central Africa, where up to 25% of the population carry the trait. In the north-eastern corner of Saudi Arabia and in a localized area of East Central India, carriers exceed 20%. Of African-Americans, 8% are heterozygous (Motulski, 1973) whereas in the Mediterranean countries the gene for HbS is much less frequent. The homozygous condition causes sickle cell anaemia. Deoxygenation of the haemoglobin variant permits the formation of rigid HbS polymers that give the red cells their typical shape and make their progression through the microcirculation difficult. Intravascular sickling is favoured by increased hydrogen ion concentration and increased temperature, the density distribution of sickle cells, their adherence to endothelial cells, the relative percentages of HbS and HbF, and by other incompletely understood factors. The clinical picture of this markedly heterogeneous disease includes infections, veno-occlusive episodes, sequestration, and haemolytic and aplastic crises. All organs and systems can suffer from the consequences of the disease, but the most dramatic complication involves the central nervous system. Stroke (**69**) which occurs in 10% of patients, spares no age group, and recurs in 70% of patients. Mortality averages 20%, while gross neurological deficits or neuropsychological defects may persist in almost half of the survivors (Ohene-Frempong,

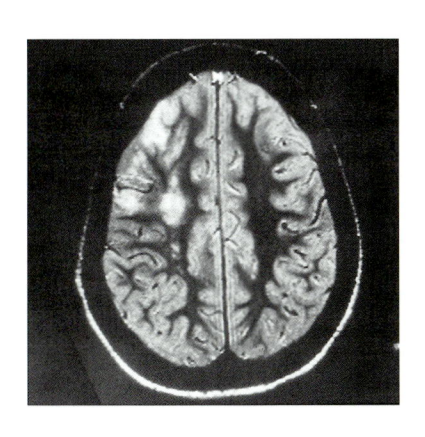

69 0T^2-weighted axial magnetic resonance image of a cerebrovascular accident in a patient with sickle cell aeaemia. The lesion, localized in the white matter of the centrum semi-ovale, is associated with an area of cortical hyperintensity in the cortex of the left fronto-lateral region. (Courtesy of Dr Ohene-Frempong.)

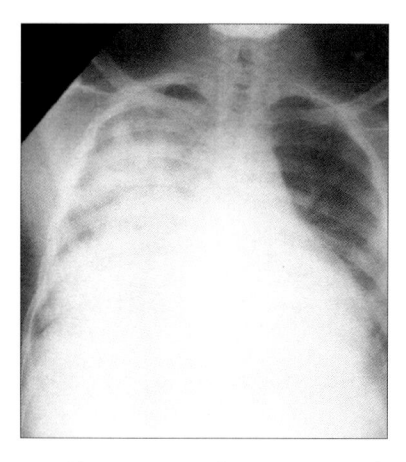

70 Chest X-ray of a patient with sickle cell anaemia and the acute chest syndrome, demonstrating lung consolidation. (Courtesy of Dr Ohene-Frempong.)

1991). Growth and sexual maturation are delayed, but the majority of patients do achieve puberty. Early in life, functional asplenia develops, and the patients are prone to the same life-threatening infections as splenectomized children. Life expectancy has greatly improved in recent years, mainly due to prompt treatment of infections. About 85% of patients survive to age 20 years (Leikin et al., 1989). The most common cause of death is infection in patients younger than 3 years, while above 3 years, stroke and acute chest syndrome (**70**) become more commonplace. Treatment is mainly symptomatic, and includes analgesic drugs, hydration, prophylaxis and therapy of the infectious episodes. Chronic transfusion therapy significantly reduces the recurrence of stroke, but can be complicated by infection, allo-immunization and, invariably, if chelation is not started, by iron overload. 5-Azacytidine (Ley et al., 1983) and hydroxyurea (Rodgers et al., 1990) have been used with some success, with the aim of increasing the percentage of HbF. However, longer trials are needed. As with the clinical course of the disease, so the cost of treatment for sickle cell anaemia varies from patient to patient, but is similar to that of patients with thalassaemia (in the order of $30 000 a year) once a programme of chronic transfusion and chelation is started.

Bone marrow transplantation

Bone marrow transplantation for sickle cell disease was successfully attempted for the first time in 1984 (Johnson et al., 1984). To our knowledge, 50 patients have been transplanted as of September 1992.

Twenty-seven patients of African origin, ranging in age from 1 to 23 years, were transplanted in Belgium (Vermylen et al., 1988, 1992; Ferster et al., 1992). Fourteen were transplanted in France (Milpied et al., 1988; Kirkpatrick et al., 1991; Bernaudin et al., 1992) and four in Italy, (Giardini et al., 1992). Five patients were transplanted in the USA (Johnson et al., 1992). In two cases, the primary indication to BMT was leukaemia (one myelogenous and one lymphoblastic), and one patient suffered from Morquio's disease. Donors were usually HLA-identical siblings. For one patient, the donor was his HLA identical, MLC (mixed lymphocyte culture)-negative father and for one her haplo-identical mother. Conditioning included cyclophosphamide (120–200 mg/kg) and busulphan (14–16 mg/kg). The patients with leukaemia received cyclophosphamide (120 mg/kg) and total body irradiation (10–11.5 Gy). Two patients also received total lymph node irradiation and a few received ATG. Graft-versus-host disease prophylaxis was with cyclosporin with or without the addition of methotrexate, or, in a few cases, prednisolone. Three patients developed limited chronic graft-versus-host disease. In the child who had received marrow from his father, a second transplant was successful after preparation with cyclophophamide, ATG and thoraco-abdominal irradiation. Stable engraftment was attained at the second attempt as was the case in the 3-year-old boy who had both sickle cell anaemia and Morquio's disease Type A (Mentzer et al., 1990) and who was transplanted from his HLA-identical, MLC non-reactive sister. One year after the second transplant, the patient had sickle trait as did his donor sister, and normal levels of white-cell N-acetylgalactosamine-6-sulphatase. However, a 22-year-old patient transplanted for acute lymphoblastic leukaemia failed to engraft, despite three attempts from two donors, and died of veno-occlusive disease of the liver, 85 days after the first transplant (Milpied et al., 1988). There were three additional deaths, due in two cases to acute graft-versus-host disease. The third patient, who had two strokes before transplant, died of a cerebrovascular accident in the immediate post-graft period. Two other patients have been transplanted following cerebrovascular accidents, in an attempt to prevent recurrence. Both, however,

Inherited Defects in Red Cell Production

had subsequent neurological events. Engraftment can be easily demonstrated by haemoglobin electrophoresis (**71, 72**). Overall results are presented in (**73**). Functional asplenia documented before grafting, disappeared in some of the patients, as shown by ^{99m}Tc scan (**74, 75**) and red cell morphology (**76, 77**). In two children who also had G6PD (glucose 6-phosphate dehydrogenase) deficiency, enzyme levels reached normal values after transplant.

In conclusion, it appears that patients with sickle cell disease do not behave differently from the experience suggested with thalassaemia. Rejection may be a slightly bigger problem, but the figures are too small to allow a definitive statement. As in thalassaemia, irradiation probably does not improve engraftment.

The decision of whether or not to transplant patients with sickle cell disease is difficult, as the course of the disease is extremely variable and

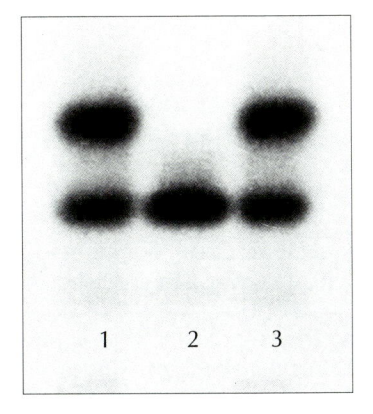

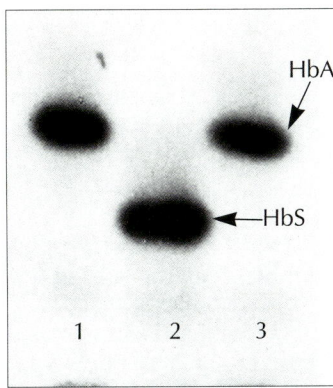

71, 72 AS donor (**71**, left), AA donor (**72**, right). Haemoglobin electrophoresis on cellulose acetate before and after bone marrow transplantation for sickle cell anaemia.
Line 1: donors. Line 2: patients (SS) before transplant. Line 3: Patients after transplant.
(Courtesy of Professor Cornu.)

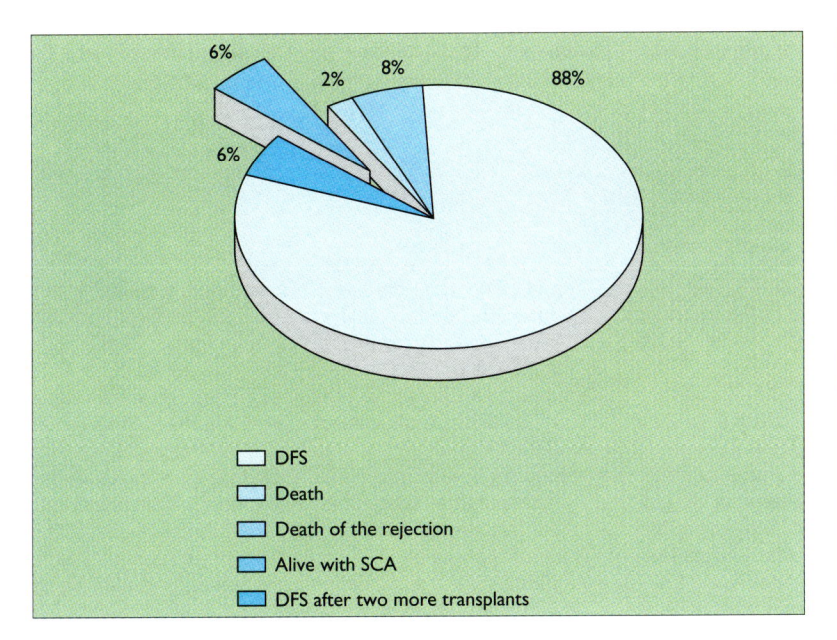

73 Results of bone marrow transplantation for sickle cell anaemia as of September 1992; 50 patients.

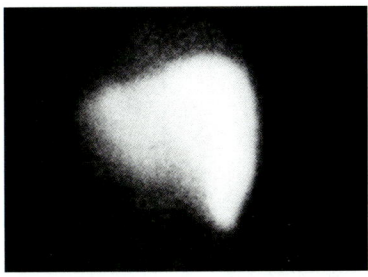

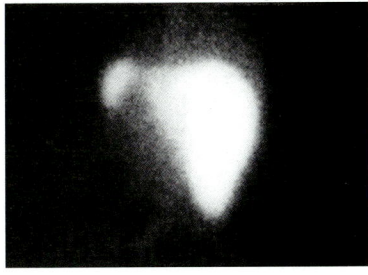

74, 75 Tc scintiscan of spleen of a patient with sickle cell anaemia: (**74**, top) before transplantation spleen is not visible; (**75**, bottom) six months after transplantation spleen function has reverted to normal. (Courtesy of Professor Fondu.)

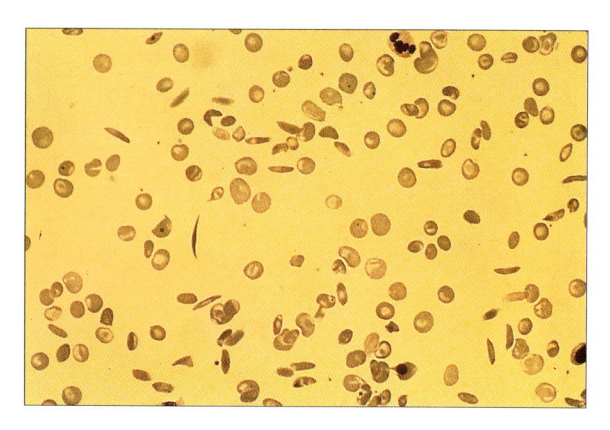

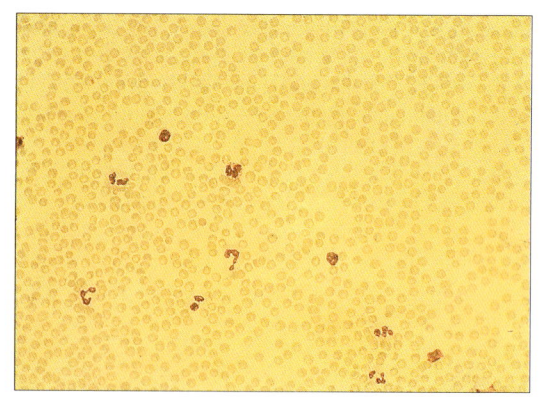

76, 77 Blood smear of a patient with sickle cell anaemia: (**76**, left) before bone marrow transplantation; (**77**, right) after bone marrow transplantation. Note the presence, before grafting, of sickled erythrocytes and Howell–Jolly bodies. Both have disappeared after transplant.

unpredictable in the first few years of life. It has been suggested (Nagel, 1991) that BMT should be considered for children presenting early with central nervous system insult, or with repetitive acute chest syndrome, the complications of which have a particularly poor prognosis. These patients, however, are the ones most likely to have severe transplant-related problems. Ideally, therefore, BMT should be performed in complication-prone children before the complications appear.

In order to make a meaningful decision on whether or not to transplant, several factors should be considered. High levels of HbF, the coexistence of α-thalassaemia-2, and the presence of at least one Senegal haplotype are considered indices of a more benign course, whereas the CAR haplotype has been reported to be an index of high morbidity (Powars, 1991). No severity score is perfect, however, and the decision of whether or not to transplant will always be somewhat arbitrary.

References

Angelucci E, Polizzi V, Lucarelli G, Muretto P. Liver iron kinetics in thalassaemia patients after bone marrow transplantation. *Prog Clin Biol Res* 1989; **309**: 291–298.

Baronciani D, Polchi P, Lucarelli G *et al*. CMV infections in thalassaemia patients after BMT. *Prog Clin Biol Res* 1989; **309**: 249–263.

Bernaudin F, Souillet G, Vannier JP. Bone marrow transplantation in 14 children with severe sickle cell disease: The French experience. *Second International Symposium on Bone Marrow Transplantation for Thalassaemia, Pesaro, September 24–27 1992*. Abstract 35.

Borgna-Pignatti C, De Stefano P, Zonta L *et al*. Growth and sexual maturation in thalassaemia major. A survey of 250 adolescents. *J Pediatr* 1985; **106**: 150–155.

Borgna-Pignatti C. Bone marrow transplantation for the haemoglobinopathies In: *Bone Marrow Transplantation in Practice*, 1992. Eds: Treleaven JG, Barrett AJ. Churchill Livingstone, London, pp. 151–159.

Cao A, Argiolu F, Sanna MA, Barella S. Il trapianto di midollo nella talassemia major. *Stato dell'arte Medico e Bambino* 1989; **1**: 33–40.

Delfini C, Polchi P, Izzi T *et al*. Bone marrow donors other than HLA genotypically identical siblings for patients with thalassaemia. *Expt Hematol* 1985; **13**: 1197–2000.

De Sanctis V, Zurlo MG, Senesi E. Insulin dependent diabetes in thalassaemia. *Arch Dis Child* 1988; **63**: 58–62.

De Sanctis V, Galimberti M, Lucarelli G *et al*. Gonadal function after allogeneic bone marrow transplantation for thalassaemia. *Arch Dis Child* 1991; **66**: 517–520.

Ferster A, De Valck C, Azzi N *et al*. Bone marrow transplantation for sickle cell anaemia. *Br J Haematol* 1992; **80**: 102–105.

Galanello R, Barella S, Maccioni L *et al*. Erythropoiesis following bone marrow transplantation from donors heterozygous for β-thalassaemia. *Br J Haematol* 1989; **72**: 561–566.

Giardini C, Galimberti M, Lucarelli G. Bone marrow transplantation in sickle cell anaemia. *Second International Symposium on Bone Marrow Transplantation for Thalassaemia, Pesaro, September 24–27 1992*. Abstract 34.

Jean G, Terzoli S, Mauri R *et al*. Cirrhosis associated with multiple transfusions in thalassaemia. *Arch Dis Child*

1984; **59**: 67–70.

Johnson FL. Bone marrow transplantation for sickle cell disease: US experience. *NIH Workshop on Bone Marrow Transplantation for Hemoglobinopathies, 1992*. Abstract 12.

Johnson FL, Look AT, Gockerman J et al. Bone marrow transplantation in a patient with sickle cell anaemia. *N Engl J Med* 1984; **311**: 780–783.

Kirkpatrick DV, Barrios NJ, Humbert JH. Bone marrow Transplantation for sickle cell anemia. *Semin Hematol* 1991; **28**: 240–243.

Lefrère JJ, Girot R. HIV infection in polytransfused thalassaemic patients. *Lancet* 1987; **2**: 686.

Leikin SL, Gallagher D, Kinney TR et al. Mortality in children and adolescents with sickle cell disease. *Pediatrics* 1989; **84**: 500–508.

Ley TJ, DeSimone J, Anagnou NP et al. 5-Azacytidine increases G-globin synthesis and reduces the proportion of dense cells in patients with sickle cell anaemia. *Blood* 1983; **62**: 370–380.

Lucarelli G, Galimberti M, Polchi P et al. Bone marrow transplantation in patients with thalassaemia. *New Engl J Med* 1990; **322**: 417–421.

Lucarelli G, Galimberti M, Polchi P et al. Bone marrow transplantation in patients with thalassaemia. *Hematol/Oncol Clin North Am* 1991; **5**: 549–556.

Mentzer W, Packman S, Wara W, Cowan M. Successful bone marrow transplantation in a child with sickle cell anaemia and Morquio's disease. *Blood* 1990; **76**: No. 10 Suppl (1) Abstract 267.

Milpied N, Harousseau JL, Garand R, David A. Bone marrow transplantation for sickle cell anaemia *Lancet* 1988; **2**: 328–329.

Motulski AG. Frequency of sickling disorders in US blacks. *N Engl J Med* 1973; **288**: 31–33.

Mozzi F, Rebulla P, Lillo F et al. and the COOLEYCARE Cooperative Group. HIV and HTLV infections in 1305 transfusion-dependent thalassaemics in Italy. *AIDS* 1992; **6**: 505–508.

Nagel RL. The dilemma of marrow transplantation in sickle cell anaemia *Semin Hematol* 1991; **29**: 180–201.

Ohene-Frempong K. Stroke in sickle cell disease: demographic, clinical and therapeutic considerations. *Semin Hematol* 1991; July 28 (3): 213–219.

Platt OS, Rosenstock W, Espeland MA. Influence of sickle hemoglobinopathies on growth and development. *N Engl J Med* 1984; **311**: 7–12.

Polchi P, Lucarelli G, Galimberti M, Moretti L. Cyclosporin in children. *Progr Clin Biol Res* 1989; **309**: 333–348.

Powars DR. Sickle cell anemia b^s-gene-cluster haplotypes as prognostic indicators of vital organ failure. *Sem Hematol* 1991; **28**: 202–206.

Rebulla P, Mozzi F, Contino G et al. Antibody to hepatitis C virus in 1305 Italian multiply transfused thalassaemics: a comparison of first and second generation tests. *Transfusion Med* 1992; **2**: 69–70.

Rodgers GP, Dover GL, Noguchi CT et al. Hematologic responses of patients with sickle cell disease to treatment with hydroxyurea. *N Engl J Med* 1990; **322**: 1037–1135.

Thomas ED, Buckner CD, Sanders JE et al. Marrow transplantation for thalassemia. *Lancet* 1982; **2**: 227–229.

Vermylen C, Fernandez Robles E, Ninane J, Cornu G. Bone marrow transplantation in 5 children with sickle cell anaemia *Lancet* 1988; **1**: 1427–1428.

Vermylen C, Cornu G. Bone marrow transplantation in sickle cell anaemia: European experience. *Second International Symposium on Bone Marrow Transplantation for Thalassemia, Pesaro, September 24–27 1992*. Abstract 33.

Weatherall DJ, Clegg JB. *The Thalassaemia Syndromes*, 1981, 3rd ed. Blackwell, Oxford.

Weiden PL, Hackman RC, Deeg HJ et al. Long-term survival and reversal of iron overload after marrow transplantation in dogs with congenital hemolytic anemia. *Blood* 1981; **57**: 66–70.

Zurlo MG, DeStefano P, Borgna-Pignatti C et al. Survival and causes of death in thalassemia major. *Lancet* 1989; **2**: 27–30.

3. Severe Aplastic Anaemia

Roberto Pasquini

Aplastic anaemia (AA) is a heterogeneous disorder of diverse aetiology characterized by pancytopenia associated with a hypocellular bone marrow. Potential pathophysiological mechanisms include deficient numbers of, or defective, haematopoietic stem cells, an abnormal bone marrow microenvironment, impairment of normal cellular interactions, and immune or non-immune suppression of marrow function. The prognosis in AA is related to the severity of pancytopenia. AA is considered severe when two or more of the following features are present: anaemia associated with a corrected reticulocyte count of less than 1%, a neutrophil count below 500/ml and a platelet count less than 20 000/µml associated with a hypocellular marrow (Camitta and Thomas, 1978). Approximately 50% of those patients receiving supportive treatment or androgen therapy will die from bleeding or infection 3–6 months from the diagnosis, and less than 20% will survive five years (Williams *et al.*, 1973). It has been recently observed that those patients with less than 200 granulocytes/ml have a very short survival, and they are now considered a distinct group designated very severe AA (SAA) (Bacigalupo *et al.*, 1988).

The true incidence of aplastic anaemia is not known and it appears to vary geographically. Recent surveys suggest that its incidence is on the order of 3–6 per million/year (Mary, 1990). Known aetiologies of AA are listed in **Table 4**.

Various treatment approaches have been adopted in an attempt to reconstitute hematopoiesis in patients with AA. These have met with variable success, as is shown in **Table 5**.

Immunosuppressive therapy with single or multiple agents is effective in improving hematopoiesis in approximately half of patients with SAA. Antihuman lymphocyte globulin (ALG) and antihuman thymocyte globulin (ATG), cyclosporin and corticosteroids are all effective in the treatment of SAA (Gluckman *et al.*, 1978; Bacigalupo *et al.* 1979; Camitta, 1983; Speck *et al.*, 1986; Young *et al.*, 1988). Partial recovery of haematopoiesis and reduction of blood transfusion needs are the most common results. Few patients have a return to normal values of their blood counts, however. Results may be superior when immunosuppressive agents are given in combination (Frickhofen *et al.*, 1991) rather than singly. Late development of clonal haematological disorders has been observed in an increasing number of patients with SAA who have done well with treatment (Tichelli *et al.*, 1988).

Allogeneic bone marrow transplantation has been shown to be superior to supportive care or androgen treatment when an HLA identical sibling donor is utilized (Bacigalupo *et al.*, 1988). Usually, complete

Table 4. Aetiological classification of the aplastic anaemias.

Acquired

Idiopathic
Secondary to:
    Drugs and chemical agents
    Radiation
    Viral infections
Paroxysmal nocturnal haemoglobinuria

Constitutional

Fanconi's anaemia
Dyskeratosis congenita
Familial aplastic anaemia

Table 5. Treatment of severe aplastic anaemia.

Immunosuppression
    Corticosteroids
    Antilymphocyte globulin (ALG)
    Antithymocyte globulin (ATG)
    Cyclosporin
    Combinations of the above agents

Bone marrow transplantation
    Syngeneic and allogeneic

Haemopoietic growth factors
    G-CSF, GM-CSF, IL-3, etc.

Miscellaneous
    Androgens and derivatives

recovery of hematopoiesis occurs, and long-term event-free survival is experienced by 60% of patients transplanted (**78**). The best results of BMT in SAA are observed in young patients who have had a short duration of disease, few prior transfusions, preparation with cyclophosphamide alone, and who have received cyclosporin immunoprophylaxis (Pasquini, 1991) (**79–81**).

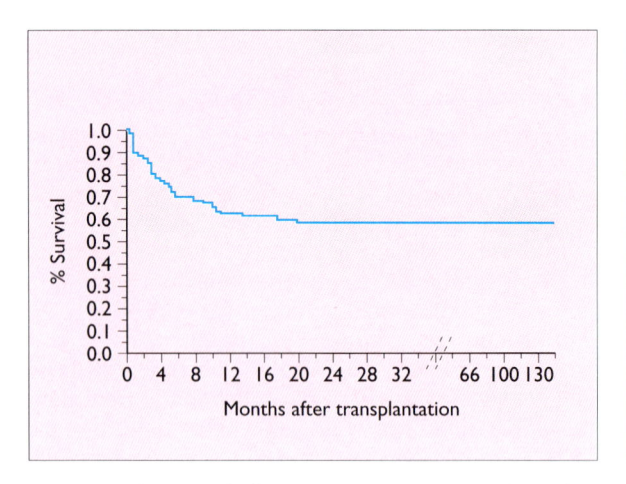

78 Overall survival of 104 SAA patients transplanted in Curitiba, Brazil (1981–1991). Kaplan–Meyer survival curves.

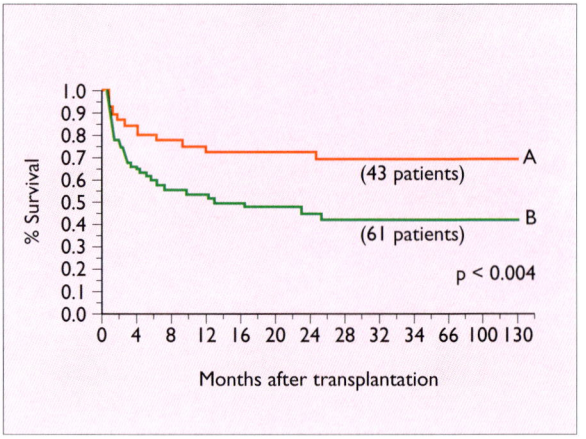

79 Kaplan–Meyer survival curves after HLA identical marrow transplantation for severe aplastic anaemia in relation to number of previous blood transfusions: **A,** less than 15 units of blood derivatives; **B,** more than 15 units of blood derivatives. (Curitiba, Brazil, 1981–1991.)

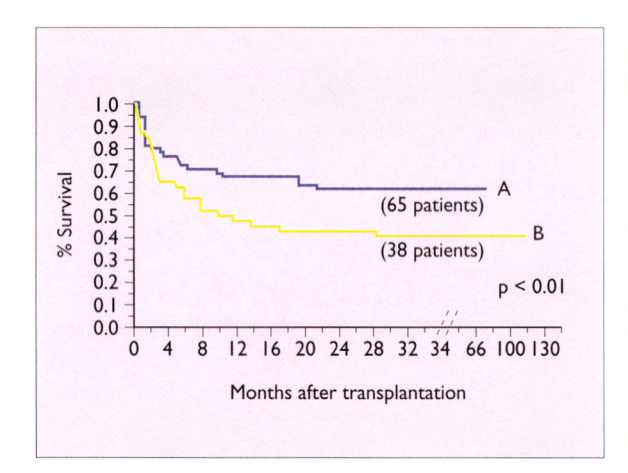

80 Kaplan–Meyer survival curves after HLA identical marrow transplantation for severe aplastic anaemia in relation to graft-versus-host disease prophylaxis. **A,** Methotrexate + cyclosporin; **B,** methotrexate. (Curitiba, Brazil, 1981–1991.)

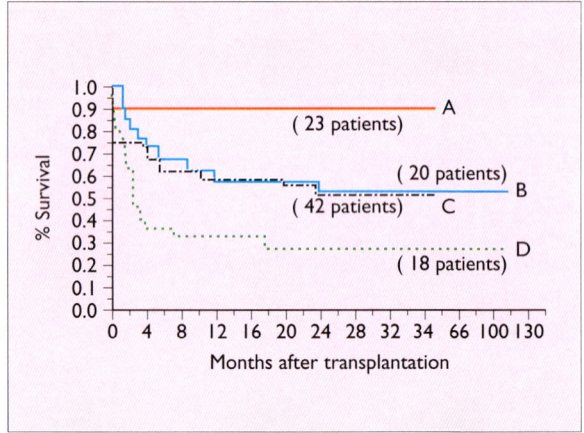

81 Kaplan–Meyer survival curves after HLA identical marrow transplantation for severe aplastic anaemia in relation to previous transfusions and graft-versus-host disease prophylaxis: **A,** less than 15 transfusions and methotrexate (MTX) + cyclosporin (CSA); **B,** less than 15 transfusions and MTX; **C,** More than 15 transfusions and MTX + CSA; **D,** more than 15 transfusions and MTX. (Brazil, 1981–1991.)

Table 6. Comparison between different treatment modalities in severe aplastic anaemia.

Status	BMT	Immunosuppression
Age (years)		
<20	Superior	Inferior
20–40	Same	Same
>40	Inferior	Superior
Neutropenia	Superior	Inferior
Clonal disease	Not reported	Common

Patients older than 30 years have more complications with transplantation, and end results with allogeneic marrow transplantation and immunosuppressive treatment alone are similar (Bacigalupo *et al.*, 1988 (**Table 6**).

The major cause of treatment failure after transplantation is death from transplant-related complications, these being primarily graft rejection, acute and chronic graft-versus-host disease and infections associated with the post-transplant immunodeficiency (**82**).

Graft failure may occur in two different forms:
1 Early, when haematological recovery is not observed within 4 weeks following transplantation or when only a partial engraftment of short duration occurs followed by complete marrow failure.
2 Late graft rejection may occur several months or years after complete haematopoietic reconstitution.

Early rejection has a poor prognosis and most patients die from complications of pancytopenia (Champlin *et al.*, 1988). A second transplant or immunosuppressive treatment can rescue more than 50% of late rejection patients (Pasquini, 1991) (**83**). Several factors correlate with the incidence of graft failure, which varies from 5 to 25% (Champlin, 1990):
1 Cyclophosphamide alone used in the preparative regimen.
2 Previous blood transfusions (Anasetti *et al.*, 1986).
3 Cell doses of <3.0 × 10⁸ nucleated bone marrow cells/kg (Storb *et al.*, 1983b).

These features may also be associated with a higher rejection rate. If radiation is added to the conditioning regimen, none of the above factors influence the rejection rate, and rejection occurs less frequently (Champlin *et al.*, 1988). Newer irradiation protocols such as total body irradiation (3–6 Gy), total lymphoid irradiation and thoraco-abdominal irradiation reduce graft failure to approximately 5%. However, interstitial pneumonia and graft-versus-host disease are more common among patients receiving any radiation as preparation for transplantation (Gluckman *et al* 1992).

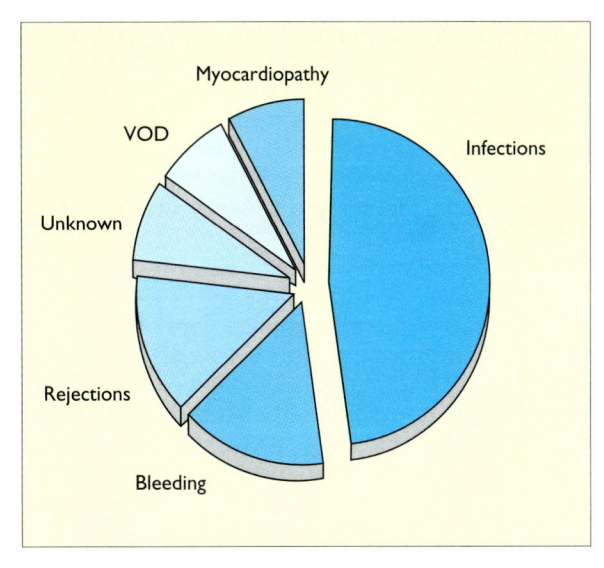

82 Cause of death in post-transplant aplastic anaemia patients. Data from fully matched allogeneic patients transplanted in Brazil (1981–1991).

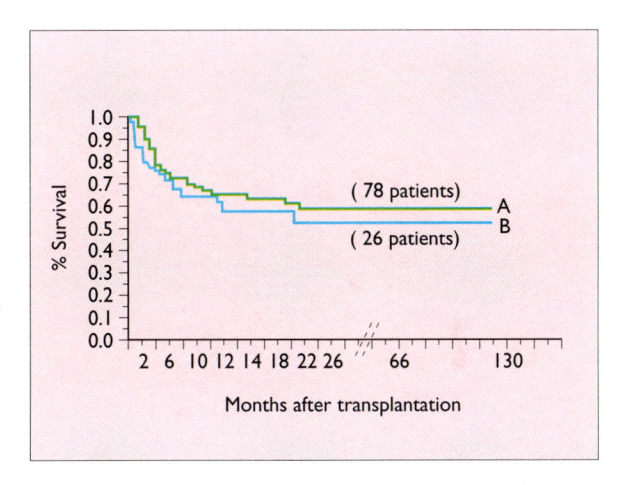

83 Kaplan–Meyer survival curves in HLA identical marrow transplantation in SAA in relation to rejection: **A**, without rejection; **B**, survival after rejection. (Brazil, 1981–1991.)

Graft-versus-host disease (GvHD) is a major complication of allogeneic transplantation and it is the major procedure-related cause of death (**84**). Older patients are more predisposed to develop both acute and chronic GvHD. The combination of methotrexate and cyclosporin has been shown to reduce the incidence and severity of GvHD and improves survival (Sullivan, 1990) (**85**). In general, 50% of patients develop acute GvHD. Chronic GvHD occurs in 30–75% and can be severe enough to prove lethal. Of long-term survivors, 10% have impaired performance status secondary to chronic GvHD (Storb *et al.*, 1983a). Although chronic GvHD occurs more frequently in patients with previous severe acute GvHD, it also develops in approximately one-third of patients not affected by acute GvHD.

Mucositis, intra-atrial catheters, neutropenia and sluggish immune reconstitution are factors that predispose to infections (Winston *et al.*, 1984). Those patients with severe neutropenia who are infected when transplanted have a very poor prognosis. Despite the lower incidence of interstitial pneumonia in aplastic anaemia patients compared with other marrow transplant patients, it is still considered a major complication because of the high attendant death rate. Cytomegalovirus is the most common cause of interstitial pneumonia in aplastic anaemia patients (Meyers, 1986).

Prolonged neutropenia, steroid treatment, and intra-atrial catheters enhance the incidence of fungal infection, particularly with *Candida* and *Aspergillus* (Bodey, 1986). Other fungi are also occasionally encountered (**86, 87**). Protozoa sometimes result in infestations. *Cryptosporidium*, *Toxoplasma*, *Trypanosoma* and *Giardia* infections have been reported (Young, 1984) (**88, 89**).

The behaviour of syngeneic bone marrow in SAA is unusual, since less than 50% of patients have sustained engraftment without conditioning therapy preceding bone marrow infusion. However, when a preparative regimen is employed, all patients engraft (Champlin *et al.*, 1984), although some will need multiple transplants (**90**).

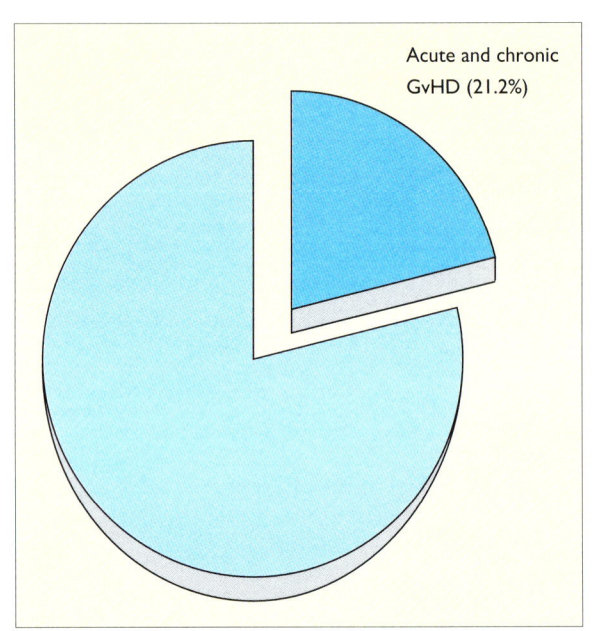

84 Graft-versus-host related mortality observed in 104 patients with severe aplastic anaemia transplanted in Curitiba-Brazil (1981–1991).

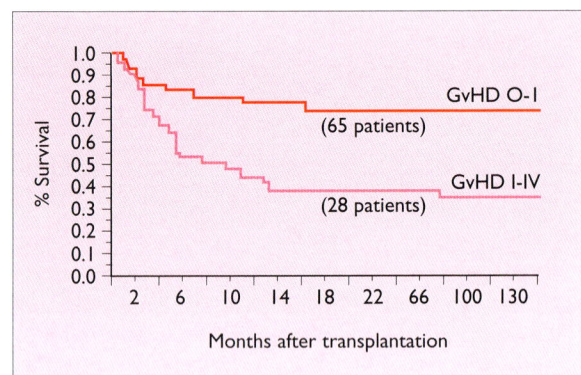

85 Kaplan–Meyer survival curves after HLA identical marrow transplantation for severe aplastic anaemia in relation to graft-versus-host disease occurrence.

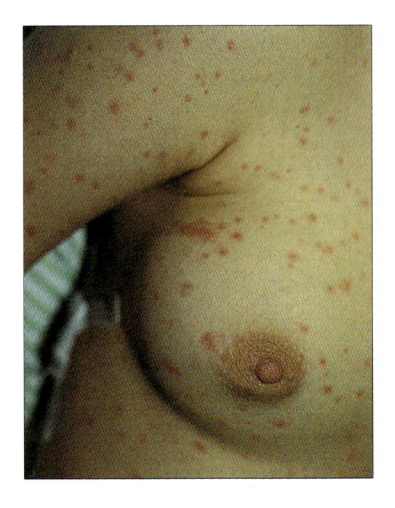

86 Skin lesions developed three weeks after marrow transplant in a patient with SAA. *Candida* sp. was found and cultured from specimen of the lesions.

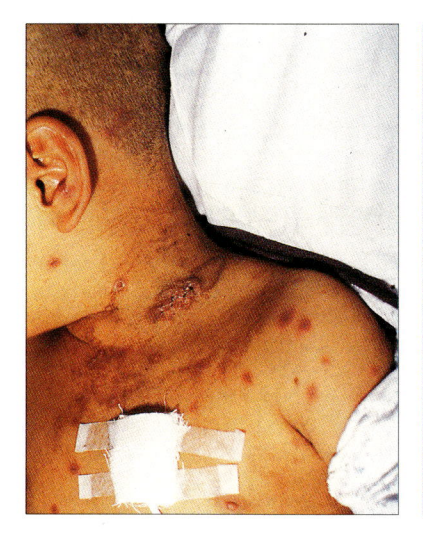

Severe Aplastic Anaemia

87 Skin lesions observed two weeks after marrow transplant in patient with SAA. *Fusarium* sp. was isolated from biopsy of the lesions.

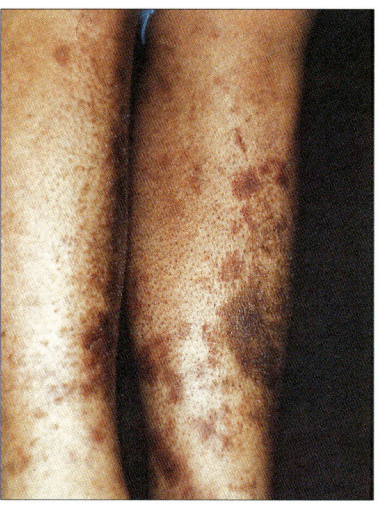

88 Skin lesions developed 15 weeks after marrow transplant for SAA in a 46-year-old female with chronic graft-versus-host disease. Histology of these lesions revealed the presence of *Trypanosoma cruzi*.

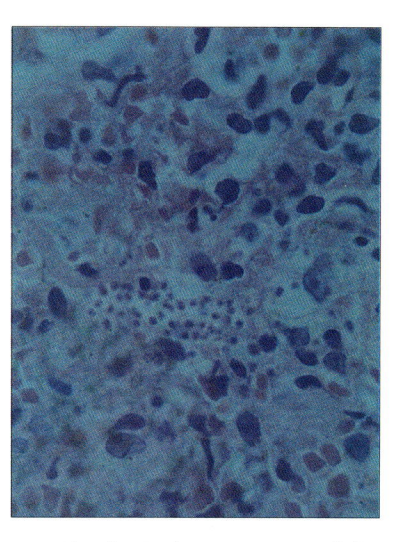

89 Histological preparation of the skin lesion shown in **88**. *Leishmania* forms of *Trypanosoma cruzi* are easily seen.

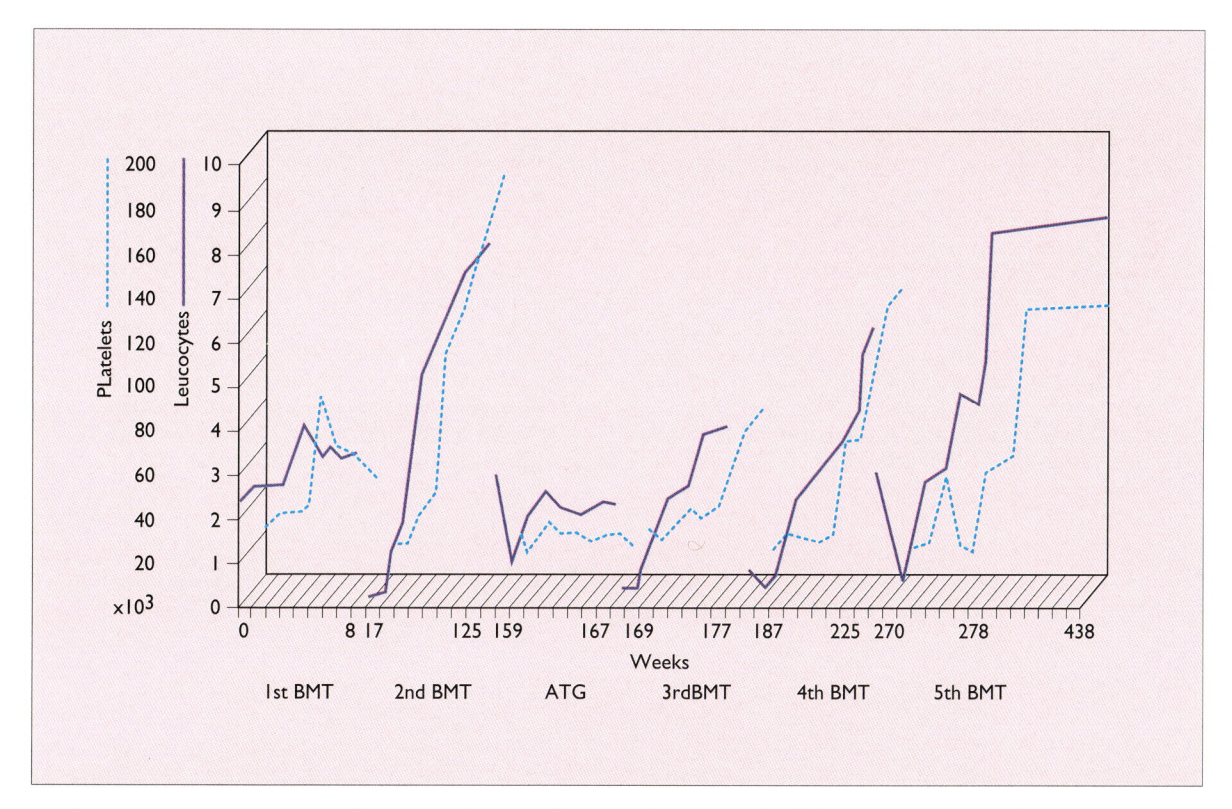

90 Syngeneic BMT. Patient aged 16 years diagnosed SAA underwent multiple bone marrow transplants. **1st** BMT: No conditioning. Only marrow infusion. **2nd** BMT: Cyclophosphamide and bone marrow. **3rd** BMT: Cyclophosphamide + ATG and bone marrow. **4th** BMT: Cyclophosphamide + ATG and bone marrow, followed by cyclosporin. **5th** BMT: Cyclophosphamide + total lymph node irradiation and bone marrow.

References

Anasetti C, Doney KC, Storb R *et al*. Marrow transplantation for severe aplastic anaemia: Long-term outcomes in fifty untransfused patients. *Ann Intern Med* 1986; **104**: 361–366.

Bacigalupo A, Giordano D, Van Lin MT *et al*., Bolus methyl-prednisolone in severe aplastic anaemia. *N Engl J Med* 1979; **300**: 501–502

Bacigalupo A, Hows J, Gluckman E *et al*., Bone marrow transplantation (BMT) versus immunosuppression for the treatment of severe aplastic anaemia (SAA): a report of the EBMT SAA working party. *Br J Haematol* 1988; **70**: 177–182.

Bodey GP. Fungal infection and fever of unknown origin in neutropenic patients. *Am J Med* 1986; **80** (suppl 5C): 112.

Camitta B, Thomas ED. Severe aplastic anaemia: a prospective study of the effect of androgens or transplantation on haematological recovery and survival. *Clin Haematol* 1978; **7**: 587–595.

Camitta B, O'Reilly RJ, Sensenbrenner L *et al*., Anti-thoracic duct lymphocyte globulin in therapy of severe aplastic anaemia. *Blood* 1983; **62**: 883–888.

Champlin RE, Feig SA, Sparkes RS, Gale RP. Bone marrow transplantation from identical twins in the treatment of aplastic anaemia: implication for the pathogenesis for the disease. *Br J Haematol* 1984; **56**: 455–463.

Champlin RE, Horowitz MM, Van Bekkum DW *et al*., Graft failure following bone marrow transplantation for severe aplastic anaemia: risk factors and treatment results. *Blood* 1988; **73**: 606–613.

Champlin RE. Bone marrow transplantation for aplastic anaemia: recent advances and comparisons with alternative therapies. In: *Bone Marrow Transplantation: Current Controversies (UCLA Symposium on Molecular and Cellular Biology)* 1990. Eds: Gale RP, Champlin RE, Alan LBS. New York, pp. 185–199.

Frickhofen N, Kaltwasser JP, Schrezenmeier H *et al*., Treatment of aplastic anaemia with antilymphocyte globulin and methylprednisolone with or without cyclosporin. *N Engl J Med* 1991; **324**: 1297–1304.

Gluckman E, Deverigie A *et al*., Treatment of severe aplastic anaemia with antilymphocyte globulin and androgens. *Exp Hematol* 1978; **6**: 679–687.

Gluckman E, Horowitz MM, Champlin RE *et al*., Bone marrow transplantation for severe aplastic anaemia: influence of conditioning and graft-versus-host disease prophylaxis regimens on outcome. *Blood*. 1992; **79**: 269–275.

Mary JY, Baumelou E, Guiguet M and the French Cooperative Group for Epidemiological Study of Aplastic Anemia. Epidemiology of aplastic anaemia in France: a prospective multicentric study. *Blood* 1990; **75**: 1646–1653.

Meyers JD. Infectious in bone marrow transplant recipients. *Am J Med* 1986; **81** (suppl 1A): 27–38.

Pasquini R. Allogeneic Bone Marrow Transplantation in Severe Aplastic Anaemia: Study of 108 Patients. Thesis. Federal University of Paran, 1991.

Speck B, Gratwhohl A, Nissen C *et al*., Treatment of severe aplastic anaemia. *Exp Hematol* 1986; **14**: 126–132.

Storb R, Prentice RL, Buckner CD *et al*., Graft-versus-host disease and survival in patients with aplastic anaemia treated by marrow grafts from HLA-identical siblings. *N Engl J Med* 1983a; **308**: 302–307.

Storb R, Prentice RL, Thomas ED *et al*., Factors associated with graft rejection after HLA-identical marrow transplantation for aplastic anaemia. *Brit J Haematol* 1983b; **55**: 573.

Sullivan KM. Chronic graft-versus-host disease. In: *Bone Marrow Transplantation: Current Controversies (UCLA Symposium on Molecular and Cellular Biology)* 1990. Eds: Gale RP, Champlin RE, Alan LBS. New York, pp.79–98.

Tichelli A, Gratwhol A, Wursch A *et al*., Late haematological complications in severe aplastic anaemia. *Br J Haematol* 1988; **69**: 413–418.

Williams DM, Lynch RS, Cartwright GE. Drug induced aplastic anaemia. *Semin Hematol* 1973 **10**: 195–223.

Winston DW, Ho, WG, Champlin RE, Gale RP. Infectious complications for bone marrow transplantation. *Exp Hematol* 1984; **12**: 205–215.

Young LS. An overview of infection in bone marrow transplant recipients. *Clin Haematol* 1984; **13**: 661–678.

Young N, Griffith P, Brittain E *et al*., A multicenter trial of antithymocyte globulin in aplastic anaemia and related diseases. *Blood* 1988; **72**: 1861–1869.

4. Primary Immunodeficiency Diseases

Jayesh Mehta

Bone marrow transplants for immune deficiency disorders constitute a small fraction of the total number of transplants reported to the International Bone Marrow Transplant Registry (Bortin et al., 1993). However, immunodeficiencies have provided a model for several advances in the field of bone marrow transplantation.

Marrow transplants for severe combined immunodeficiency disease (SCID) and the immunological component of the Wiskott–Aldrich syndrome were the first successful sibling allografts performed (Gatti et al., 1968; Bach et al., 1968). The first marrow transplant from a histocompatible unrelated donor was performed in a patient with SCID (O'Reilly et al., 1977). The earliest T cell-depleted transplants from HLA-incompatible donors were performed in patients with SCID (Reinherz et al., 1982).

This chapter is an overview of bone marrow transplantation in the treatment of primary immunodeficiency disorders. Details of bone marrow transplantation in individual disorders have been dealt with elsewhere (Lenarsky and Parkman, 1990; Parkman, 1991; Morgan, 1992). Congenital disorders of the monocyte–macrophage system including osteopetrosis have also been included.

Table 7 shows the various congenital immunodeficiency disorders which have been corrected by allogeneic bone marrow transplantation. The classification is based upon the scheme outlined by a WHO working party (Eibl et al., 1989). **Table 8** shows disorders of the monocyte–macrophage system which have been corrected by bone marrow transplantation.

Table 7. Congenital immunodeficiency diseases* treated by bone marrow transplantation, based on WHO.

A. Combined immunodeficiencies

Severe combined immunodeficiency
X-linked
Autosomal recessive (Swiss-type agammaglobulinaemia)
Adenosine deaminase deficiency
Purine nucleoside phosphorylase deficiency
MHC Class II deficiency
Reticular dysgenesis
Omenn syndrome

B. Predominantly antibody deficiencies

X-linked agammaglobulinaemia
Common variable immunodeficiency (CVID)

C. Other well-defined immunodeficiency syndromes

Wiskott–Aldrich syndrome
Ataxia telangiectasia
DiGeorge syndrome

D. Syndromes associated with immunodeficiency

Chromosome abnormalities
Fanconi's anaemia
X-linked lymphoproliferative disorder

E. Defects of phagocytic function

Chronic granulomatous disease
Leukocyte adhesion defect
Chédiak–Higashi syndrome

* see other diseases in Table 8.

Table 8. Congenital diseases of the myeloid and monocyte–macrophage lineages treated by bone marrow transplantation*.

Infantile genetic agranulocytosis (Kostmann syndrome)
Neutrophil actin deficiency
Neutrophil membrane gp180 deficiency
Familial haemophagocytic lymphohistiocytosis
Osteopetrosis

* see also Table 7.

The nature of stem cell engraftment required for correction

Complete engraftment of the donor marrow (i.e. lymphoid as well as myeloid lineage) is not essential in all cases, and the type and extent of engraftment required to correct the clinical manifestations of the disease depends upon the nature of the underlying defect.

SCID is a clinical entity characterized by lack of antigen-specific B and T cell-mediated immunity, and is the result of any of several primary defects. The primary defect ranges from absence of pluripotent stem cells (reticular dysgenesis), on the one hand, to the presence of phenotypically normal T cells capable of responding to mitogenic stimulation but not to specific antigenic stimulation on the other. Defects at the level of the pluripotent stem cell or the lymphoid stem cell result in absent T as well as B cells, whereas defects occurring later in T-cell differentiation result in normal B cells with absent or abnormal T cells. Individual disorders have been described comprehensively elsewhere (Eibl et al., 1989).

Correction of reticular dysgenesis requires engraftment of both lymphoid and haematopoietic lineages as both types of stem cells are deficient. Correction of most disorders with selective lymphoid stem cell defects can be achieved with lymphoid engraftment alone. SCID due to interleukin-1 (IL-1) deficiency is an exception where monocytes and macrophages are also incapable of IL-1 production and therefore require replacement. Another exception is major histocompatibility complex (MHC) Class II deficiency where correction of the defect in antigen presentation requires engraftment of a normal monocyte–macrophage system that is capable of Class II histocompatibility expression as well.

The first successful transplant for Wiskott–Aldrich syndrome was only partially successful because only lymphoid engraftment was achieved with correction of the immunological abnormalities (Bach et al., 1968). However, complete correction was achieved with complete engraftment (Parkman et al., 1978). Correction of the disorders of the monocyte–macrophage system and osteopetrosis requires complete engraftment of the donor marrow.

Conditioning regimens

Pretransplant conditioning regimens comprise myelo-ablative therapy to destroy the recipient's haematopoietic system to create 'space' for donor cells, and immunosuppressive therapy to permit durable engraftment without immune-mediated rejection of the donor marrow.

Complete engraftment of the donor lympho-haematopoietic system can be achieved in reticular dysgenesis by infusion of the donor marrow without any prior conditioning therapy. The correction of immunodeficiency due to absence of lymphoid stem cells can usually be corrected by infusion of the donor marrow that results in lymphoid engraftment alone: the haematopoietic elements continue to be of recipient origin. Pretransplant myelo-ablation is necessary in MHC Class II deficiency and IL-1 deficiency, as complete correction of these disorders additionally requires a normal haematopoietic system.

The degree of immunosuppression required to achieve engraftment is usually proportional to the patient's immunocompetence and degree of HLA mismatch with the donor. Most patients with adenosine deaminase (ADA) deficiency can be successfully transplanted without pretransplant conditioning by simple marrow infusion. However, non-engraftment occurs in some patients who can later be successfully transplanted with prior cytoreduction. It is known that exogenous ADA can induce T-lymphocyte differentiation. Thus, infused donor bone marrow may be a source of the deficient enzyme which may stimulate low levels of immunological function within the recipient, resulting in graft rejection.

Cyclophosphamide as a single drug for immunosuppression may be useful in cases where myeloablation is unnecessary. Total body irradiation (Halberg *et al.*, 1990) or busulphan (Kapoor *et al.*, 1981) are added for myelo-ablation where complete engraftment is essential. Total body irradiation is technically difficult and undesirable in very young children due to its long-term adverse effects on growth and development. The combination of busulphan and cyclophosphamide has now become the standard conditioning regimen for this group of diseases.

With the exception of partial leukocyte adhesion deficiency, all the disorders of the myeloid lineage, including those of the monocyte–macrophage lineage, have normal immune function. This results in normal resistance to acceptance of marrow allografts, making a full cytoreductive conditioning regimen mandatory. Morbidity and mortality are consequently significant.

Familial haemophagocytic lymphohistiocytosis is an autosomal recessive disorder characterized by uncontrolled proliferation of histiocytes in lymphoid tissues, liver, bone marrow and the central nervous system. The biological behaviour is similar to that of a malignant disorder. While conventional cytotoxic chemotherapy only rarely results in long-term survival, an allograft from a histocompatible donor may be curative (Blanche *et al.*, 1991). Etoposide and methotrexate are very active in this disease, and conditioning usually includes etoposide, with intrathecal methotrexate being employed peritransplant.

Graft rejection

Graft rejection or failure is not a significant occurrence with histocompatible sibling grafts for immunodeficiencies. It is, however, the single most important cause of failure of T-cell depleted histoincompatible grafts. Graft failure in patients with other diseases transplanted with T cell-depleted marrow is mediated by recipient-derived CD8+ cells. This does not usually occur in immunodeficiency diseases due to the basic nature of the disease. However, occasionally in cases of IL-2 deficiency and ADA deficiency, provision of exogenous factor by the normal bone marrow may result in endogenous production of cytotoxic T lymphocytes which can mediate graft rejection.

The presence of normal natural killer cell activity and/or the absence of IL-1 production in SCID patients correlates with lack of engraftment when no pretransplant cytoreduction is used (Sahdev *et al.*, 1989; O'Reilly *et al.*, 1989). This can, however, be overcome by using a conditioning regimen which is myelo-ablative as well as immunosuppressive. Increasing pretransplant immunosuppression with monoclonal antibodies when using T cell-depleted marrow has improved engraftment rates considerably compared to historic controls (Fischer *et al.*, 1991).

Graft-versus-host disease

With matched sibling donors, the incidence of acute and chronic graft-versus-host disease (GvHD) in patients with SCID is very low even when no posttransplant immunosuppression is routinely used. This is in marked contrast to other diseases where lack of post-transplant immunosuppression after the transplantation of unmanipulated fully matched sibling marrow is associated with hyperacute GvHD and high mortality (Sullivan *et al.*, 1986).

The incidence of GvHD following T cell-depleted haplo-identical transplants is related to the degree of T-cell depletion. The incidence of GvHD is higher when the donor marrow has been depleted of T cells by antibody-mediated lysis than when T cells have been removed by physical methods. The maximum experience has been with the agglutination–rosetting technique where T lymphocytes are agglutinated using soybean lectin, and removed by E-rosette formation with sheep red blood cells. Over 100 patients with SCID have been transplanted using this technique (O'Reilly *et al.*, 1989). T-cell depletion with monoclonal antibodies to mature T-lymphocyte differentiation antigens (CD3) does not eliminate GvHD completely. Monoclonal antibodies to pan-T-lymphocyte antigens (CD5, CD2) result in more complete elimination of GvHD.

Use of alternative sources of normal stem cells

Alternative sources of normal haematopoietic stem cells are necessary since histocompatible sibling donors are available for only a minority of patients with SCID. The alternatives that have been explored include histo-incompatible family donors, matched unrelated volunteer donors, fetal tissues and umbilical cord blood.

The earliest bone marrow transplants from matched unrelated donors were performed in patients with immunodeficiencies (O'Reilly *et al.*, 1977; Foroozanfar *et al.*, 1977). This remains a risky procedure, but 50% survival is seen in patients with immunodeficiencies (Filipovich *et al.*, 1992; Kernan *et al.*, 1993).

Fetal liver contains pluripotent haematopoietic progenitor cells that are capable of reconstituting lethally irradiated recipients with a reduced risk of graft-versus-host disease. Despite complete HLA incompatibility between transplanted stem cells and host cells, functional activities of donor-derived T lymphocytes are not restricted. Correction of congenital immunodeficiencies has been attempted by infusion of histo-incompatible fetal liver with or without fetal thymus (Keightley *et al,*. 1975; Touraine *et al.*, 1987). *In utero* infusion of fetal liver cells has been reported to correct SCID (Touraine *et al.*, 1992).

Umbilical cord blood collected at birth contains enough haematopoietic progenitor stem cells to effect engraftment. Due to the high proliferative capacity of neonatal haematopoietic progenitors and the relative immunological functional immaturity of neonatal lymphocytes, cord blood cells could be used for matched unrelated or partially mismatched transplants. At least one patient with an immunodeficiency disorder (X-linked lymphoproliferative disorder) has received a cord blood transplant with prompt engraftment and development of chimaerism with minimal GvHD (Gluckman *et al.*, 1992).

Recovery of immune function post-transplant

When no conditioning regimen is employed, donor T cells can be detected 2–3 weeks post-transplant with histocompatible unmanipulated grafts (Keever *et al.*, 1989). However, B-lymphocyte chimaerism is not detectable in a number of patients, especially those who have host B cells at the outset. Full T- and B-cell function develops in approximately 6 months.

With T cell-depleted haplo-identical grafts, however, full T- and B-cell function may take over a year to develop when conditioning chemotherapy is used (Wijnaendts *et al.*, 1989). Immunological recovery is prolonged because it is dependent upon recapitulation of normal fetal ontogeny by the donor lymphoid stem cells within the recipient. Without prior conditioning, immune reconstitution may take even longer, and B-cell function may not develop at all. A number of these patients remain hypoimmunoglobulinaemic and require regular replacement therapy. They are also prone to autoimmune phenomena, especially haemolytic anaemia.

Successful bone marrow transplantation results in the reversal of the skeletal abnormalities seen in infantile osteopetrosis (Coccia *et al.*, 1980). While progression of neurological defects is prevented, reversal of major existing defects does not occur. It is important therefore to undertake the procedure as soon as possible. T cell-depleted grafts from mismatched family donors have been employed successfully in patients without matched sibling donors (Orchard *et al.*, 1987; Fischer *et al.*, 1991).

B-lymphocyte proliferative disease

Up to 30% of patients allografted with T cell-depleted histo-incompatible marrow develop Epstein–Barr virus (EBV)-associated polyclonal B-lymphocyte proliferation which is usually donor in origin (Shapiro et al., 1988; Fischer et al., 1990). This syndrome is commoner in patients transplanted for severe immunodeficiency disorders compared to those receiving similar T cell-depleted histo-incompatible allografts for other diseases. SCID patients with EBV-associated lymphomas rarely respond to chemotherapy, and the prognosis is very poor.

The frequency of EBV-associated lymphomas with the soybean lectin E rosette formation technique is significantly less than with techniques removing mature T cells alone. The former also removes B cells from the graft, reducing the probability of introducing EBV into the recipient.

Results

Of 80 patients transplanted for SCID from 1968 to 1977, 18 survived (Kenny and Hitzig, 1979). With the earlier diagnosis and greatly improved supportive care available now, the overall survival of SCID patients receiving a matched sibling allograft has improved to around 70% (O'Reilly et al., 1984; Fischer et al., 1990). Good-risk patients (younger than 6 months, no evidence of active pulmonary infection at the time of transplant) have a probability of cure of around 90% (Fischer et al., 1990). Overall survival after T cell-depleted mismatch transplants from family donors is in the region of 50% (O'Reilly et al., 1989; Fischer et al., 1990).

Allografting from unrelated donors continues to be a high-risk procedure with a significantly higher risk of GvHD, graft failure and serious infections. Overall survival is 50% with relatively short follow-up (Filipovich et al., 1992; Kernan et al., 1993).

While matched sibling allografts cure 80% of patients with the Wiskott–Aldrich syndrome (O'Reilly et al., 1984), the results of haplo-identical T cell-depleted transplants have been relatively poor with less than 25% surviving. The number of transplants carried out for all other disorders is too small for any useful comments to be made.

Alternative therapy

The immunodeficiency in ADA deficiency is at least partially correctable by administration of purified bovine ADA conjugated with polyethylene glycol (PEG-ADA). This replacement therapy can lead to reconstitution of immunity. While it may provide an alternative to mismatch transplants, a matched sibling allograft remains the treatment of choice. Problems with PEG-ADA therapy include production of antibodies to the bovine enzyme, and the need for life-long treatment.

Purine nucleoside phosphorylase (PNP) deficiency is another specific enzyme deficiency to be described in association with a severe immunodeficiency. Theoretically, enzyme replacement in this disease could have a role, but no suitable PNP preparation is available.

Common variable immunodeficiency with predominantly antibody deficiency responds to intravenous immunoglobulin replacement therapy, and bone marrow transplantation is indicated only under exceptional circumstances.

Though successful marrow transplants have been performed for infantile genetic agranulocytosis (Rappeport et al., 1980), recombinant human granulocyte colony-stimulating factor (G-CSF) has been found to increase the granulocyte count and to diminish susceptibility to infection. Presently, this offers a much safer alternative to bone marrow transplantation, especially in patients without matched sibling donors. As transplants become safer, the advantage of a curative procedure over the safety of long-term administration of growth factors will require consideration.

The decreased microbicidal activity seen in chronic granulomatous disease due to defective oxygen metabolism has been corrected with HLA-matched sibling (Rappeport et al., 1982) and unrelated (Foroozanfar et al., 1977) marrow transplants. Antimicrobial prophylaxis with trimethoprim–sulphamethoxazole and itraconazole with or without dicloxacillin extends the infection-free intervals in many patients. Administration of γ-interferon corrects the cytochrome *b* content partially in some patients and restores phagocytic activity to almost normal for up to 5 weeks. This may be the treatment of choice in patients who are poor-risk candidates for bone marrow transplantation. The defective gene responsible for chronic granulomatous disease has also been identified and cloned, resulting in the possibility of gene therapy in the future.

Gene therapy

Insertion of a normal copy of a defective gene into the cells of the patient has the potential of restoring these cells to normal function, and can theoretically be ideal therapy for many genetic disorders. Gene transfer on primitive haematopoietic progenitor cells obtained from autologous bone marrow or peripheral blood stem cells has the advantage of *ex vivo* treatment and delivery of gene therapy only to somatic cells. The potential targets for this therapy are all genetic diseases that are fully correctable by allogeneic bone marrow transplantation. Retroviral-mediated gene transfer into haematopoietic precursors often results in short-term transduction *in vivo* due to transfer into proliferating committed progenitor cells rather than into uncommitted primitive progenitors.

Identification and cloning of the gene responsible for the condition is essential for development of gene therapy. Genes for only four primary immunodeficiencies have been cloned so far: ADA deficiency, purine nucleosidase phosphorylase deficiency, chronic granulomatous disease and leukocyte adhesion defect.

There are a number of other conditions that must be fulfilled for gene therapy to be effective (Blaese, 1993). When the gene has been identified, its function must be fully understood. The gene must then be delivered to the target cells, possibly at a specific time within the cell cycle, and possibly at a specific location within the cell. Gene expression may require very tight control, taking into account time within cell cycle, response to messenger molecules, and synchronization with the expression of other genes within the cell. High-efficiency gene transfer will be needed to prevent residual defective or deficient cells from interfering with the function of normal cells. Cytoreduction may be necessary to destroy residual abnormal cells, as may development of a method to stop the production of an abnormal product.

Clinical cure occurs with engraftment of allogeneic T cells alone in ADA-deficient SCID patients. Patients without an HLA-matched donor benefit clinically and immunologically from enzyme replacement therapy with PEG-ADA.

Two patients have so far been treated with periodic infusions of autologous culture-expanded T cells genetically corrected by insertion of a normal ADA gene using retroviral-mediated gene transfer (Blaese, 1993). The first patient was anergic, lymphopenic, and deficient in antibody responses and isohaemagglutinins experiencing recurrent infections after two years of PEG-ADA treatment. The second child had less severe disease, but was deficient in isohaemagglutinins and antibody responses to recent environmental exposures, with depressed cellular immune responses. After multiple infusions of corrected T cells, both have demonstrated a substantial increase in the number of circulating T cells and the ADA activity in her peripheral blood T cells. This has been associated with the development of positive delayed-type hypersensitivity skin tests, an increase in the level of isohaemagglutinins, the regrowth of tonsils, and a decreased number of infectious illnesses. The improvement has persisted during suspension of treatment for more than 6 months.

References

Bach FH, Albertini RJ, Joo P et al. Bone-marrow transplantation in a patient with the Wiskott–Aldrich syndrome. *Lancet* 1968; **2**: 1364–1366.

Blaese RM. Development of gene therapy for immunodeficiency: adenosine deaminase deficiency. *Pediatr Res* 1993; **33**: S49–S55.

Blanche S, Caniglia M, Girault D et al. Treatment of haemophagocytic lymphohistiocytosis with chemotherapy and bone marrow transplantation: a single-center study of 22 cases. *Blood* 1991; **78**: 51–54.

Bortin MM, Horowitz MM, Rowlings PA et al. Progress report from the International Bone Marrow Transplant Registry. *Bone Marrow Transplant* 1993; **12**: 97–104.

Coccia PF, Krivit W, Cervenka J et al. Successful bone-marrow transplantation for infantile malignant osteopetrosis. *N Engl J Med* 1980; **302**: 701–708.

Eibl M, Griscelli C, Seligmann M et al. Primary immunodeficiency diseases: Report of a WHO sponsored meeting. *Immunodefic Rev* 1989; **1**: 173–205.

Filipovich AH, Shapiro RS, Ramsay NK et al. Unrelated donor bone marrow transplantation for correction of lethal congenital immunodeficiencies. *Blood* 1992; **80**: 270–276.

Fischer A, Landais P, Friedrich W et al. European experience of bone-marrow transplantation for severe combined immunodeficiency. *Lancet* 1990; **336**: 850–854.

Fischer A, Friedrich W, Fasth A et al. Reduction of graft failure by a monoclonal antibody (anti-LFA-1 CD11a) after HLA nonidentical bone marrow transplantation in children with immunodeficiencies, osteopetrosis, and Fanconi's anaemia: a European Group for Immunodeficiency/European Group for Bone Marrow Transplantation report. *Blood* 1991; **77**: 249–256.

Fischer AM, Simon F, Le Deist F et al. Prospective study of the occurrence of monoclonal gammopathies following bone marrow transplantation in young children. *Transplantation* 1990; **49**: 731–735.

Foroozanfar N, Hobbs JR, Hugh-Jones K et al. Bone-marrow transplant from an unrelated donor for chronic granulomatous disease. *Lancet* 1977; **1**: 210–213.

Gatti RA, Meuwissen HJ, Allen HD et al. Immunological reconstitution of sex-linked lymphopaenic immunological deficiency. *Lancet* 1968; **2**: 1366–1369.

Gluckman E, Devergie A, Thierry D et al. Clinical applications of stem cell transfusion from cord blood and rationale for cord blood banking. *Bone Marrow Transplant* 1992; **9** (suppl 1): 114–117.

Halberg FE, Wara WM, Weaver KE et al. Total body irradiation and bone marrow transplantation for immunodeficiency disorders in young children. *Radiother Oncol* 1990; **18** (suppl 1): 114–117.

Kapoor N, Kirkpatrick D, Blaese RM et al. Reconstitution of normal megakaryocytopoiesis and immunologic functions in Wiskott–Aldrich syndrome by marrow transplantation following myeloablation and immunosuppression with busulfan and cyclophosphamide. *Blood* 1981; **57**: 692–696.

Keever CA, Small TN, Flomenberg N et al. Immune reconstitution following bone marrow transplantation: comparison of recipients of T-cell depleted marrow with recipients of conventional marrow grafts. *Blood* 1989; **73**: 1340–1350.

Keightley RG, Lawton AA, Cooper M. Successful fetal liver transplantation in a child with severe combined immunodeficiency. *Lancet* 1975; **2**: 850–853.

Kenny AB, Hitzig WH. Bone marrow transplantation for severe combined immunodeficiency disease. Reported from 1968 to 1977. *Eur J Pediatr* 1979; **131**: 155–177.

Kernan NA, Bartsch G, Ash RC et al. Analysis of 462 transplantations from unrelated donors facilitated by the National Marrow Donor Program. *N Engl J Med* 1993; **328**: 593–602.

Lenarsky C, Parkman R. Bone marrow transplantation for the treatment of immune deficiency states. *Bone Marrow Transplant* 1990; **6**: 361–369.

Morgan G. Bone marrow transplantation for immunodeficiency syndromes. In: *Bone Marrow Transplantation in Practice*, 1992, Eds: Treleaven J, Barrett J. Churchill Livingstone, Edinburgh, pp. 119–135.

Orchard PJ, Dickerman JD, Mathews CH et al. Haploidentical bone marrow transplantation for osteopetrosis. *Am J Pediatr Hematol Oncol* 1987; **9**: 335–340.

O'Reilly RJ, Dupont B, Pahwa S et al. Reconstitution in severe combined immunodeficiency by transplantation of marrow from an unrelated donor. *N Engl J Med* 1977; **297**: 1311–1318.

O'Reilly RJ, Brochstein J, Dinsmore R, Kirkpatrick D. Marrow transplantation for congenital disorders. *Semin Hematol* 1984; **21**: 188–221.

O'Reilly RJ, Keever CA, Small TN, Brochstein J. The use of HLA-non-identical T-cell-depleted marrow transplants for correction of severe combined immunodeficiency disease. *Immunodefic Rev* 1989; **1**: 273–309.

Parkman R. The biology of bone marrow transplantation for severe combined immune deficiency. *Adv Immunol* 1991; **49**: 381–410.

Parkman R, Rappeport J, Geha R et al. Complete correction of the Wiskott–Aldrich syndrome by allogeneic bone-marrow transplantation. *N Engl J Med* 1978; **298**: 921–927.

Rappeport JM, Parkman R, Newburger P et al. Correction of infantile agranulocytosis (Kostmann's syndrome) by allogeneic bone marrow transplantation. *Am J Med* 1980; **68**: 605–609.

Rappeport JM, Newburger PE, Goldblum RM et al. Allogeneic bone marrow transplantation for chronic granulomatous disease. *J Pediatr* 1982; **101**: 952–955.

Reinherz EL, Geha R, Rappeport JM et al. Reconstitution after transplantation with T-lymphocyte-depleted HLA haplotype-mismatched bone marrow for severe combined immunodeficiency. *Proc Natl Acad Sci USA* 1982; **79**: 6047–6051.

Sahdev I, O'Reilly R, Hoffman MK. Correlation between interleukin-1 production and engraftment of transplanted bone marrow stem cells in patients with lethal immunodeficiencies. *Blood* 1989; **73**: 1712–1719.

Shapiro RS, McClain K, Frizzera G *et al*. Epstein–Barr virus associated B cell lymphoproliferative disorders following bone marrow transplantation. *Blood* 1988; **71**: 1234–1243.

Sullivan KM, Deeg HJ, Sanders J *et al*. Hyperacute graft-v-host disease in patients not given immunosuppression after allogeneic marrow transplantation. *Blood* 1986; **67**: 1172–1175.

Touraine JL, Roncarolo MG, Royo C, Touraine F. Fetal tissue transplantation, bone marrow transplantation and prospective gene therapy in severe immunodeficiencies and enzyme deficiencies. *Thymus* 1987; **10**: 75–87.

Touraine JL, Raudrant D, Rebaud A *et al*. *In utero* transplantation of stem cells in humans: immunological aspects and clinical follow-up of patients. *Bone Marrow Transplant* 1992; **9** (suppl 1): 121–126.

Wijnaendts L, Le Deist F, Griscelli C, Fischer A. Development of immunologic functions after bone marrow transplantation in 33 patients with severe combined immunodeficiency. *Blood* 1989; **74**: 2212–2219.

5. Leukaemias, Lymphomas and Myeloma

John Luckit and Jennifer Treleaven

Leukaemias

Acute myeloid leukaemia (AML)

Acute myeloid leukaemia is a heterogeneous malignant disorder of the haemopoietic cells. The incidence rises with age from 1 per 100 000/year in childhood to 10 per 100 000/year in those over 70 years. AML can be divided into 7 main categories based on morphology and cytochemistry as proposed by the French, American and British (FAB) group (Bennett et al., 1985) (**Table 9**). Immunology, cytogenetics and electron microscopy allow further identification and subclassification of leukaemia cells. Some of these subtypes may be associated with a particularly poor outcome after chemotherapy alone. M5, for example, is associated with the presence of extramedullary disease (**91**) and gum hypertrophy, which may represent an increased tumour load and hence render the disease less sensitive to the effects of chemotherapy. Other subtypes, for example M3 (**92**), are associated with a more favourable outcome, and in some series up to 40% of patients are disease-free five years from diagnosis after chemotherapy alone (Cunningham et al., 1989). The use of bone marrow transplantation, itself associated with a relatively high morbidity and mortality, is therefore possibly

Table 9. FAB morphological classification of acute myeloid leukaemia.

M0 Acute myeloid leukaemia with minimal evidence of myeloid differentiation
M1 AML without maturation
M2 AML with maturation
M3 Acute hypergranular promyelocytic leukaemia
M4 Acute myelomonocytic leukaemia
M5 Acute monocytic/monoblastic leukaemia
M6 Erythroleukaemia
M7 Acute megakaryoblastic leukaemia

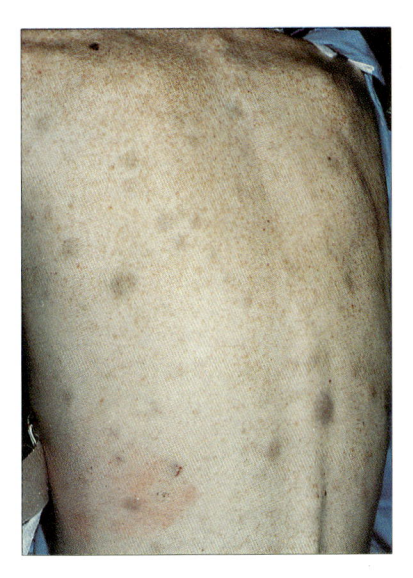

91 Skin infiltration in monocytic leukaemia.

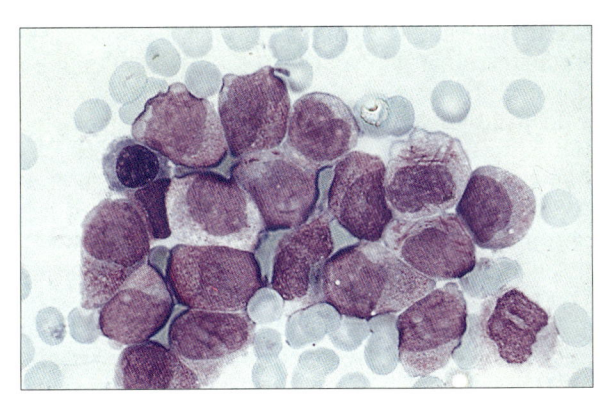

92 Acute promyelocytic leukaemia (M3) showing classical Auer rods in the leukaemia blast cells.

not indicated for this particular subgroup of AML patients. Overall, however, the FAB classification has not been found to be significantly useful as a predictive factor for outcome after chemotherapy alone. FAB type has been shown to significantly correlate neither with remission rates after conventional chemotherapy (Swirsky et al., 1986) nor reliably with outcome after chemotherapy with or without allogeneic transplantation (Tallman et al., 1989). However, cell surface phenotype may be of use to define the very poor-risk leukaemias. For example, CD34 positivity (Geller et al., 1990), implies pluripotent stem cell disease, in which case patients may lack any normal stem cells.

Table 10. Myelodysplastic syndrome. FAB classification.

Refractory anaemia
Refractory anaemia with ring sideroblasts (RARS)
Refractory anaemia with excess of blasts (RAEB)
Chronic myelomonocytic leukaemia
Refractory anaemia with excess of blasts in transformation

Myelodysplastic syndromes

Myelodysplastic syndromes are morphologically classified as shown in **Table 10**. In patients of an appropriate age, allogeneic bone marrow transplantation is the treatment of choice since all of these syndromes eventually metamorphose into acute myeloid leukaemia, and treatment with chemotherapy alone is usually even more unsatisfactory than is the case with *de novo* acute myeloid leukaemia.

Conventional chemotherapy

There have been few major changes in induction chemotherapy strategies over the past decade, and the best post-induction therapy for AML is yet to be clearly defined. Relapse remains the major cause of treatment failure and, to a large extent, this reflects the narrow therapeutic window between anti-leukaemic activity and toxicity of the available treatment options.

Overall, between 60 and 75% of adults with *de novo* AML attain a first remission. Successful remission induction is strongly age related, and becomes less common in patients older than 50 years (Rees et al., 1986). Without further chemotherapy, the median time to relapse for first remission patients is commonly less than one year.

Both relapse and long-term survival probabilities can be considerably improved with additional 'consolidation' chemotherapy, usually given as two or three courses of sufficient intensity to produce pancytopenia (Champlin et al., 1987). Maintenance chemotherapy has not generally been found to prolong remission, a situation at variance with that seen with acute lymphoblastic leukaemia, although a small number of studies which use intermittent intensive chemotherapy to marrow aplasia have demonstrated an advantage in their maintenance group (Dutcher et al., 1988). Overall, survival figures as low as 6% have been reported (Brineker et al., 1990) but the majority of studies report 15–25% long-term survivors after successful first remission induction. With modern chemotherapy protocols 25–40% of adults (aged over 16 and under 40 years) achieve three years of leukaemia-free survival.

When relapse occurs, the likelihood of attaining a second remission is approximately 50% and the probability of a prolonged remission is extremely low. Allogeneic bone marrow transplantation in first remission from an HLA-identical sibling is thus the current most successful approach for preventing leukaemia relapse and increasing the probability of long-term disease-free survival and potential cure. In this situation, 40–70% disease-free survival rates (**93**) are to be anticipated. This approach is, however, limited by age constraints and the availability of a matched sibling donor. Only 10–15% of patients with a median age at presentation of approximately 50 years are candidates for allograft.

Similar survival rates have been reported for transplants from related partially HLA-matched donors but for HLA-matched unrelated donors the survival is <20%. More recently, however, the Seattle group have shown a similar probability of relapse-free survival at one year for unrelated and sibling donor transplants (41 vs. 46%).

In an attempt to reduce transplant-related toxicity, intensified graft-versus-host disease prophylaxis using a combination of cyclosporin and methotrexate has been shown to reduce acute but not chronic graft-versus-host disease. This measure is, however, associated with an increased relapse rate (Buckner et al., 1989).

Autologous bone marrow transplantation (ABMT) may be effective for selected patients. However, the same major drawback remains, that is, the presence of minimal residual disease and the absence of the graft-versus-leukaemia effect associated with allogeneic BMT. *In vitro* bone marrow purging or the use of peripheral blood stem cells (PBSC) (Reiffers et al., 1990) may circumvent the former problem but at present autologous transplantation remains investigational.

93 Probability of leukaemia-free survival after matched sibling allograft in first remission according to age. (Courtesy International Bone Marrow Transplant Registry, Wisconsin, USA.)

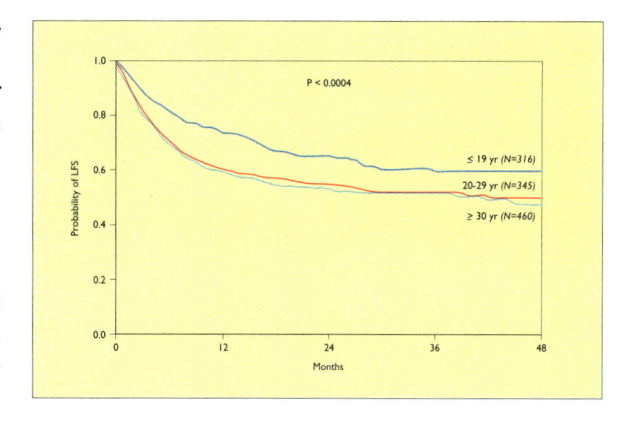

Acute lymphoblastic leukaemia (ALL)

In adults, acute lymphoblastic leukaemia carries a much poorer prognosis than is the case in childhood, with only approximately 20% of patients remaining disease-free after five years with chemotherapy alone (Hoelzer and Gale, 1987). The reasons for this are not entirely clear, except for the fact that certain poor prognostic features such as Philadelphia chromosome positivity occur more commonly with advancing age. Adult patients should therefore probably undergo allogeneic bone marrow transplantation in first remission of their disease if a suitable donor is available and if they are of an appropriate age, although some centres still retain this form of treatment for second remission patients, in view of the relatively high procedural morbidity and mortality associated with allogeneic bone marrow transplantation.

With children, the position is less clear. Overall, the disease carries a good prognosis with chemotherapy alone if certain specific risk factors are absent at diagnosis. These include some chromosome abnormalities of the leukaemic cells such as the presence of the Philadelphia chromosome, the presence of the B-cell phenotype, boys with very high counts at presentation, and disease which has already relapsed after conventional chemotherapy (**Table 11**). The proponents of aggressive chemotherapy alone claim that results from this are as good as those seen following bone marrow transplantation, in that the higher procedural mortality offsets the higher relapse rate after chemotherapy alone. As data have accumulated on BMT for ALL, it has now become possible to compare results of BMT series with those seen after chemotherapy alone (Horowitz *et al.*, 1991). While BMT has a higher probability of curing poor risk ALL, the higher procedural mortality has brought the disease-free survival into the same range as that achieved by chemotherapy alone (Herzig *et al.*, 1987). Thus, the place of BMT in ALL has remained controversial. Proponents of BMT emphasize the low chance of long term survival following chemotherapy alone in relapsed ALL and in ALL presenting with poor prognosis features, while proponents of chemotherapy have drawn attention to the increasing success achieved with new, more intensive and better designed protocols, which, it is claimed, may ultimately rule out the need for BMT with few exceptions (Pinkel, 1987). More recently, Chessells *et al.* (1992) looked at 144 children with poor-risk ALL undergoing the UK ALL X chemotherapy programme, of whom 34 proceeded to BMT. BMT was carried out at a median time of 17 weeks from diagnosis (range 9–50

Table 11. Poor prognostic indices in acute lymphoblastic leukaemia.

Infants
Males
Some chromosomal translocations (t9;22 and t4;11)
High initial leucocyte count (>100¥109/l)
Cell phenotype (B-cell ALL)
Presence of extramedullary disease
Relapsed disease

weeks). The event-free survival in UK ALL X for patients age 1–15 years with a white cell count at diagnosis of greater than $100 \times 10^9/l$ is 50% at five years. In this particular study, the five-year event-free survival was 69% for the BMT arm and 52% for the chemotherapy alone arm, a difference which was not statistically significant. All patients had entered remission by 15 weeks from diagnosis. Chessells *et al.* found there to be more relapses in the chemotherapy group and more treatment-related deaths in the BMT group, and noted that some prognostic features in this patient series were more important than others (**Table 12**), in particular, sex, white count at diagnosis and age at diagnosis.

McCarthy *et al.* (1992) subsequently pointed out that the 69% five-year event-free survival in BMT arm may not be statistically better than the 52% seen in the chemotherapy arm, but the BMT arm has a plateau survival curve not seen in the chemotherapy arm. In 1988 they had reported 8 out of 9 children 7–16 years old surviving disease-free 4.5–13 years after BMT (89% actuarial survival).

As many patients deemed to merit a bone marrow transplant have no HLA-compatible sibling donor, autografting in remission is commonly considered as an alternative. Blaise *et al.* in 1990 examined a group of high-risk ALL patients comparable in terms of age, initial presentation of ALL, and induction chemotherapy. Twenty-five received an allograft from an HLA-matched sibling and 22 underwent auto-BMT. The probability of relapse was 9% for the allograft patients and 52% for the autograft patients. Disease-free survival was 71% in the allograft group and 40% for the autograft group, which, although not statistically significant, suggested that early allografting is preferable to autografting in high-risk ALL.

As is the case with the other haematological malignancies, younger patients in first remission at the time of transplant suffer less leukaemia relapse and less toxicity than patients in later stages of their disease (**94**). This should therefore be taken into consideration if BMT is potentially a treatment option.

The following four statements sum up the situation concerning BMT in ALL as it stands at present, although patient selection may well be problematic (Barrett, 1991).

1. BMT is particularly appropriate in ALL of stem cell origin.
2. Autologous BMT in patients with stem cell origin ALL is more likely to result in relapse of the disease.
3. Both autologous and allogeneic BMT may have a role in the eradication of ALLs of poor prognosis because of their rapid proliferation rate (B–ALL; T–ALL).
4. It is also possible that there may be a role for continuing maintenance therapy with weekly methotrexate and daily 6-mercaptopurine after autografting (Tiley *et al.*, 1993).

Relapse after BMT has emerged as a major problem (Barrett *et al.*, 1986). As prognostic criteria for outcome of chemotherapy have become more reliable, an increasing number of patients with poor-risk ALL achieving first remission have undergone HLA identical sibling BMT. The behaviour of ALL and its response to treatment support the concept that it behaves either as a 'slow' good prognosis disease, or a 'fast' high relapse risk disease. As Butturini *et al.* pointed out in 1987, both chemotherapy and allogeneic BMT confer leukaemia-free survivals of about 45% for patients whose first

Table 12. Factors influencing outcome after chemotherapy (Chessells et al., 1992).

Important	Less-important factors
Male sex	Age
Leukocyte count at diagnosis	Cell type
Bone marrow status at day 29	Ploidy

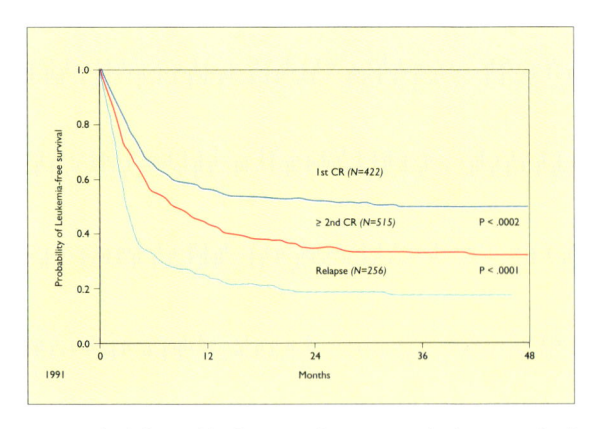

94 Probability of leukaemia-free survival after matched sibling allograft for acute lymphoblastic leukaemia according to disease status at transplant. (Courtesy International Bone Marrow Transplant Registry, Wisconsin, USA.)

relapse occurs off maintenance chemotherapy, but only 15% for relapses occurring on maintenance, facts which would emphasize the concepts of 'slow' and 'fast' disease.

Analyses of BMT for relapsed ALL have highlighted the similar outcome achieved for adults and children, the impact of on-treatment relapse as a predictor for poor transplant outcome (threefold increased risk of relapse post-BMT for on-chemotherapy relapses), and the relative lack of impact of any presentation disease features. Also of significance is the relatively small difference in outcome seen after BMT in second, third, fourth or even subsequent remissions. The relatively good survival of these multiply relapsing patients probably reflects the fact that they are a selected group of patients with slow disease who have remained survivors after chemotherapy but who have not been cured.

The place of BMT in childhood ALL remains, therefore, controversial, although the presence of the poor risk features outlined in **Table 11** may be an indication for it to take place if a matched sibling donor is available while the patient is in first remission. Only time and randomized, controlled trials will ultimately reveal the position of autografting, allografting and chemotherapy in the more nebulous diagnostic areas.

Chronic granulocytic leukaemia (CGL)

Chronic granulocytic leukaemia is a clonal disorder of the pluripotent stem cell. It is commonest in the middle aged (40–60 years) and has an annual incidence of approximately 1/100 000 (Jones and Goldman, 1987).

The disease is characterized by the presence of the Philadelphia (Ph´) chromosome; chromosome 22 is shortened, secondary to a reciprocal translocation between chromosomes 9 and 22. In this translocation the Ableson proto-oncogene (ABL) from the long arm of chromosome 9 is juxtaposed to the breakpoint cluster region (BCR) on chromosome 22 to form a chimaeric BCR/ABL gene (**95**). This new gene transcribes an 8.5-kb messenger RNA (mRNA) instead of the normal 6- or 7-kb mRNA associated with ABL and is translated into a protein of 210 kDA (p210). Unlike the normal 145-kDA ABL product, the p210 protein has a much higher tyrosine kinase activity. This altered enzymatic activity, and evidence that the BCR/ABL product can transform haemopoietic cells, strongly implicates its role in the genesis of CGL. Further evidence for this comes from studies of the analogous product of the viral oncogene, V-abl. The tyrosine kinase encoded by V-abl causes B-cell leukaemia in susceptible mice and therefore it is highly likely that the product of BCR/ABL is important in causing human CGL.

CGL usually follows a prolonged chronic phase (3–5 years) that eventually proceeds to accelerated phase and finally a blastic transformation (blast crisis) to acute leukaemia, which may be myeloid or lymphoid in type. No chemotherapy is curative, since only the blood count is suppressed without eradicating the Philadelphia-positive cells. α-interferon may effect haematologic remission in up to 70% of cases and complete suppression of the Philadelphia chromosome in up to 23% of cases. Although this Ph´ negativity is not sustained in most cases, a number of trials are now in progress to assess whether survival is prolonged in those who have shown cytogenetic response. However, bone

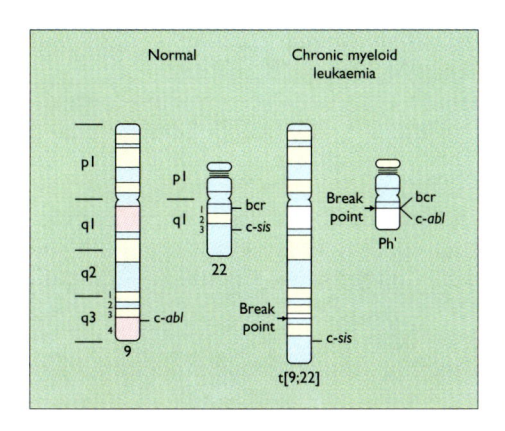

95 Diagrammatic representation of the 9;22 chromosome translocation in chronic myeloid leukaemia.

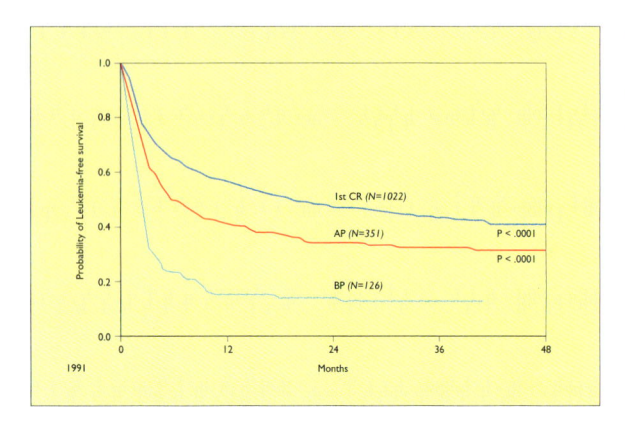

96 Probability of leukaemia-free survival after matched sibling allograft for chronic myeloid leukaemia, according to disease status at the time of transplant. (Courtesy International Bone Marrow Transplant Registry, Wisconsin, USA.)

marrow transplantation remains the only option affording probable cure, and it must be carried out while patients are in chronic phase of the disease, or relapse risk is greatly increased (**96**).

To reduce the chances of patients succumbing to transplant-related problems, attempts have been made to attenuate the course of graft-versus-host (GvHD) disease by using T-cell depletion of donor marrow with or without additional cyclosporin and/or methotrexate. Very high rates of disease relapse were seen in the patients who had suffered no GvHD, again highlighting the concept of a graft-versus leukaemia effect coexisting with GvHD (Apperley *et al.*, 1988) It is possible, however, that more selective removal of cells such as the CD8-positive T lymphocytes that mediate GvHD will result in a similar reduction in GvHD without compromising the graft-versus-leukaemia effect.

The only curative treatment for CGL at present is allogeneic BMT, preferably from an HLA-matched sibling. It is the treatment of choice for younger patients (<40 years) in chronic phase and should ideally be performed within one year of diagnosis as delay may permit acceleration or blastic transformation prior to transplant, thereby increasing the chances of subsequent relapse.

Various conditioning regimes have been used, the best known of which is the Seattle combination of cyclophosphamide and total body irradiation (TBI). However, newer preparative regimens such as busulphan and cyclophosphamide (Copelan *et al.*, 1989) and VP-16/TBI are under evaluation and appear promising. World-wide, the results of allografting in the chronic phase of CGL show that approximately 50% of patients are long-term disease-free survivors. This is reduced to a 15–20% long-term survival for BMT in accelerated or blastic phase(**96**).

The probability of relapse is about 10% and 45% for those transplanted in chronic and accelerated phases, respectively. Relapsed patients may be treated with further chemotherapy appropriate to the type of relapse (i.e. myeloid or lymphoid) or by a second transplant from the original donor, excluding the use of irradiation in the conditioning therapy (Cullis *et al.*, 1992a). An interesting approach used by some centres is treatment with donor-derived leukocytes harvested by leukopheresis with or without interferon. With such an approach, assuming a graft-versus-leukaemia effect of donor lymphocytes (Cullis *et al.*, 1992b; Kolb *et al.*, 1990), some patients have been restored to Ph′ negativity.

About two-thirds of patients with CGL have no HLA-identical sibling or are too old to undergo allogeneic BMT with all its attendant problems. For such patients (a) autologous bone marrow or peripheral blood stem cell (PBSC) transplant or (b) matched unrelated donor (MUD) bone marrow transplant are alternative procedures.

Bone marrow or PBSC autotransplantation in chronic phase has surprisingly led to persistent Ph′-negative haematopoiesis in some cases (Brito-Babapulle *et al.*, 1988; Butterini *et al.*, 1990). Such results may be improved in the future by *in vitro* manipulations including long-term cell culture (Barnett *et al.*, 1990) or use of marrow treated with γ-interferon before re-infusion (Arcese *et al.*, 1990), or use of α-interferon to maintain Ph′ negativity. Using matched but unrelated donors, the incidence of graft failure and GvHD is greater but a two-year disease-free survival of about 40% has been achieved (Ash *et al.*, 1990; McGlave *et al.*, 1990).

Present treatment trends are directed towards improving the situation with matched but unrelated bone marrow transplantation, and towards developing better techniques for maximizing the survival advantage of Philadelphia-chromosome-negative cells so that these can potentially be exploited in the autografting situation (Goldman, 1990).

Lymphomas

Lymphomas are a heterogeneous group of malignant conditions arising from the lymphatic system, conventionally divided into Hodgkin's and non-Hodgkin's lymphomas. In recent years, bone marrow transplantation has been increasingly used for the treatment of malignant lymphomas. In over 90% of cases autografting has been used, employing apparently lymphoma-free marrow to 'rescue' bone marrow function after high-dose chemoradiotherapy. Currently, in excess of 2000 patients from Europe and the USA have undergone an autografting procedure. However, as this is a relatively new treatment approach, follow-up time after the procedure is still relatively short, making adequate evaluation of the technique untenable.

The issues of importance in autografting for both Hodgkin's and non-Hodgkin's lymphoma are:
- Appropriate patient selection and timing of the transplantation procedure.
- How to optimise conditioning therapy.
- Whether or not to purge bone marrow prior to infusion.
- Appropriate use of peripheral blood stem cells.
- The role of growth factors and biological response modifiers.
- Minimizing toxicity of the procedure and long-term side effects.

Principles of dose escalation

Autologous BMT (ABMT) involves the use of high-dose chemo/radiotherapy and infusion of bone marrow harvested prior to commencement of high-dose therapy to 'rescue' bone marrow function. Animal models have demonstrated that for drug-sensitive tumours, a definite and sometimes steep dose–response curve exists, especially for radiation therapy and therapy with alkylating agents. Clinical studies support dose escalation in Hodgkin's disease and non-Hodgkin's lymphoma (Frei and Canellos, 1980), and it has been shown that in some haematological malignancies, intensive chemo/radiotherapy with allogeneic BMT can be curative in a small proportion of end-stage patients (Thomas, 1982). Dose escalation studies with cyclophosphamide and total body irradiation (TBI), and etoposide and TBI (Appelbaum and Buckner 1986) have been undertaken with both allogeneic/syngeneic and autologous bone marrow transplants, and the main conclusions are as follows:
- Since myelosuppression can be overcome by bone marrow rescue, the non-haemopoietic toxicities of the agents used are the dose-limiting factors.
- Different alkylating agents are commonly synergistic in their antitumour actions.

Thus, there is a ceiling to the quantity of any cytotoxic agent which can be used, secondary to its non-haematological toxicities.

Hodgkin's lymphoma

In Europe, the incidence of Hodgkin's lymphoma is 3/100 000 per year. There is a bimodal distribution with a major peak around the age of 25 years and a smaller peak in old age. The disease is commoner in males. Hodgkin's disease usually arises in the lymph nodes and most commonly presents as a painless swelling. Some patients have 'B' symptoms (fever, night sweats, unexplained weight loss), or they may experience generalized pruritus or alcohol-induced pain in involved lymph nodes.

The presence of Sternberg–Reed binucleated giant cells with large owl's eyes nuclei is diagnostic of the disease. Hodgkin's lymphoma is subclasified into four types:

1. Lymphocyte predominant (LP).
2. Nodular sclerosing (NS)
3. Mixed cellularity (MC)
4. Lymphocyte depleted (LD).

Nodular sclerosing is the most common type, and, together with mixed cellularity accounts for 90% of cases in Western countries.

The disease spreads stepwise to adjacent lymph nodes, and treatment decisions are made on extent of spread. The Ann Arbor anatomical staging classification was developed to distinguish those who would benefit from radiotherapy alone from those requiring systemic therapy. However, the recognition that tumour burden has an impact on outcome has led to modifications of this and resulted in the Cotswold staging classification (**Tables 13** and **14**).

Patients with advanced disease (stages III and IV) are treated with combination chemotherapy, and complete remission is attained in 70–90% of patients. Relapse occurs in about one-third of these, and approximately 10–15% are rescued by further combination chemotherapy. If relapse occurs more than 12 months after initial treatment with chemotherapy, there is a 90% probability of achieving a second complete remission. If, however, relapse occurs early less than 12 months after cessation of initial chemotherapy, or if the disease is primarily resistant, 'salvage' treatment with by non-cross-resistant chemotheraputic agents (e.g. ABVD for previous MOPP-type treatment) may be given, although the prognosis is poor with five-year survival rates of less than 10%. The results of such 'salvage' chemotherapy can be improved to 20–40% by high-dose chemotherapy and autologous BMT. Patients who are primarily resistant or who have relapsed early should be considered for such procedures.

Allogeneic BMT (Armitage, 1989) and autologous PBSC transplantation (Kessinger et al., 1989; Korbling et al., 1990) are alternatives for those with bone marrow involvement or poor marrow function, although again, experience in these diseases with these treatments is, to date, small and follow-up time short.

The use of haematopoietic growth factors, in particular G-CSF (Taylor et al., 1989) and GM-CSF (Devereux et al., 1989) to accelerate haematopoietic recovery following either peripheral blood stem cell or bone marrow autografting is becoming more prevalent. Most studies indicate that aplasia time can be shortened by a number of days, at least in terms of return of a peripheral blood neutrophil count. However, these growth factors have little effect on platelet recovery.

Table 13. Cotswold staging of Hodgkin's disease.

Stage I	Involvement of a single lymph region or structure
Stage II	Involvement of two or more lymph node regions on the same side of the diaphragm (the mediastinum is considered as a single site, whereas hilar lymph nodes are considered bilaterally). The number of anatomical site should be indicated by a subscript (e.g. II3).
Stage III	Involvement of lymph node regions or structures on both sides of the diaphragm
Stage III.1	With or without involvement of splenic, hilar, coeliac or portal nodes
Stage III.2	With involvement of para-aortic, iliac and mesenteric nodes
Stage IV	Involvement of one or more extranodal sites in addition to a site for which the designation 'E' has been used

Table 14. Designations applicable to any disease stage.

A	No symptoms
B	Fever (>38°C, night sweats, unexplained weight loss (>10% within the preceding 6 months)
X	Bulky disease (a widening of the mediastinum by more than one-third, or the presence of a nodal mass >10 cm
E	Involvement of a single extranodal site that is contiguous or proximal to the known nodal site
CS	Clinical stage
PS	Pathological stage as determined by laparotomy

Non-Hodgkin's lymphoma

The non-Hodgkin's lymphoma (NHL) working formula classification is shown in **Table 15**. High-dose chemo/radiotherapy and autologous BMT for the treatment of relapsed low-grade NHL has been evaluated by only a few centres, and a relatively small number of patients has been treated (Colombat et al., 1989). There are several problems associated with the use of marrow transplantation in this disease:
- Long natural history of indolent NHL.
- High frequency of bone marrow involvement at diagnosis.
- Decreased marrow reserve.
- Potential prolonged engraftment time as a result of previous therapy,
- Resistance to therapy following multiple relapses.

At a median follow-up time of 3 years, the projected disease-free survival is approximately 50%, so to date it is impossible to assess whether this approach has a beneficial outcome because of the short follow-up period.

Although most patients achieve complete remission (CR) after conventional therapy, the median duration of CR is between 12 and 24 months. Disease-free survival is only 25% at 5 years.

Patients with histological conversion to a more aggressive form of the disease who are still responsive to salvage therapy may be further salvaged by high-dose therapy and ABMT, and better results may be obtained in such patients than is the case with conventional chemotherapy.

Aggressive non-Hodgkin's lymphoma

In current practice, essentially all high- and intermediate-grade patients (with the exception of those that are staged by laparotomy to Stage I) receive combination chemotherapy. In patients with Stage III and Stage IV disease, the CR rate with CHOP chemotherapy is 53%, and 30% of patients are apparently cured. The results with localized disease are considerably better, but in the British National Lymphoma Institute (BNLI) series, the long-term survival of patients clinically staged at Stage II was approximately 50% (Linch and Vaughan-Hudson, 1988). Thus, a large proportion of patients still die of their disease and considerable efforts have been made over the last decade to improve these results with more aggressive approaches to therapy, and in particular, dose intensification. The most extreme example of dose intensification is autologous BMT (ABMT) (Chopra et al., 1990), possibly useful because approximately 50% of patients will either fail first-line treatment and require further treatment or relapse after complete remission, therefore requiring salvage therapy. However, it is not possible to assess at this stage whether such aggressive regimens confer any more benefit long-term than the older regimens.

Patients with disease retaining chemosensitivity may show a CR rate of about 30%, and salvage chemotherapy may be useful in achieving a state of minimal disease prior to intensive chemo/radiotherapy and ABMT. However, it is unclear whether conventional salvage therapy is better than ABMT in relapsed patients.

Autologous BMT in NHL as salvage therapy

Compared to salvage therapy with conventional dose chemotherapy, initial pilot sudies with ABMT suggest better disease-free survival in chemosensitive patients (Gribben et al., 1989). The procedure-related death rate in this group of transplant patients is in the order of 10%. Patients with primary refractory disease have an innate resistance which cannot be overcome by dose intensification. Treatment strategies for these unfortunate patients are yet to be developed.

Autologous BMT for NHL in first remission as consolidation treatment

It has been suggested that some patients with small non-cleaved cell lymphoma (SNCCL) and lymphoblastic lymphoma, as well as those with peripheral T-cell lymphoma, with poor prognosis at presentation, should be considered for high-dose chemo/radiotherapy and ABMT as consolidation treatment.

In adults with lymphoblastic lymphoma, high CR rates of between 70% and 95% can be achieved using intensive multi-drug chemotherapy protocols, similar to those used in acute lymphoblastic leukaemia.

Table 15. Non-Hodgkins lymphoma working formula classification.

Low Grade

   Small lymphocytic
   Follicular predominantly small cleaved cell
   Follicular mixed small cleaved and large cell

Intermediate Grade

   Follicular predominantly large cell
   Diffuse small cleaved cell
   Diffuse mixed small cleaved and large cell
   Diffuse large cell

High Grade

   Large cell, immunoblastic
   Lymphoblastic
   Small non-cleaved; Burkitt's lymphoma

Long-term disease-free survivals in the order of 56% at 3 years (Coleman et al., 1986) and 45% (Slater et al., 1986) have been reported. There is, however, a subgroup of patients who have a poor prognosis with conventional dose chemotherapy. Such poor prognostic features are definable and includes those with the following features at diagnosis:
- A raised lactic dehydrogenase and either a tumour mass ≥10 cm, or two or more extranodal sites, or Stage III or IV disease.
- A normal lactic dehydrogenase, but tumour mass ≥10 cm, and two or more extranodal sites, and stage II or IV disease.

This group of patients should be considered for high-dose chemo/radiotherapy and ABMT as consolidation.

Even in this poor prognosis group, however, overall survival is 41% on first-line chemotherapy, and the advantages of exposing these patients to further treatment have not, to date, been shown.

Multiple myeloma

The vast majority of patients presenting with this disease are over 60 years of age at diagnosis, and thus by virtue of their age ineligible for a transplantation procedure. However, for those in the younger age groups, both allogeneic and autologous bone marrow transplantation have been attempted, although again follow-up times are relatively short thus making data interpretation difficult.

The first reported allograft for myeloma was carried out by the Seattle team using a syngeneic donor (Osserman et al., 1982). A second similar report (Fefer et al., 1982) then followed. However, even major centres have carried out relatively few allogeneic transplants for myeloma, and heterogeneity of the patient population makes it possible to draw only limited conclusions from individual series.

Analysis of pooled data by the European or International Transplant Registries is therefore particularly important. In 1987, the first report from the European Bone Marrow Transplantation (EBMT) group described 14 patients, some of whom had been reported elsewhere (Tura et al., 1986; Gahrton et al., 1986). At the time of reporting, there had been 2 transplant-related deaths and 2 deaths from early relapse. Of the 10 surviving patients, five were in complete remission 9–34 months post-BMT, including two who had previously been refractory to treatment. Four patients were well with minimal disease 6–13 months post-BMT.

By 1990, data on 93 patients had been reported to the EBMT (Gahrton et al., 1990).The overall long-term survival was 41% for all patients, and 43% for those transplanted with identical donors. Patients transplanted electively following first-line treatment fared much better than those transplanted later in the course of their disease. For early, elective transplantation, the survival curve reached a plateau at 60% projected long-term survival, and stage at diagnosis had a profound influence on results.

Data concerning allogeneic transplants conditioned with BuCy (busulphan cyclophosphamide) was updated by Bensinger et al. in 1990, and currently, the potential to increase dose of Cy is under evaluation.

Allogeneic BMT in myeloma carries a high mortality. A realistic estimate of long-term transplant-related death approaches 40–50% of all patients. In patients transplanted early in the course of their disease, mortality is less, but is certainly higher than that seen in acute leukaemia patients transplanted in remission, or in chronic myeloid leukaemia patients transplanted in chronic phase. This may partly reflect the higher average age of myeloma patients, but is probably due also to the high incidence of active disease, clinical or subclinical renal impairment, and the increased susceptibility to infection. Previous radiotherapy to the thoracic region may increase the risk of pneumonitis, and previous transfusions may increase probability of cytomegaloviral seropositivity at BMT.

In spite of the high risk of allogeneic BMT, however, results are encouraging, in that a proportion of patients with advanced disease enter long-term remission.

Autografting in myeloma is perhaps a more popular high-dose therapy strategy, particularly in view of the fact that patients tend to be older at presentation and hence are not candidates for allografting. Results are encouraging, but toxicity is still a major problem. High-dose melphalan (HDM) with or without total body irradiation (TBI) or other drugs has been the commonest conditioning therapy,

In contrast to patients with leukaemia in remission, the bone marrow in myeloma patients is usually contaminated with plasma cells even after response to treatment. While marrow from such patients contains adequate normal haemopoietic progenitor cells and can successfully be used to shorten cytopenia time after intensive therapy, re-infusion of myeloma cells may prejudice the response to such treatment. This has led some groups to explore methods of *ex vivo* purging, while others have used intensive initial chemotherapy in an attempt to eradicate myeloma cells prior to harvesting and ABMT (*in vivo* purging).

Using HDM alone (Selby *et al.*, 1988), it was observed that a single dose of 140 mg/m² induced remission in 87% of untreated patients and 66% of previously treated patients. Of previously untreated patients, 27% achieved complete remission. However, toxicity was high, with 17% treatment-related early deaths and response duration was disappointingly short (median 18 months), even in patients who had achieved complete remission. It was concluded that although ABMT reduced toxicity of HDM, this alone was of limited value in patients with advanced disease. An attempt was subsequently made to induce more frequent and durable remissions by adding TBI (8.5 Gy in five fractions) to HDM (140 mg/m²) (Barlogie *et al.*, 1987). Median remission duration was 15 months. Data on HDM with TBI were further updated in 1990 (Jagannath *et al.*, 1990) with special reference to prognostic factors.

High β_2-microglobulin at ABMT and non-IgG isotype were identified as poor prognostic factors, and the results indicated that ABMT could not be recommended for patients with resistant relapse or those with a combination of high β_2-microglobulin and non-IgG isotype. It is probable, therefore, that even the addition of TBI does not result in a high frequency of durable responses. It was noted that the number of plasma cells in re-infused marrow had no obvious effect on remission duration, suggesting that failure to eradicate disease in patients was the major problem.

Following these observations, it seemed logical to carry out ABMT earlier in the course of the disease, having achieved initial response where possible, so as to reduce the amount of myeloma in the patient and in harvested marrow. This has been the approach used by the Royal Marsden and St Bartholomew's group (Gore *et al.*, 1989; McElwain *et al.*, 1989). Patients are treated initially with VAMP (vincristine and adriamycin by infusion with high-dose methylprednisolone). Those who achieve a plasma-cell reduction to below 30% proceed to harvest and ABMT after single-agent HDM at a dose of 200 mg/m². Those who fail to achieve this degree of tumour reduction receive HDM (140 mg/m²) without ABMT. At a median follow-up time of 1.2 years, 5 of 25 patients in CR had relapsed and 10 of 12 in partial remisssion (PR) had evidence of disease progression. The projected median response duration from the time of HDM was 12 months in the patients who achieved PR. These data confirm earlier observations that ABMT reduces mortality of HDM. However, the evidence that durable responses will be obtained even with a dose of 200 mg/m² is not as yet convincing.

An alternative approach to the problem of re-infusion of myeloma cells during ABMT has been the use of peripheral blood as a source of stem cells, on the grounds that these are less likely to be contaminated with myeloma cells, and with the advent of recombinant GM-CSF, it became possible to augment the post-chemotherapy peak in circulating CFU-GM approximately fivefold (Socinski *et al.*, 1988). As far as myeloma is concerned, peripheral blood stem cell transplantation (PBSCT) is an attractive alternative to ABMT because cells can be harvested even in patients with extensive marrow infiltration.

Marit *et al.* (1990) reported 8 patients who received peripheral blood stem cells (PBSC) alone and 5 others who received additional marrow. One patient received HDM alone as conditioning and the remainder HDM and TBI. All patients had significant tumour regression, and eight entered CR. Four relapsed from 5 to 18 months post-transplant and 9 remained in CR or with Stage I disease at 4–14 months post-ABMT. However, patients receiving PBSC alone are not separated from those who received additional marrow. Thus, it is impossible to discern any difference in response duration between the two groups.

The MD Anderson group have reported a series of 11 patients treated with PBSCT (Ventura *et al.*, 1990). All had advanced refractory disease. PBSC were collected after Cy (1 g/m²). Two patients died with pneumonitis. Of the remaining nine, response (>75% reduction in tumour mass) was observed in four and improvement in three. However, response duration was short (median 7 months).

High-dose cyclophosphamide used to recruit stem cells does not cause the prolonged aplasia seen after HDM and can be safely given without stem cell support, and in general, higher doses of Cy promote higher CFU-GM peaks. However, GM-CSF used to enhance stem cell harvesting may not be appropriate in view of the evidence that it is a growth factor for myeloma cells, and it is possible that use of rhGM-CSF to increase yields of PBSC might result in increased numbers of circulating myeloma stem cells.

References

Appelbaum FR, Buckner R. Overview of the clinical relevance of autologous bone marrow transplantation. *Clin Haematol* 1986; **15**: 1–19.

Apperley JF, Mauro F, Goldman JM *et al*. Bone marrow transplantation for chronic myeloid leukaemia in chronic phase: importance of a graft-versus-leukaemia effect. *Br J Haematol* 1988; **69**: 239–245.

Arcese W, Mauro FR, Alimena G *et al*. Interferon therapy for Ph′ positive CML patients relapsing after T-cell depleted allogeneic bone marrow transplantation. *Bone Marrow Transplant* 1990; **5**: 309–315.

Armitage JO. Bone marrow transplantation in the treatment of patients with lymphoma. *Blood* 1989; **73**: 1749–1758.

Ash RD, Casper JT, Chitambar CR *et al*. Successful allogeneic transplantation of T-cell depleted bone marrow from closely HLA-matched unrelated donors. *N Engl J Med* 1990; **322**: 485–494.

Barlogie B, Alexanian R, Dicke KA *et al*. High-dose chemoradiotherapy and autologous bone marrow transplantation for resistant multiple myeloma. *Blood* 1987; **70**: 869–872.

Barnett MJ, Eaves CJ, Phillips GL. Autografting in CML with cultured marrow:consistent restoration of Philadelphia (Ph′) negative haematopoiesis in patients selected by prior assessment of their marrow *in vitro*. *Blood* 1990; **76** (suppl 1): 526a (Abstract 2096).

Barrett AJ, Joshi R, Kendra J *et al*. Prediction and prevention of relapse of acute lymphoblastic leukaemia after bone marrow transplantation. *Br J Haematol* 1986; **64**: 179–185.

Barrett AJ. Progress in allogeneic and autologous BMT for acute lymphoblastic leukaemia (ALL). *Bone Marrow Transplant* 1991; **7** (suppl 2): 59–61.

Bennett JM, Catovsky D, Daniel MT *et al*. Proposed revised criteria for the classification of acute myeloid leukemia: a report of the French–American–British co-operative group. *Ann Intern Med* 1985; 103: 620–625.

Bensinger WI, Buckner CD, Clift R *et al*. Marrow transplantation for multiple myeloma using busulphan and cyclophosphamide. *Blood* 1990; **76** (suppl 1): 527a.

Blaise D, Gaspard MH, Stoppa AM *et al*. Allogeneic or autologous bone marrow transplantation for acute lymphoblastic leukaemia in first complete remission. *Bone Marrow Transplant* 1990; **5**: 7–12.

Brineker H, Christensen BE. Long term survival and late relapses in acute leukaemia in adults. *Brit J Haematol* 1990; **74**: 156–160.

Brito-Babapulle F, Bowcock SJ, Marcus RE. Autografting for patients with CML in chronic phase: PBSC may have a finite capacity for maintaining haemopoiesis. *Br J Haematol* 1988; **73**: 7–81.

Buckner CD, Clift RA. Clinical studies of allogeneic marrow transplantation in patients with acute non-lymphoblastic leukaemia. *Bone Marrow Transplant* 1989; **4** (suppl 3): 83–84.

Butterini A, Rivera GK, Bortin MM, Gale RP. Which treatment for childhood acute lymphoblastic leukaemia in second remission? *Lancet* 1987; **1**: 429–432.

Butturini A, Keating A, Goldman JM, Gale RP. Autotransplants in chronic myelogenous leukaemia: strategies and results. *Lancet* 1990; **1**: 1255–1258.

Champlin R, Gale RP. Review article. Acute myelogenous leukaemia: recent advances in therapy. *Blood* 1987; **68**: 1551–1562.

Chessells JM, Bailey C, Wheeler K, Richards SM. Bone marrow transplantation for high-risk childhood lymphoblastic leukaemia in first remission: experience in MRC UK ALL X. *Lancet* 1992; **340**: 565–568.

Chopra R, Goldstone AH, Linch DC *et al*. High dose combination chemotherapy and autologous bone marrow transplantation: minimum three year follow-up of 50 patients with Hodgkin's and non-Hodgkin's lymphoma. *Br J Haematol* 1990; **74** (suppl 1): 79.

Coleman CN, Picozzi VJ, Cox RS. Treatment of lymphoblastic lymphoma in adults. *J Clin Oncol* 1986; **4**: 1628–1637.

Colombat P, Biron P, Binet C *et al*. High-dose chemotherapy with autologous bone marrow transplantation in low-grade non-Hodgkin's lymphoma. In: *Proceedings of the Fourth International Symposium on Autologous Bone Marrow Transplantation, University of Texas, 1989*. Eds: Dicke K, Spitzer G, Jagannath S *et al*., University of Texas, pp. 317–327.

Copelan EA, Grever MR, Kapoor N, Tutschka PJ. Marrow transplantation following busulphan and cyclophosphamide for chronic myelogenous leukaemia in accelerated or blastic phase. *Br J Haematol* 1989; **71**: 487–491.

Cullis JO, Schwarer AP, Hughes TP *et al*. Second transplants for patients with chronic myeloid leukaemia after original transplant with T-depleted donor marrow: feasibility of using busulphan alone for re-conditioning. *Br J Haematol* 1992a; **80**: 33–39.

Cullis JO, Jiang YZ, Schwarer AP *et al*. Donor leukocyte infusions in the treatment of chronic myeloid leukemia in relapse following allogeneic bone marrow transplantation. *Blood* 1992b; **79**: 1379–1381.

Cunningham I, Gee TS, Reich LM *et al*. Acute promyelocytic leukaemia: treatment results during a decade at the Memorial Hospital. *Blood* 1989; **73**: 1116–1122.

Devereux S, Linch DC, Gribben JG *et al*. GM-CSF accelerates neutrophil recovery after autologous bone marrow transplantation for Hodgkin's disease. *Bone Marrow Transplant* 1989; **4**: 49–54.

Dutcher JP, Wiernik PH, Markus S *et al*. Intensive maintenance therapy improves survival in adult acute nonlymphocytic leukaemia: an eight-year follow-up. *Leukaemia* 1988; **2**: 413–419.

Fefer A, Greenberg PD, Cheever MA *et al*. Treatment of multiple myeloma with chemoradiotherapy and identical twin bone marrow transplantation. *Proc Am Soc Clin Oncol* 1982; **1**: C731.

Frei E, Canellos GP. Dose: A critical factor in cancer chemotherapy. *Am J Med* 1980; **69**: 585–594.

Gahrton G, Ringden O, Lonnquist B et al. Bone marrow transplantation in three patients with myeloma. *Acta Med Scand* 1986; **219**: 523–527.

Gahrton G, Belanger B, Cavo M et al. Allogeneic bone marrow transplantation in multiple myeloma—an EBMT Registry study. *Bone Marrow Transplant* 1990; **5** (suppl 2): 2.

Geller RB, Zahurak M, Hurwitz C et al. Prognostic importance of immunophenotyping in adults with acute myelocytic leukaemia: the significance of the stem-cell glycoprotein CD34 (My10). *Br J Haematol* 1990; **76**: 340–347.

Goldman JM. Options for the management of chronic myeloid leukemia—1990. *Leukemia Lymphoma* 1990; **3**: 159–164.

Gore ME, Selby PJ, Viner C et al. Intensive treatment of multiple myeloma and criteria for complete remission. *Lancet* 1989; **2**: 879–882.

Gribben JG, Goldstone AH, Linch DC et al. Effectiveness of high dose combination chemotherapy and autologous bone marrow transplantation for patients with non-Hodgkin's lymphomas who are still responsive to conventional dose chemotherapy. *J Clin Oncol* 1989; **7**: 1621–1629.

Herzig RH, Bortin MM, Barrett AJ et al. Bone marrow transplantation in high risk acute lymphoblastic leukaemia in first and second remission. *Lancet* 1987; **1**: 786–789.

Hoelzer D, Gale RP. Acute lymphoblastic leukaemia in adults: recent progress, future directions. *Semin Haematol* 1987; **24**: 27–39.

Horowitz MM, Messerer D, Hoelzer D et al. Chemotherapy compared with bone marrow transplantation for adults with acute lymphoblastic leukaemia in first remission. *Ann Intern Med* 1991; **115**: 13–19.

Jagannath S, Barlogie B, Dicke K et al. Autologous bone marrow transplantation in multiple myeloma: identification of prognostic factors. *Blood* 1990; **76**: 1860–1866.

Jones L, Goldman J. Management of chronic leukaemias. *Med Internat* 1987; **40**: 1653–1657.

Kessinger A, Armitage JO, Smith DM et al. High dose therapy and autologous peripheral blood stem cell transplantation for patients with lymphoma. *Blood* 1989; **74**: 1260–1265.

Kolb HJ, Mittermuller J, Clemm Ch et al. Donor leukocyte transfusions for treatment of recurrent chronic myelogenous leukemia in marrow transplant patients. *Blood* 1990; **76**: 2462–2465.

Korbling M, Holle R, Haas R et al. Autologous blood stem cell transplantation in patients with advanced Hodgkin's disease and prior radiation to the pelvic site. *J Clin Oncol* 1990; **8**: 978–982.

Linch DC, Vaughan-Hudson B. The management of Hodgkin's disease and the non-Hodgkin's lymphomas. In: *Recent Advances in Haematology*, 1988, Vol 5. Ed: Hoffbrand AV. Churchill Livingstone, London, pp. 211–243.

Marit G, Boiron JM, Reiffers J. Autologous blood stem cell transplantation (ABSCT) in high-risk multiple myeloma. *Bone Marrow Transplant* 1990; **5** (suppl 2): 42.

McCarthy D, Poynton C, Barrett AJ. Bone marrow transplantation for high-risk childhood lymphoblastic leukaemia. *Lancet* 1992; **340**: 1045.

McElwain TJ, Selby PJ, Gore ME et al. High dose chemotherapy and autologous bone marrow transplantation for myeloma. *Eur J Haematol* 1989; **43** (suppl 51): 152–156.

McGlave PB, Beatty P, Ash R, Hows JM. Therapy for chronic myelogenous leukemia with unrelated donor bone marrow transplantation: results in 102 cases. *Blood* 1990; **75**: 1728–1732.

Osserman EF, Di Re LB, Di Re J, Sherman WH et al. Identical twin transplantation in multiple myeloma. *Acta Haematol (Basel)* 1982; **68**: 215–223.

Pinkel D. Curing children of leukemia. *Cancer* 1987; **60**: 1683–1691.

Rees JK, Gray RG, Swirsky D, Hayhoe FGJ. Principal results of the Medical Research Council's 8th Acute Myeloid Leukaemia Trial. *Lancet* 1986; **2**: 1236–41.

Reiffers J, Marit G, Boiron JM et al. Autologous blood stem cell transplantation in acute leukemia: present status and future directions. *Bone Marrow Transplant* 1990; **5** (suppl 1): 48–49.

Selby P, Zulian G, Forgeson G et al. The development of high dose melphalan and of autologous bone marrow transplantation in the treatment of multiple myeloma: Royal Marsden and St Bartholomew's Hospital studies. *Hematol Oncol* 1988; **6**: 173–179.

Slater DE, Mertelsmann R, Kaziner B. Lymphoblastic lymphoma in adults. *J Clin Oncol* 1986; **4**: 57–67.

Socinski M, Cannistra SA, Elias A et al. Granulocyte–macrophage colony-stimulating factor expands the circulating haemopoietic progenitor cell compartment in man. *Lancet* 1988; **1**: 1194–1198.

Swirsky DM, de Bastos M, Parish SE et al. Features affecting outcome during remission induction of acute myeloid leukemia in 619 patients. *Br J Haematol* 1986; **64**: 435–453.

Tallman MS, Kopecky KJ, Amos D et al. Analysis of prognostic factors for the outcome of marrow transplantation or further chemotherapy for patients with acute nonlymphoblastic leukemia in first remission. *J Clin Oncol* 1989; **7**: 326–337.

Taylor K, Jagannath S, Spitzer G. Recombinant human granulocyte colony-stimulating factor hastens granulocyte recovery after high-dose chemotherapy and autologous bone marrow transplantation in Hodgkin's disease. *J Clin Oncol* 1989; **7**: 1791–1799.

Thomas ED. The role of marrow transplantation in the eradication of malignant disease. *Cancer* 1982; **49**: 1963–1969.

Tiley C, Powles RL, Treleaven JG et al. The feasibility and efficiency of combined maintenance chemotherapy and autologous bone marrow transplantation for treatment of first remission acute lymphoblastic leukaemia. *Bone Marrow Transplant* 1993; **12**: 449–457.

Tura S. Bone marrow transplantation in multiple myeloma: current status and future perspectives. *Bone Marrow Transplant* 1986; **1**: 17–20.

Ventura GJ, Barlogie B, Hester JP et al. High dose cyclophosphamide, BCNU and VP16 with autologous blood stem cell support for refractory multiple myeloma. *Bone Marrow Transplant* 1990; **5**: 265–268.

6. Solid Tumours

Joseph A Sparano, Nicolae Ciobanu and Rasim Gucalp

Autologous bone marrow transplantation (ABMT) accelerates haematopoietic recovery in patients with solid tumours treated with high-dose chemotherapy (HDC) (Cheson, 1989). The *in vivo* administration of haematopoietic colony-stimulating factors, such as granulocyte–macrophage colony stimulating factor (GM-CSF), further accelerates haematopoietic recovery by significantly shortening the duration of severe granulocytopenia, thereby resulting in a reduced frequency of documented infections, diminished antibiotic and parenteral nutrition usage, and shortened hospital stay (Nemunaitis,1991). Other haematopoietic growth factors, such as interleukin-3 and stem cell growth factor, or PIXY-321 and interleukin-6, expand the stem cell population and stimulate megakaryocytopoiesis respectively, thereby raising expectations that they may be useful in further accelerating both granulocyte and platelet recovery in patients treated with HDC/ABMT (Groopman *et al.*,1989). Recent evidence also suggests that *in vitro* incubation of marrow allografts with haematopoietic growth factors prior to marrow re-infusion may further hasten haematopoietic recovery (Naparstek, 1992). Finally, preliminary evidence suggests that the re-infusion of autologous, peripheral blood-derived stem cells in combination with GM-CSF accelerates both granulocyte and platelet recovery in patients receiving high-dose chemotherapy administered alone or with ABMT (Shea *et al.*, 1992; Huan *et al.*, 1992). Therefore, with continued improvement in supportive care, it is anticipated that the morbidity, mortality, and cost of HDC/ABMT will be substantially reduced.

Considerable evidence suggests that graft-versus-host disease prevents relapse in patients with acute or chronic leukaemia who undergo allogeneic bone marrow transplantation (i.e. graft-versus-leukaemia effect) (Sullivan, 1988). Graft-versus-host disease occurs infrequently in patients receiving ABMT, however. While prospective trials comparing autologous versus allogeneic bone marrow transplantation in patients with solid tumours have not been performed, a case-controlled analysis revealed no evidence for a graft-versus-tumour effect in patients with non-Hodgkin's lymphoma who received allogeneic bone marrow transplantation, except in a subgroup of patients with lymphoblastic lymphoma (Chopra *et al.*, 1992). Therefore, given the absence of clear evidence for a graft-versus-tumour effect, the substantial morbidity and mortality associated with graft-versus-host disease, and the low likelihood of having an HLA-identical sibling donor, most patients with solid tumours receive autologous rather than allogeneic bone marrow transplantation after treatment with HDC.

In order for HDC/ABMT to be a tenable strategy in patients with solid tumours, the tumour should be inherently drug-sensitive at standard drug doses, there should be *in vitro, in vivo,* or clinical evidence supporting a dose–response treatment effect, and haematologic toxicity should be the dose-limiting toxic effect of the drugs to be employed in the preparative regimen. Therefore, most clinical trials of HDC/ABMT in patients with solid tumours have included diseases which are either potentially curable (e.g. germ cell tumours) or moderately responsive (e.g. breast and ovarian carcinoma) to standard chemotherapy, and have led to some encouraging results which will prompt further investigation. Trials in patients with inherently drug-resistant neoplasms (e.g. lung and colon carcinomas) have not yielded promising results (Cheson *et al.*, 1989).

Preclinical evidence supporting a dose–response effect

The seminal studies of Schabel demonstrated the dose–response effect for cytotoxic drugs; a doubling of the dose of cyclophosphamide in animals with L1210 leukaemia led to a four-log reduction in tumour burden (Schabel, 1975). Other studies have confirmed the dose–response effect *in vitro* and *in vivo* for cytotoxic drugs, particularly alkylating agents (Frei *et al.*, 1989). Other means of assessing dose–response relationship include the *in vitro* human tumour cloning assay (Von Hoff *et al.*, 1986) and the *in vivo* excision assay (Frei *et al.*, 1989). With the former technique, human tumour specimens are grown *in vitro*, exposed to varying drug concentrations, and tumour colony-forming units are analysed, facilitating calculation of dose–response effect. With the latter technique, mice with transplantable tumours treated with cytotoxic drugs undergo tumour excision 24 hours after drug exposure; the excised tumour is grown in a quantitative clonal assay. Both techniques have substantiated the dose–response effect for cytotoxic drugs in general, and for alkylating agents in particular.

Table 16. Drugs amenable to dose escalation.

Drug	Conventional dose* (mg/m²)	ABMT dose (mg/m²) *	Dose-limiting toxicity	Reference
Alkylating agents				
Cyclophosphamide	500–1500 mg	7500 mg†	Cystitis Myocarditis Pneumonitis	Smith et al. 1983
Ifosphamide	5000–12 000 mg	18 000 mg†	Renal insufficiency	Elias et al. 1990
Cisplatin	40–80 mg	240 mg†	Nephrotoxicity Ototoxicity	Ozols et al. 1984
Carboplatin	300–400 mg	2000 mg	Peripheral neuropathy Hepatotoxicity Nephrotoxicity Ototoxicity	Shea et al. 1989
Thiotepa	12–30 mg	1135 mg	Mucositis Neurological toxicity	Wolff et al. 1989
Busulphan	2–4 mg/kg	16 mg/kg	Stomatitis VOD***	Bensinger et al. 1992
BCNU	240–300 mg	1000 mg	Pneumonitis VOD***	Phillips et al. 1983
Melphalan	40 mg	260 mg	Mucositis	Lazarus et al. 1985
Methchlorethamine	6 mg	0.3–2.0 mg/kg**	Neurological toxicity	Sullivan et al. 1982
Chlorambucil	2 mg	6 mg/kg	Neurological toxicity	Ciobanu et al. 1987
Plant alkaloids				
Etoposide	240–500 mg	2400 mg	Mucositis	Wolff et al. 1983
Plant antibiotics				
Mitoxantrone	14 mg	75 mg**	Mucositis	Mulder et al. 1989a
Mitomycin C	10 mg	90 mg	Hepatic toxicity	Sarna et al. 1982

* Dose per square metre except where indicated.
** Used in combination with cyclophosphamide.
† May not require autologous bone marrow support.
*** Veno-occlusive disease.

Drugs amenable to dose escalation

Not all drugs which exhibit a dose–response effect *in vitro* are suitable for dose escalation requiring autologous bone marrow support. An agent whose major dose-limiting toxicity is haematologic at conventional doses is best suited for escalation. Numerous Phase I trials evaluating drug escalation with autologous stem cell support have been performed. In general, drug escalation continued until non-haematologic toxicity became dose-limiting, and investigators accepted a greater degree of haematologic toxicity than normally achieved in trials employing conventional drug dosing. Alkylating agents are the class of drugs which are best suited for escalation due to their predominantly haematologic toxicity and due to the *in vitro* and *in vivo* evidence demonstrating their dose-dependent antineoplastic effects (**Table 16**). The non-cell cycle-specific cytotoxic effect of alkylators also makes them attractive agents to escalate, since most tumour cells are not actively cycling at the time of drug exposure. Other drugs with important activity not belonging to the alkylating agent class of drugs

Table 17. Selected Phase I trials of combination chemotherapy plus ABMT.

Drug combination	Maximum tolerable doses (mg/m^2)	Dose-limiting toxicity	Toxic death*	*Reference
Cisplatin Cyclophosphamide Carmustine	165 5625 600	Multi-organ toxicity: VOD, hypertension, refractory thrombocytopenia	1/19 (5%)	Peters *et al.* 1986
Cisplatin Etoposide Carmustine	200 2400 600	Stomatitis, oesophagitis enteritis, pulmonary	5/79 (6%)	Lazarus *et al.* 1992
Cyclophosphamide Etoposide Carmustine	7200 2000 450	Interstitial pneumonitis with >600 mg/m^2 of carmustine	2/40 (5%)	Wheeler *et al.* 1990
Cyclophosphamide Thiotepa	7500 7500	Stomatitis, enteritis, infection	1/18 (6%)	Williams *et al.* 1987
Cyclophosphamide Carboplatin Thiotepa	6000 800 500	Stomatitis, oesophagitis, cardiac and pulmonary	2/22 (9%)	Eder *et al.* 1990
Cyclophosphamide Carboplatin Mitoxantrone	90 mg/kg 1500 75	Mucositis, enteritis, renal insufficiency	2/14 (14%)**	McKenzie *et al.* 1991
Ifosfamide Carboplatin Etoposide (or teniposide)	7500 1000 1250 (or 750)	Nephropathy Oesophagitis	6/44 (13%)	Lotz *et al.* 1991
Ifosfamide Carboplatin Etoposide	16000 1800 1500	Renal, cardiac, CNS dysfunction	0/37 (0%)	Wilson *et al.* 1992

* Toxic deaths occurring at the maximum tolerated dose or below.
** Includes all patients treated.

include etoposide (a plant alkaloid) and mitoxantrone (a plant antibiotic).

Phase I studies of high-dose drug combinations have also been performed which have employed drugs with non-overlapping toxicities. Examples of commonly employed treatment regimens are outlined in **Table 17**. Infection, mucositis, enteritis, pneumonitis, and veno-occlusive disease of the liver are the major life-threatening toxic effects of such therapy, but virtually every organ system may be affected (Cheson et al., 1989). Haematopoietic recovery is variable and is often delayed in patients with who receive purged bone marrow or who have received extensive prior chemotherapy or irradiation. For example, the median time to granulocyte recovery (>500 granulocytes/mm^3) was 21 days (range, 10–51 days), the median time to platelet transfusion independence (platelets >20 000/mm^3 without platelet transfusions) was 23 days (range 10–81 days), and the median period of hospitalization was 32 days (range 22–113 days) in 29 patients with advanced breast cancer treated with high-dose carboplatin (800 mg/m^2), cyclophosphamide (6000 mg/m^2) and thiotepa (500 mg/m^2) (Antman, 1992). Since it is has long been recognised that the risk of infection increases with more severe and/or prolonged granulocytopenia (Bodey et al., 1966), efforts to reduce treatment-related toxicity have focused on accelerating haematopoietic recovery with haematopoietic growth factors and peripheral-blood stem cells. However, recent studies have suggested other means by which regimen-related toxicity can be ameliorated. For example, pentoxifylline, a haemorrheologic agent which is known to inhibit production of tumor necrosis factor-α, reduced the frequency of mucositis, veno-occlusive disease and renal insufficiency, and diminished parenteral nutrition use and hospital stay in a cohort of patients treated with allogeneic or autologous bone marrow transplantation compared with a historical control group (Bianco et al., 1991). While efforts to ameliorate regimen-related toxicity continue, it is important that carefully controlled trials identify treatment regimens which have an acceptable degree of regimen-related toxicity. Despite the completion of carefully performed clinical trials designed specifically to identify tolerable treatment regimens, as well as improved patient selection and methods to accelerate haematopoietic reconstitution and reduce treatment-related morbidity, approximately 5–10% of patients treated with HDC/ABMT die due to treatment-related complications.

Clinical evidence supporting a dose–response effect

Retrospective analysis of available data suggests a dose–response effect for combination chemotherapy in producing objective response in patients with advanced adenocarcinoma of the ovary and breast (Hryniuk and Bush, 1984; Levin and Hryniuk, 1987). Relapse-free survival and survival are also improved in patients with advanced or operable breast cancer who receive more dose-intense regimens (Hryniuk and Bush, 1984).

Dose intensification without autologous bone marrow support has been prospectively studied in a limited number of trials in patients with solid tumours. In advanced breast cancer, two prospective clinical trials have been performed comparing two treatment regimens of differing dose intensity. In one trial, 66 patients with advanced breast cancer were randomly assigned to receive high-dose cyclophosphamide (600 mg/m^2), methotrexate (40 mg/m^2), and 5-fluorouracil (600 mg/m^2) (CMF) given intravenously once every three weeks with dose escalation if minimal toxicity occurred, and 67 patients were assigned to receive low-dose CMF (300 mg/m^2, 20 mg/m^2 and 300 mg/m^2, respectively) (Tannock et al., 1988). The response rate was significantly higher for patients who received high-dose CMF (30%) compared with patients who received low-dose CMF (11%). Vomiting, conjunctivitis, granulocytopenia, thrombocytopenia and partial or complete alopecia were significantly more common in the high-dose arm, but a quality-of-life analysis that related to the effect of breast cancer (e.g. pain) or general health (e.g. mobility) showed a trend to higher values, or less symptoms, in patients treated with high-dose CMF. Despite the fact that patients who failed low-dose CMF were crossed over to high-dose CMF, a study design which often obscures any survival advantage for a particular treatment, there was still a survival advantage for the high-dose arm (median survival 15.6 months) compared with the low-dose arm (12.8 months). However, the interval from relapse to randomization, an important prognostic variable, was significantly longer in patients in the high-dose arm (2.4 months versus 1.4 months); when the survival analysis was corrected for this imbalance, there was still a trend, but no longer a significant difference, favouring the high-dose arm. This is an extremely important observation which is of particular importance in evaluating the results of HDC/ABMT trials because of the inherent delay in implementing such therapy. There are multiple reasons for such delay, which include the time required for referral to the appropriate centre, screening, and the logistics of scheduling the bone marrow harvest and/or the transplant procedure (Berman et al., 1992). Therefore, even a seemingly small delay from the diagnosis of recurrent disease to implementation of therapy may select a patient population which is inherently more likely to survive longer, potentially confounding the interpretation of HDC/ABMT trials in patients with solid tumours, as has already been recognized to occur in patients with acute leukaemia who are selected to undergo autologous or allogeneic bone marrow transplantation (Berman et al., 1992).

In another prospective, randomized study of dose intensification in patients with advanced breast cancer, conventional dose 5-fluorouracil (500 mg/m^2, days 1, 8), Adriamycin (50 mg/m^2 day 1), and cyclophosphamide (500 mg/m^2, day 1, repeated every 28 days) (FAC) combination was compared with a high-dose FAC combination requiring supportive care measures that included total protective isolation and prophylactic antibiotics; the high-dose FAC regimen consisted of 5-fluorouracil (500 mg/m^2/day) via continuous i.v. infusion for 5 days combined with escalating doses of Adriamycin (60–80 mg/m^2) and cyclophosphamide (1000–1500 mg/m^2, day 1) (Hortobagyi et al., 1987). There was no significant improvement in response or survival with high-dose FAC; moreover, high-dose FAC was substantially more toxic. Unlike the previous trial reported by Tannock et al., in which the high-dose arm actually represented a conventional dose regimen, the high-dose arm in the current study employed a maximally tolerable regimen (without haematopoietic growth factor support, which was not available at the time of the study), and included Adriamycin, the single most active agent in the treatment of advanced breast cancer. Therefore, while these prospective trials suggest that there may a dose–response effect favouring intermediate (i.e. conventional dose) or high-dose chemotherapy regimens over low-dose regimens, there may be a shoulder on the dose–response curve above which further drug escalation achievable without autologous bone marrow support does not result in improved outcome. Autologous bone marrow transplantation may facilitate further drug escalation above this apparent shoulder on the dose–response curve.

In operable breast cancer, disease-free survival and survival were significantly improved in patients who received high-dose FAC compared with low-dose FAC in a prospective, randomized trial, the former of which was twofold more dose intensive than the latter (Budman et al., 1992). As in the trial reported by Tannock et al., however, the low-dose arm employed a less than conventional dose of FAC, while the high-dose arm employed a conventional dose of FAC, again failing to answer the question of whether intensification above a conventional dose level could result in improved survival.

Prospective trials involving dose intensification without autologous bone marrow support in patients with solid tumours other than carcinoma of the breast have also been limited. A high-dose regimen consisting of cisplatin (200 mg/m^2), etoposide (500 mg/m^2), vinblastine (0.2 mg/kg) and bleomycin (30 units weekly) was no more active than a conventional dose regimen containing cisplatin (100 mg/m^2), vinblastine (0.3 mg/kg) and bleomycin (30 units weekly) in patients with poor-prognosis germ cell tumours (Nichols et al., 1991). Likewise, another trial found that high-dose vinblastine (0.4 mg/kg) combined with cisplatin and bleomycin was no more active that intermediate-dose vinblastine (0.3 mg/kg) in patients with germ cell tumours, yet was substantially more toxic (Stoter et al., 1986). In ovarian carcinoma, one study which compared intermediate-dose cisplatin (75 mg/m^2) plus hexamethylmelamine with low-dose cisplatin (37.5 mg/m^2) plus hexamethylmelamine found a significantly higher response rate for patients receiving intermediate-dose cisplatin (61% versus 47%) (Wiernik et al., 1992).

Hence, while retrospective analysis of published data suggests a clinically meaningful dose–response relationship for cytotoxic therapy of solid tumours, the results of prospective trials suggest that there may be a threshold above which further intensification without autologous bone marrow support does not yield improved outcome. By ameliorating haematological treatment-related toxicity, autologous bone marrow re-infusion may facilitate further intensification above this threshold.

High-dose chemotherapy plus autologous bone marrow transplantation for the treatment of solid tumours

Breast cancer

Advanced breast cancer

In one of the first HDC/ABMT trials breast cancer, 22 patients with Stage IV breast cancer who had not received prior chemotherapy for advanced disease were treated with high-dose cisplatin (165 mg/m^2), cyclophosphamide (5625 mg/m^2) and carmustine (600 mg/m^2) (Peters et al., 1992). Sixteen patients (73%) had an objective response, including 12 patients (54%) who had a complete response (CR), the latter of which was substantially higher than the 10% CR rate observed in conventional chemotherapy trials (Eddy, 1992). Furthermore, three patients (14%) followed for 4–7 years were alive and progression-free with no other treatment administered. However, the median response duration was 7 months, the median survival was 10 months, and five patients (23%) died due to treatment-related complications. Others have observed comparable findings when employing HDC/ABMT as initial therapy for patients with advanced breast cancer (**Table 18**) (Antman et al., 1992). In an attempt to improve this result, 18 clinical trials involving 268 patients with advanced breast cancer have been performed employing HDC/ABMT after a period of cytoreduction with dose-intensive treatment regimens not requiring stem cell support (**Table 19**). When the results of these studies are combined, CR occurred in 39% after induction chemotherapy, and 59% after HDC/ABMT. Twenty-eight percent remain in continuous CR with variable periods of follow-up ranging from 1–42+ months. Approximately 10% of patients died due to treatment-related complications.

The high CR rate for induction chemotherapy in these studies reflects the dose-intensive nature of non-transplant chemotherapy that these patients received; it may also reflect selection bias for patients with minimal tumour burden which is inherent in such trials. The CR rate was higher for patients receiving induction therapy prior to HDC/ABMT than in patients receiving HDC/ABMT as the first treatment for metastatic disease. Thus, treatment with HDC/ABMT, whether used as initial therapy for patients with advanced breast cancer or in patients responding to standard chemotherapy, has resulted in 15–25% of patients remaining alive and progression-free for periods exceeding 2 years, and uncommon event in patients treated with standard therapy.

In another overview analysis of the data, comparison of HDC/ABMT with standard chemotherapy resulted in a fourfold increase in CR rate, a twofold increase in overall response rate, but no improvement in response duration or proportion of patients surviving 2 years (Eddy, 1992). Therefore, unlike some potentially curable diseases such as lymphoma and germ cell tumours, where the achievement of CR has resulted in the cure of most such patients, the majority of patients with breast cancer who have a CR appear destined to die of progressive breast cancer. The modest gains achieved in patients with advanced breast cancer treated with HDC/ABMT occur at the cost of a 12% treatment-related death rate, compared with 1% treatment-related death rate for standard

Table 18. Summary of high-dose combination chemotherapy plus ABMT trials in patients with advanced breast cancer.

Timing of HDC/ABMT treatment of patients	Response after induction*		Response after BMT*		Continuous CR	Toxic death
	CR	PR	CR	PR		
As initial therapy 53	–	–	25%	67%	17%	9%
After induction chemo. 268	39%	90%	59%	90%	28%	10%

* CR = complete response; PR = partial response.

Table 19. Selected clinical trials of high-dose chemotherapy plus ABMT in patients with ovarian cancer.

Drugs (mg/m²)	(n)	Comment	Toxic death	Reference
Single agents				
Melphalan (140)	14	36% disease-free (median follow-up 43 months)	0	Dauplat et al. 1989
Melphalan (140)	35	45% progression-free (median follow-up 23 months)	3 (9%)	Viens et al. 1990
Melphalan (140)	11	45% Disease-free survival > 36 months	0	Dufuor et al. 1991
Thiotepa (> 900)	10	Six patients had objective response	not reported	Herzig et al. 1988
Combinations				
Chlorambucil (6 mg/kg) Vinblastine (0.6 mg/kg) Etoposide (1200)	3	One CR (10 months) CNS toxicity precluded further study	0	Ciobanu et al. 1987
Cyclophosphamide (7000) Etoposide 900–1500	8	5/5 patients with microscopic disease responded	0	Mulder et al. 1989b
Cyclophosphamide (5625) Thiotepa (300) Cisplatin (90) (intraperitoneal)	12	6 patients had documented response but only two are progression-free	3 (25%)	Shpall et al. 1990
Cyclophosphamide (90–120 mg/kg) Carboplatin (1500) Mitoxantrone (30–75)	17	60% CR rate. One-third alive and progression-free (4+ to 22+ months)	2 (12%)	McKenzie et al. 1991; Stiff 1992

97–99 Breast Cancer. 39-year-old female with widely spread metastatic breast cancer (brain, retinal, chest and bone metastases), refractory to several conventional salvage regimens. Treated in October 1990 with BCNU 250 mg/m²/day on days −6, −5, −4, cisplatin 40 mg/m²/day on days −7 through to −3 and thiotepa (250 mg/m²/day) on days −5 and −4. Pretransplant radiation therapy given to bony lesions, brain and retinal metastases. Enjoyed two years free of disease progression.

97 Pre-ABMT chest CT. Axial section at mid-hilum level demonstrates central right middle mass of 1.5 cm in transverse diameter.

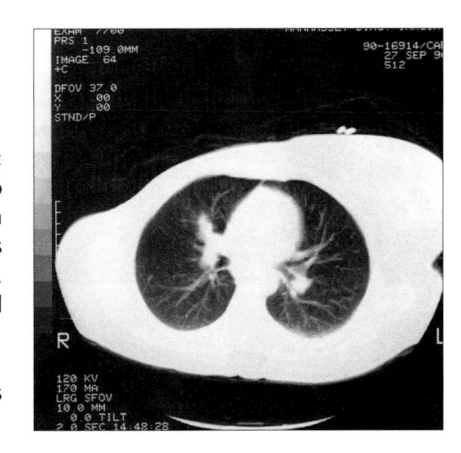

Bone Marrow Transplantation

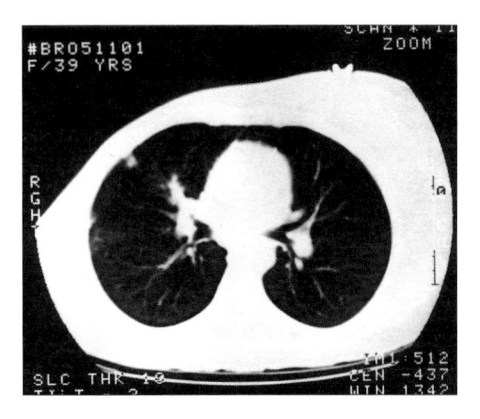

98 Post-ABMT chest CT 1. Follow-up CT scan shows no significant change in size of the right middle lobe mass. There is a small (0.7 cm diameter) peripheral nodule at the right anterior chest wall (present on the previous scan only at a slightly different level).

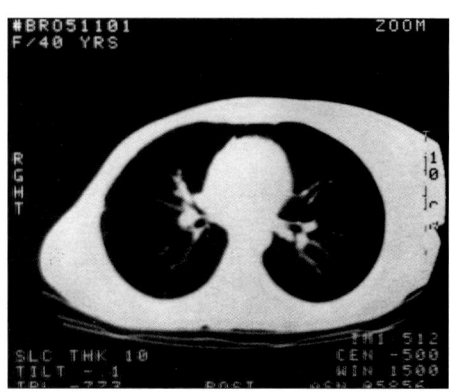

99 Post-ABMT chest CT 2. The central right middle lobe lesion is now 1.2 cm in diameter and the peripheral nodule has decreased in size (0.2 × 0.5 cm).

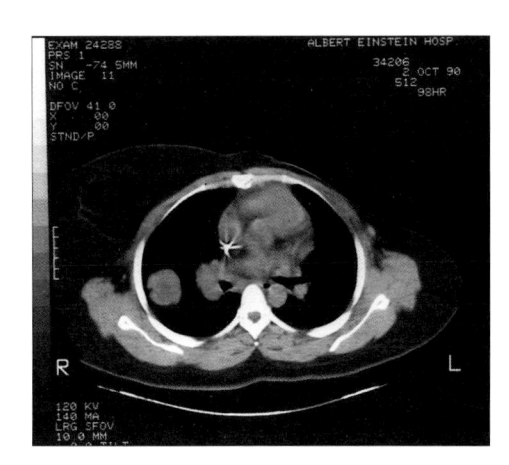

100–102 Breast cancer. 41-year-old female with metastatic breast cancer. Treated with melphalan (180 mg/m^2) and etoposide (3000 mg/m^2 with ABMT). She reached complete remission post-ABMT. Eight months later had a brain recurrence and died with progressive disease.

100 Pre-ABMT chest CT. CT scan through the mid-hilum demonstrates a 3-cm right middle lobe mass and right hilar adenopathy. The patient is post-mastectomy.

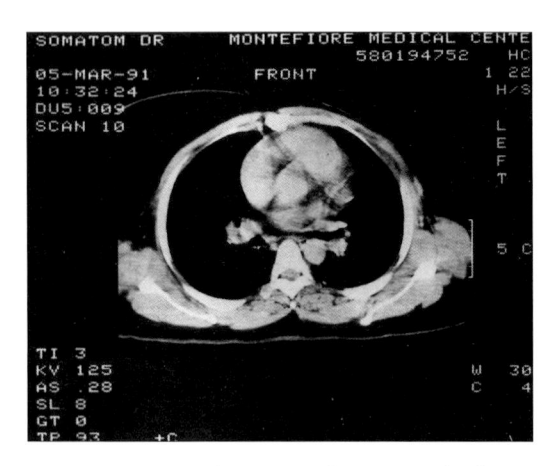

101 Post-ABMT chest CT. Follow-up study shows resolution of the lung mass and decrease in size of the hilar adenopathy.

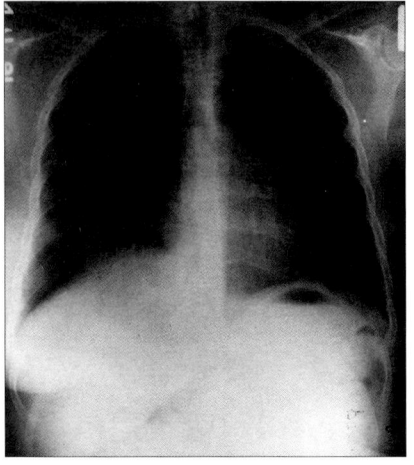

102 Post-ABMT Chest X-ray. Chest X-ray confirms complete resolution of the right middle lobe mass.

chemotherapy. Finally, when appraising both the clinical and financial considerations of this treatment strategy in patients with advanced breast cancer using a decision tree analysis, HDC/ABMT was determined to be of modest efficacy in improving survival but at an untenable cost (Hillner et al., 1992). Nevertheless, the results of these studies are sufficiently encouraging to continue to investigate this treatment approach in patients with advanced breast cancer.

High-risk operable breast cancer

HDC/ABMT has also been studied in patients with operable breast cancer at high risk for relapse despite treatment with conventional adjuvant chemotherapy. One hundred and two patients with high-risk operable breast cancer registered in a pilot trial to receive high-dose cisplatin, carmustine and cyclophosphamide plus ABMT after four cycles of standard FAC chemotherapy; 85 patients completed the full treatment course (Peters et al., 1992). Patients were required to have at least 10 axillary lymph nodes involved by tumour. After a median follow of 24 months (range 10–58 months), 10 patients have relapsed, including five systemic and five local relapses. The estimated Kaplan–Meier event-free survival was 72%, compared a 38% event-free survival in a historical control group treated with conventional therapy who had survived for at least five months without relapse. Randomized clinical trials are presently ongoing to confirm the improved outcome suggested by the pilot trial.

Ovarian carcinoma

The median survival for patients with advanced ovarian carcinoma is about two years; while the majority of patients respond to cisplatin- (or carboplatin) based therapy, only 15% have histologically confirmed CR, and only 4% survive progression-free for 10 years (Hoskins et al., 1992). Intraperitoneal chemotherapy administration, while producing response and palliation in some patients with residual disease following primary therapy, has not had a clearly enhanced curability (Ozols 1991). Given the inherent drug sensitivity of ovarian adenocarcinoma, and the evidence suggesting a dose–response relationship in this disease, HDC/ABMT is a reasonable strategy to consider in such patients.

A limited number of trials involving HDC/ABMT have been performed in patients with ovarian carcinoma (**Table 19**). Melphalan has been the most extensively studied drug in this setting. Fourteen patients with microscopic (five patients) or macroscopic (nine patients) residual disease at second-look laparotomy after responding to cisplatin-based chemotherapy received high-dose melphalan (140 mg/m^2) plus ABMT (Dauplat et al., 1989). There were no treatment-related deaths. After a mean follow-up of 43 months, five patients (36%) continued to be disease-free, an outcome superior to that expected for such patients. Likewise, 35 patients received high-dose melphalan ($\geq$140 mg/m^2) after second-look laparotomy following cisplatin-based chemotherapy (Viens et al., 1990). With a median followup of 23 months, 15 patients (43%) were alive and progression-free. Finally, 11 patients received high-dose melphalan (140 mg/m^2) plus ABMT as consolidation therapy after achieving response to cisplatin-based chemotherapy, five of whom had received abdominal radiotherapy prior to melphalan plus ABMT (Dufour et al., 1991). Five patients were alive and progression-free more than 3 years after HDC/BMT. Thiotepa, another alkylating agent, has been studied as a single agent in 10 patients at doses up to 900 mg/m^2; six patients responded to therapy (Herzig 1988). These studies indicate that the administration of high-dose alkylating agents plus ABMT in patients with advanced ovarian carcinoma responding to cisplatin-based chemotherapy is feasible and safe; furthermore, approximately one-third of patients with disease at second look laparotomy, a finding associated with a poor prognosis with standard therapy, achieved sustained progression-free survival lasting 2 or more years. Patients with bulky disease, however, do not appear to benefit from such an approach.

Information regarding other drugs or drug combinations in ovarian carcinoma is more limited. Three patients received high dose chlorambucil (6 mg/kg), vinblastine (0.6 mg/kg), and etoposide (1200 mg/m^2); while one patient had a CR of 10 months duration, transient central nervous system toxicity consisting of tremour, myoclonus and seizures prevented further investigation (Ciobanu, 1987). Eight patients received cyclophosphamide (7 mg/m^2) and etoposide (900–1500 mg/m^2) plus ABMT (Mulder et al., 1989b). Five patients had persistent microscopic residual disease at second-look laparotomy after standard chemotherapy, and three patients had bulky disease (>5 cm). While none of three patients with bulky disease responded, all five patients with microscopic disease had CR documented by laparotomy or laparoscopy. In another trial, eight patients received cyclophosphamide (5625 mg/m^2) and thiotepa (300 mg/m^2) plus ABMT; six patients had pathologically documented 75% or greater tumour response which persisted for a median 6 months (range 3–9 months) (Shpall et al., 1990). Finally, 17 patients with recurrent or resistant ovarian cancer received high-dose cyclophosphamide (120 mg/kg), carboplatin (1,500 mg/m^2) and mitoxantrone (75 mg/m^2); CR occurred in 60% and approximately one-third remained in CR from 4+ to 22+ months. Patients with non-bulky disease and those responding to salvage chemotherapy prior to HDC/ABMT fared better (McKenzie et al., 1991; Stiff, 1992)

Thus, few clinical trials have been published regarding HDC/ABMT in patients with advanced ovarian carcinoma. High-dose melphalan plus ABMT appears to be safe and may benefit approximately one-third of patients who achieve disease control. Only patients with non-bulky disease appear to benefit from therapy. Preliminary results from some trials involving drug combinations appear encouraging and merit further study.

103–104 Ovarian cancer. 59-year-old woman with refractory ovarian carcinoma treated with high-dose busulphan (16mg/kg) plus ABMT.

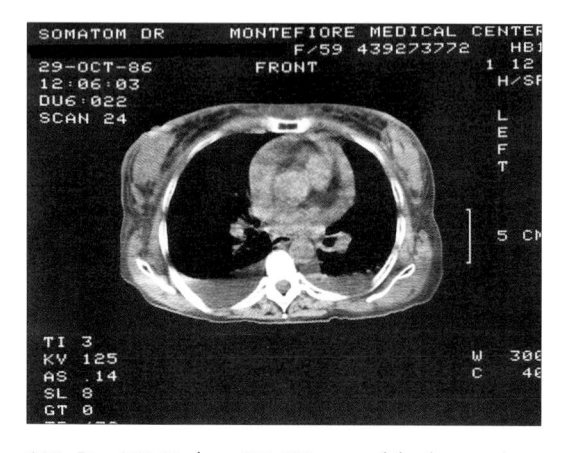

103 Pre-ABMT chest CT. CT scan of the lower chest demonstrates bilateral pleural effusions and pericardial effusion.

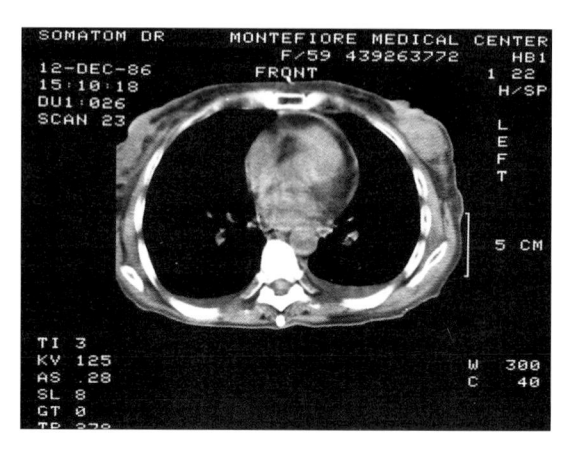

104 Post-ABMT chest CT. Resolved pericardial effusion and nearly completely resolved pleural effusions.

Germ cell tumours

While malignant germ cell tumours are eminently curable for the majority of men (and women) treated with standard cisplatin-based chemotherapy, the prognosis for patients with relapsed or resistant disease is poor. Current research has focused on reducing treatment-related morbidity for patients with good prognostic features, and improving treatment for patients with poor prognostic features by intensification or by the addition of active new agents, such as ifosfamide, to primary therapy. While clinical trials of HDC/ABMT in patients with testicular carcinoma have generally included only patients with disease which has relapsed or been resistant to standard chemotherapy, HDC/ABMT may represent a reasonable alternative to standard therapy if that procedure were associated with acceptable morbidity and mortality.

The long-term outcome for 40 patients with testicular carcinoma who were treated with one or two courses of high-dose carboplatin (900–2000 mg/m^2) and etoposide (1200 mg/m^2) plus ABMT at a single treatment centre has been reported (Broun et al., 1992) **(Table 20)**. Seven patients (18%) died due to treatment-related complications. Twelve patients (30%) had a CR. Five patients of the CRs have relapsed and died at a median of 18 months, and one patient died of treatment-related leukaemia at 27.5 months without evidence of recurrent germ cell tumour. Therefore, six patients (15%) achieved long-term remission (median 35+ months, range 28+ to 51+ months), all of whom received two courses of therapy. Complete response occurred less frequently in patients who were cisplatin-refractory, and did not

Table 20. Selected clinical trials of high-dose chemotherapy plus ABMT in patients with germ cell tumours.

Drugs (mg/m2)	Patients(n)	Complete response	Survival	Toxic death	Reference
Carboplatin (900–2000) Etoposide (1200) Ifosfamide * 10 g/m²	40	12 (30%)	2-year disease-free survival 15%	7 (18%)	Broun et al. 1992
Carboplatin (1500) Etoposide (1200)	40	9 (23%)	1-year disease-free survival (13%)	3 (13%)	Nichols et al. 1992
Carboplatin + Etoposide	88	22 (25%)	10 durable complete responses(11%)	14 (16%)	Motzer et al. 1992
Carboplatin + Etoposide + Ifosfamide (or Eyclophosphamide)	149	50 (34%)	33 durable complete responses(22%)	11 (7%)	
Cisplatin (200) Etoposide (1750) Cyclophos pharmide. (6400)	44 **	24 (54%)	2-year disease-free survival 60%	4 (9%)	Baume et al. 1990

* 3 patients received ifosfamide.
** 16 patients treated in first complete response or partial response with poor risk features.

105–112 Testicular cancer. 42-year-old man with recurrent embryonal cell carcinoma treated with high-dose carboplatin (1500 mg/m²) and etoposide (1200 mg/m²) plus ABMT × 2.

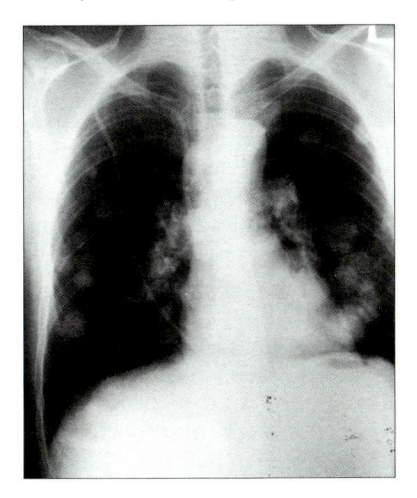

105 Pre-ABMT Chest X-ray. Chest X-ray demonstrates multiple large bilateral metastases and bilateral hilar adenopathy.

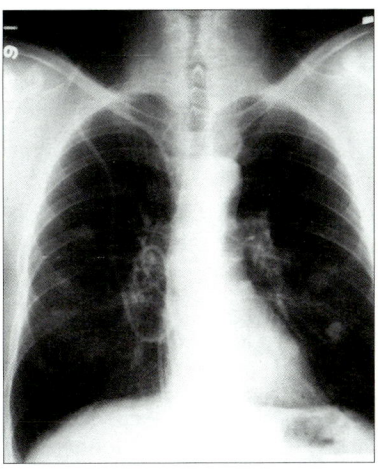

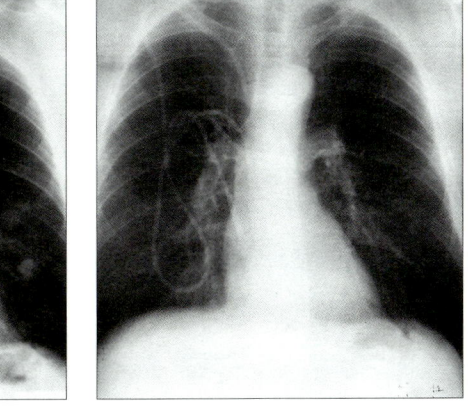

106, 107 Gradual resolution of metastatic disease. The α-fetoprotein was elevated prior to the 1st ABMT, but decreased to within normal limits. Two year's after the procedure an isolated pelvic metastasis was resected. The patient is alive and disease-free 43 months post treatment.

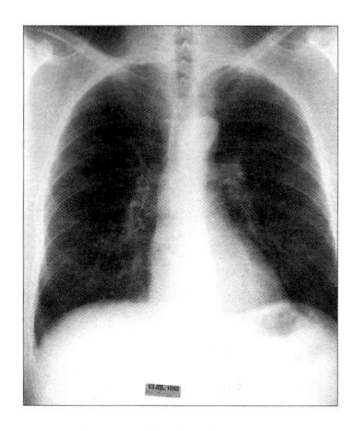

108 Post-ABMT X-ray: complete resolution of all metastatic disease 6 months post-ABMT. The lung nodules regressed gradually during this time.

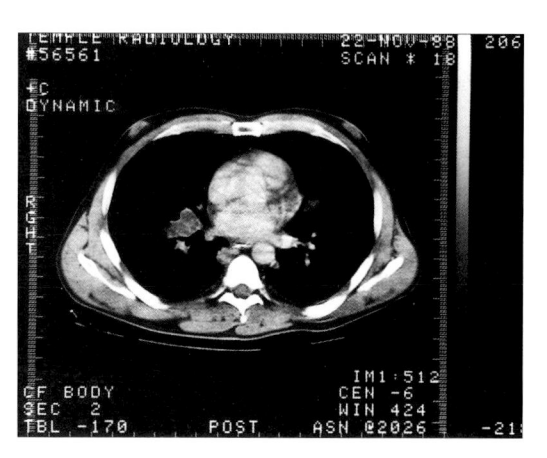

109 Pre-ABMT chest CT. Axial CT scan through the lower hilar region demonstrates right hilar adenopathy and scattered bilateral metastatic lesions.

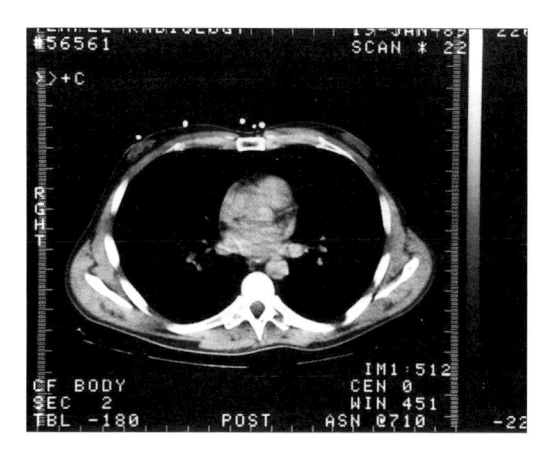

110 Post-ABMT chest CT. The hilar adenopathy is nearly completely resolved. Reduction in size and number of bilateral metastatic lesions.

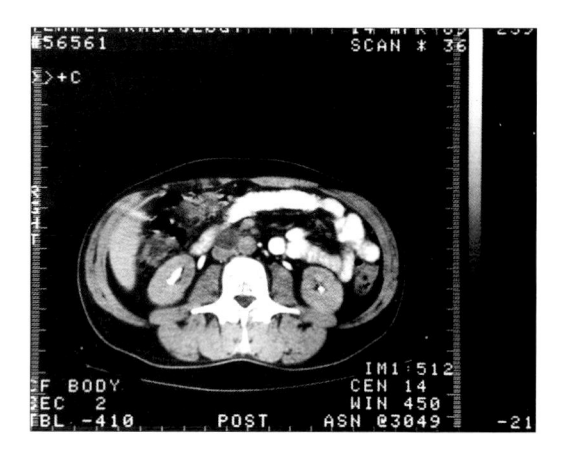

111 Pre-ABMT abdominal/pelvic CT. Axial CT section at the level of the lower pole of the kidneys demonstrates a 2.4 × 2 cm adenopathy in the aorto-caval region.

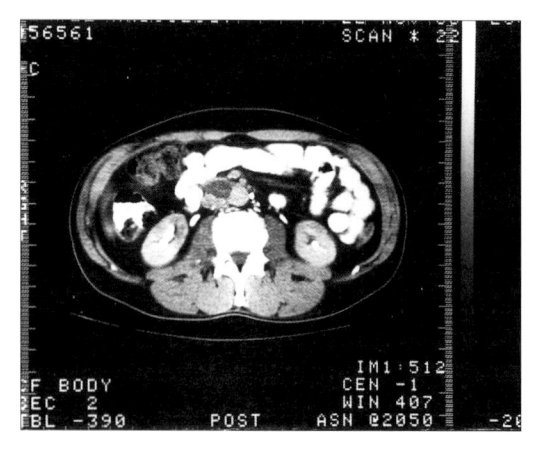

112 Post-AMBT abdominal/pelvic CT. Follow-up demonstrates no change in size of above lesion.

occur in any of the eight patients with primary mediastinal cell tumours. Thirteen of the 14 patients who had a partial response died of progressive disease. A similar outcome has been reported in a multicentre trial performed by the Eastern Cooperative Oncology Group (Nichols et al., 1992). Forty patients with relapsed or refractory germ cell tumours received carboplatin (1500 mg/m^2) and etoposide (1200 mg/m^2) plus ABMT; responding patients received a second treatment. There were nine complete responses (23%), with five patients (13%) remaining alive and disease-free for a median of 18+ months (range 12–21+ months). Five patients (13%) died due to treatment-related complications.

Solid Tumours

113–116 Testicular cancer. 45-year-old very obese man with Stage IV testicular cancer refractory to conventional salvage chemotherapy underwent a single course of high-dose etoposide 400 mg/m^2/day and carboplatin 500 mg/m^2/day given on days −7, −5 and −3 in January 1990. Currently in non-maintained progression free survival with normal markers.

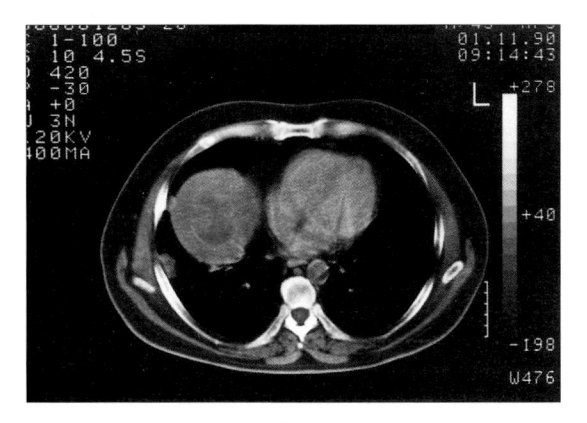

113 Pre-ABMT CT. Axial CT scan through the dome of the liver shows a 6 × 3.5 cm non-homogeneous lesion of the dome of the liver.

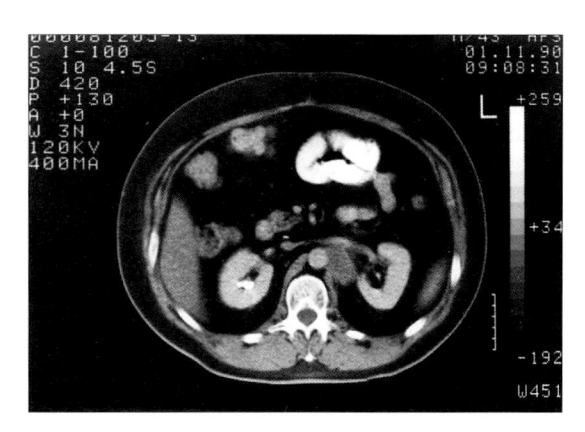

114 Pre-ABMT CT. Section at the level of the left renal vein demonstrates 2.7 × 3.4 cm left paraortic adenopathy.

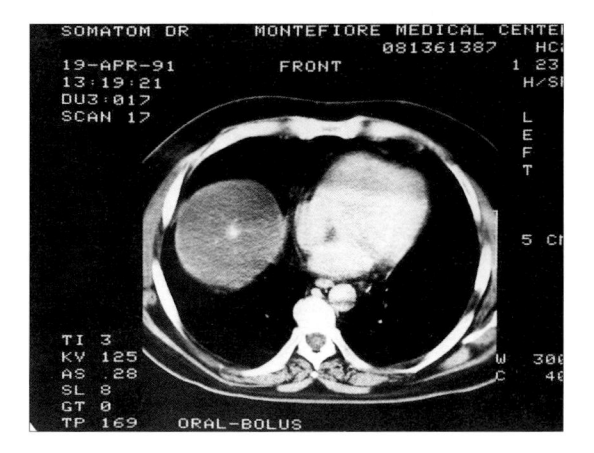

115 Post-ABMT CT. Follow-up CT of the abdomen demonstrates diffuse fatty infiltration of the liver. The metastatic lesion in the dome of the liver is seen as a 1.5 × 1 cm focus of increased density.

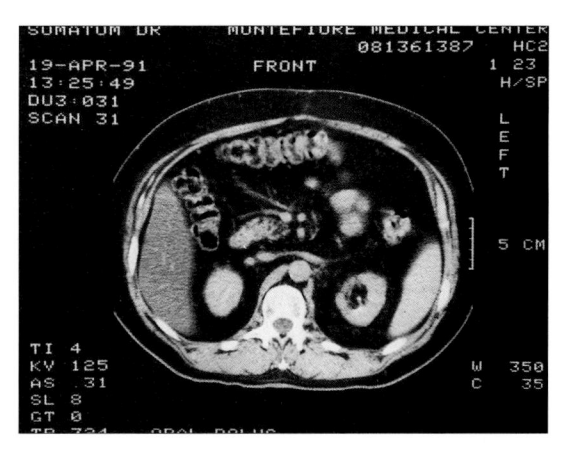

116 Post-ABMT CT. Near complete resolution of para-aortic adenopathy.

Clinical trials which have included a combination of carboplatin (or cisplatin), etoposide plus an oxazaphosphorine have yielded improved results (Motzer and Bosl, 1992). Of 149 patients treated with the aforementioned combination, CR occurred in 50 patients (34%), of whom 33 patients (22%) achieved durable remissions. Treatment-related death occurred in 11 patients (7%), comparable to the experience in patients treated with carboplatin and etoposide only.

Although it is difficult to draw definitive conclusions regarding the effectiveness of HDC/AMBT relative to standard regimens in the treatment of patients with relapsed germ cell tumours, analysis of the inversion rate, or the occurrence of clinically significant remission (≥12 months) which last longer than the initial remission, may facilitate such a comparison. While standard salvage chemotherapy only rarely produces inversion in patients with relapsed or resistant disease, inversion occurred in 17.5% of patients treated with HDC/ABMT, suggesting that this approach was capable of curing a proportion of patients who were otherwise destined to die of progressive tumour (Broun *et al.*, 1992). The high mortality rate associated with treatment, as well as the inability to salvage patients with resistant disease, however, underscores the limitation of this procedure in such patients. With improved supportive care and patient selection, a more prudent approach might be to employ this procedure in patients responding to standard chemotherapy who have poor prognostic features. Employing such an approach, Baume et al. (1990) treated 44 patients with high-dose cyclophosphamide (6400 mg/m^2), cisplatin (200 mg/m^2) and etoposide (1750 mg/m^2), of whom 26 were treated in first complete or partial response and had poor prognostic features; the two-year disease-free survival for this group was 60%. Based on this preliminary data, randomized trials comparing standard chemotherapy with HDC/ABMT in patients with poor prognosis germ cell tumors are now ongoing.

Melanoma

Advanced melanoma is a relatively chemotherapy-resistant disease, though a few agents such as dacarbazine, cisplatin, carmustine and procarbazine produce an objective response in approximately 10% of patients. Dose escalation of alkylating agents plus ABMT has led to higher response rates than that achieved with conventional chemotherapy (**Table 21**). High objective response rates have been reported with high-dose melphalan (60%), carmustine (38%) and thiotepa (41%). CR occurred in approximately 10%, the median response duration was approximately six months, and approximately 10% of patients remained progression-free for more than one year. Response was less likely to occur in patients previously treated with chemotherapy.

High-dose combination chemotherapy regimens have also been studied in advanced melanoma. Objective response occurred in 60% of patients treated with dacarbazine plus melphalan (Thatcher et al., 1989) and in 58% of patients treated with cisplatin, carmustine, cyclophosphamide and melphalan (Shea et al., 1989). In the former study,

Table 21. Selected clinical trials of high-dose chemotherapy plus ABMT in advanced melanoma.

Drugs (mg/m^2)	Patients (n)	Complete response	Partial response	Response duration (months)	Toxic death	Reference
Single agents						
Melphalan (140)	20	2 (10%)	10 (50%)	5 (4–11)	3 (15%)	Lazarus et al. 1985
Carmustine (1200)	29	4 (14%)	7 (24%)	6 (1.5–29+)	20% *	Philips et al. 1983
Thiotepa (180–1575)	71	4 (6%)	25 (35%)	3 (1–31+) 10% disease-free survival > 1 year	15 (21%)	Wolff et al. 1989
Combination						
Cyclophosphamide (1500–7500) Cisplatin (75–180) Carmustine (150–750) + Melphalan	19	1 (5%)	10 (53%)	5 (1–23)	0	Shea et al. 1988
Dacarbazine (2500–10 500) Melphalan (30–130)	27	5 (19%)	11 (41%)	Median survival 6 months	4 (15%)	Thatcher et al. 1989
Cisplatin (200) Carmustine 1050	11	2 (18%)	1 (9%)	CR 2, 19+ PR 8+	1 (9%)	Ciobanu 1988

* 20% of 139 patients with various tumour types died due to treatment-related complications in this Phase I and II study.

Solid Tumours

117–119 Melanoma. 35-year-old male with widespread metastatic melanoma, rapidly progressing after interleukin-2/LAK immunotherapy, treated in March 1987 with BCNU (300 mg/m^2/day) on days −6, −5 and −4 and cisplatin (40 mg/m^2/day) on days −7 to −3. Remained in complete remission for four months until his death in July 1987 from pneumococcal pneumonia. No melanoma at autopsy.

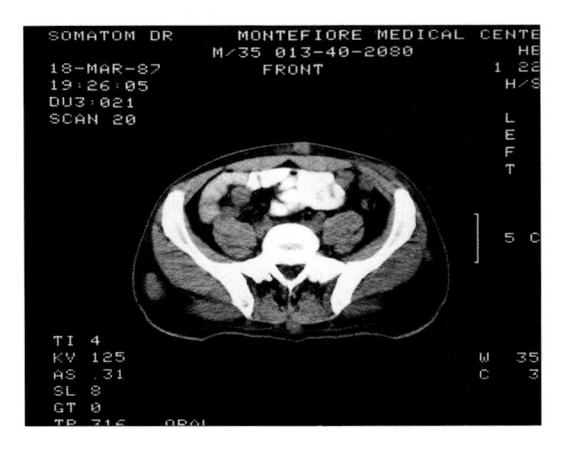

117 Pre-ABMT abdominal/pelvic CT. Axial CT section through mid pelvis demonstrates multiple subcutaneous tissue nodules.

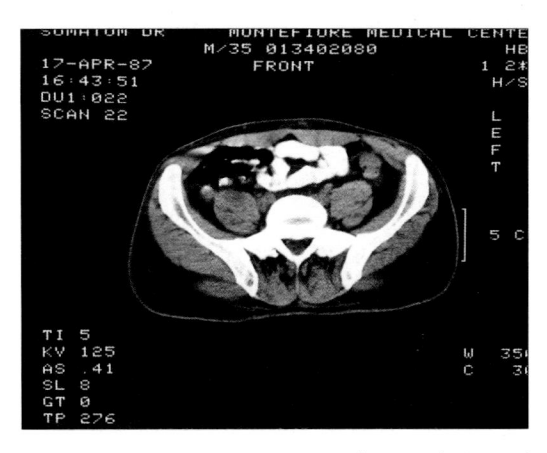

118 Post-ABMT CT 1. Near complete resolutions of all previously visualized nodules. Minimal thickening of the left anterior lateral abdominal wall remains.

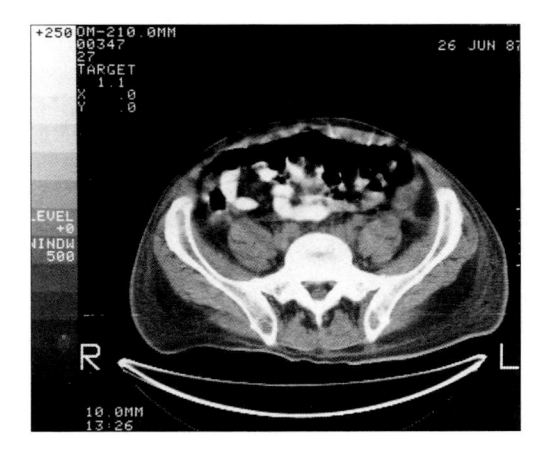

119 Post-ABMT CT 2. Complete resolution of all subcutaneous nodules.

response occurred with equal frequency in patients with or without prior therapy, and in patients with or without visceral organ involvement.

Information regarding patients who fail biological therapy is limited. Eleven patients who failed treatment with high-dose interleukin-2 administered either alone or in combination with lymphokine-activated killer cells received high-dose cisplatin and carmustine plus ABMT (Ciobanu et al., 1988). Two patients had a CR which persisted for 3 and 19+ months, while one patient had a PR which persisted for 8 months. Sites of response included the liver, skin and lymph nodes.

Therefore, HDC/ABMT appears capable of producing tumour regression in a substantial proportion of patients with advanced melanoma, a disease characterized by a low response rate to standard chemotherapy. A minority of patients experience disease control exceeding one year, which may reflect selection bias rather than the effect of treatment. The experience with HDC/ABMT in patients with advanced melanoma illustrates that, while the procedure may frequently produce objective response in patients with drug-resistant tumours, the remissions are usually partial in nature and of brief duration.

Bone Marrow Transplantation

120–124 Melanoma. 47-year-old male with metastatic melanoma. Treated with BCNU and cisplatin (same regimen as above). Entered a good partial remission of six months duration.

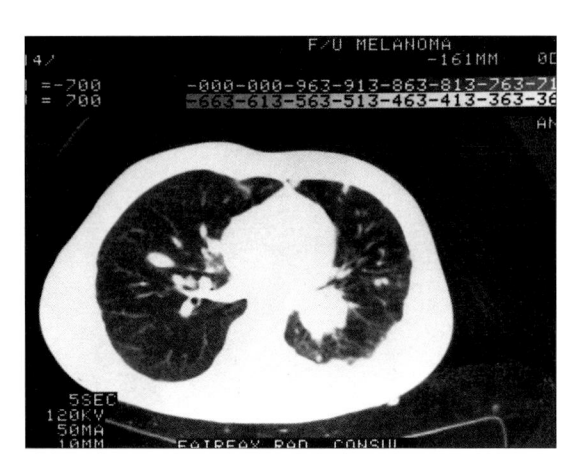

120 Pre-ABMT chest CT. Chest CT through inferior hilum shows a 5 × 6 cm infrahilar mass and a few small scattered nodules in the left lung and the right middle area. There is evidence of left pleural disease.

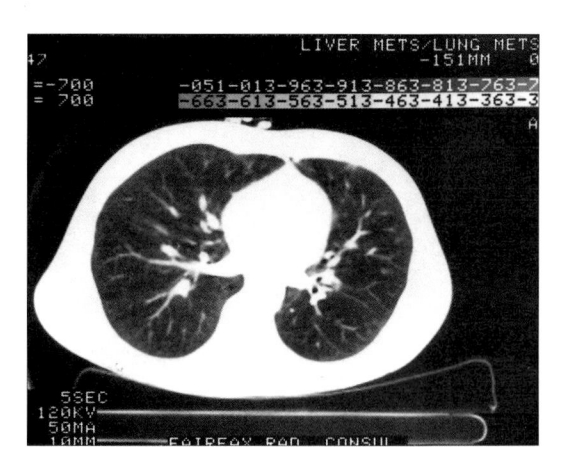

121 Post-ABMT chest CT. Chest CT shows complete resolution of the left infrahilar mass, of the left lung nodules and left pleural disease. The right middle lobe nodule has decreased in size.

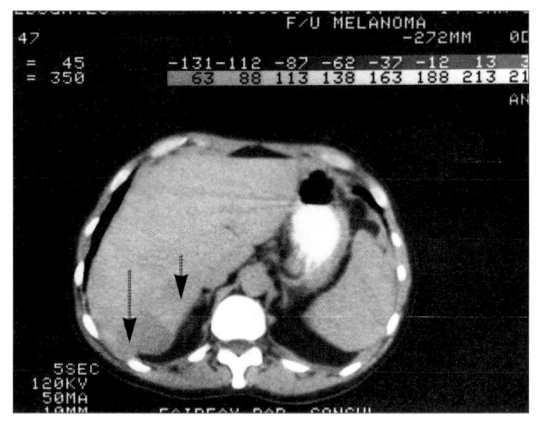

122 Pre-ABMT. Axial sections via a contrast enhanced CT scan through the liver demonstrate at 6 × 4.5 cm low-density mass in the posterior segment of the right hepatic lobe (long arrow). A second small lesion is present anterior to the large one (short arrow).

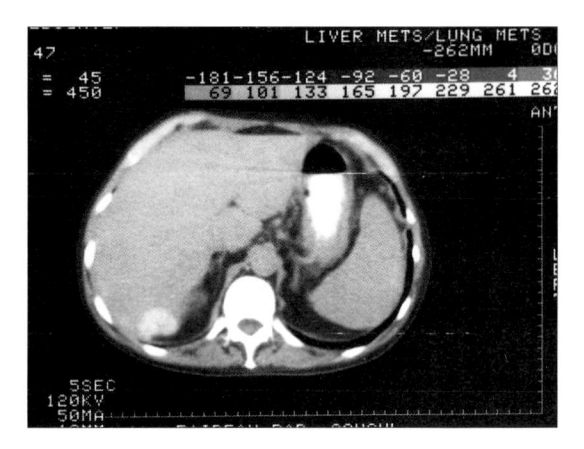

123 Post-ABMT 1. The lesion has decreased in size to 3.5 × 2 cm and become calcified. The smaller lesion is no longer visible.

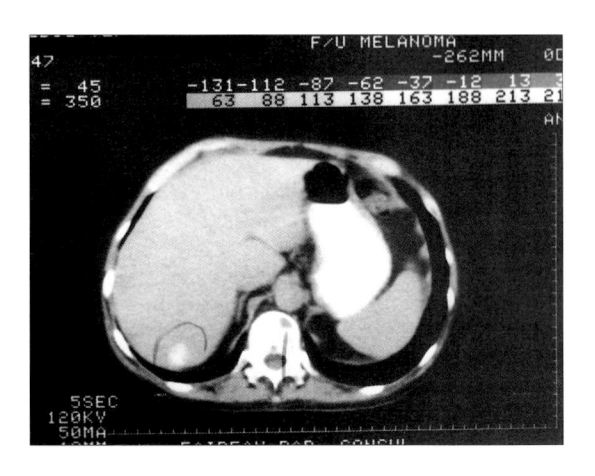

124 Post-ABMT 2. Further decrease in the size of the lesion.

Brain tumours

Administration of carmustine to patients with Grade III or IV astrocytoma after surgical resection and postoperative radiation therapy improves survival compared with patients receiving surgery and radiation therapy alone; however, median survival is only 12 months, only 20% survive 2 years, and few survive longer than 3 years (Black, 1991).

Intensification of carmustine with ABMT has been investigated in a number of trials (**Table 22**). Thirty-six patients with Grade III or IV astrocytoma received high-dose carmustine (1050 mg/m^2) plus ABMT followed by whole-brain irradiation (60 Gy) after surgical resection, 27 of whom had progressive disease after prior therapy, and nine of whom were treated after primary surgery (Philips et al., 1986). Twelve patients (44%) in the progressive disease group responded. Two patients in the progressive disease group and three patients in the adjuvant group have had prolonged progression-free survival (median 60 months, range 27–84 months), an unusual occurrence in such patients. Two of the long-term survivors developed dementia. Likewise, in another trial involving 25 patients with Grade III or IV astrocytoma treated with high dose carmustine (1050 mg/m^2) plus whole-brain radiation therapy (60 Gy) after primary surgery, the projected median survival was 26 months, significantly better than the median survival for a historical control group (Johnson 1989). Four patients (16%) died due to treatment-related complications. In the largest trial involving HDC/ABMT in patients with malignant gliomas, 89 patients with no prior therapy and nine patients who had relapsed after prior therapy received high-dose carmustine (800 mg/m^2) plus ABMT as an out-patient, followed by whole-brain irradiation (24 Gy) and a boost to the tumour bed (21 Gy) (Biron, 1991). Twenty patients had Grade III astrocytoma, 75 had Grade IV astrocytoma, and three were of uncertain histological type. Response data were not provided due to inherent difficulty in assessing tumour response in patients with cerebral tumors. Median survival was 13 months for patients with Grade III tumours and 11 months for Grade IV tumours. Features associated with improved outcome included young age (<50 years) and good performance status (0, 1 or 2). Treatment-related death occurred in 7%.

Table 22. Selected clinical trials of high-dose chemotherapy plus ABMT in patients with malignant astrocytoma.

Drugs (mg/m^2) and radiation dose	Patients (n)*	Age	Median survival and comments	Toxic death	Reference
Carmustine (1050–1350)	36 (27)	37	All patients 4 months Adjuvant, 16 months	6 (17%)	Philips et al. 1986
Carmustine (1050), 60 Gy	25 (0)	46	All patients 26 months. Survival significantly longer than in matched historical control group	4 (16%)	Johnson et al. 1987
Carmustine (800), 45 Gy	89 (9)	48	Grade III, 11 months. Grade IV, 13 months. Patients with good PR (0, 1, 2) had median survival of 17 months and 21% 3 year progression-free survival	7 (7%)	Biron 1991
Thiotepa (750–900), 60 Gy	21	–	6 patients had non-maintained complete responses	–	Ahmed et al. 1992
Thiotepa (900) Etoposide (1500) Carmustine (1500) (or carboplatin, 1500)	61	55 (n <21)	6 patients had complete responses. Most had failed prior therapy	13 (21%)	Finlay et al. 1991

* Patients treated in adjuvant setting after initial surgery.

125–131 Glioma. 19-year-old male with recurrent malignant astrocytoma who presented in March 1989 with grand mal seizures. Treated with BCNU (300 mg/m^2/day) days –6, –5, –4 cisplatin (40 mg/m^2/day on days –7 to –3 and thiotepa (250 mg/m^2/day) on day –5. Currently without evidence of disease. (Pathologically proven CR.) Sixty months after surgery, high-dose BCNU and cisplatin plus ABMT.

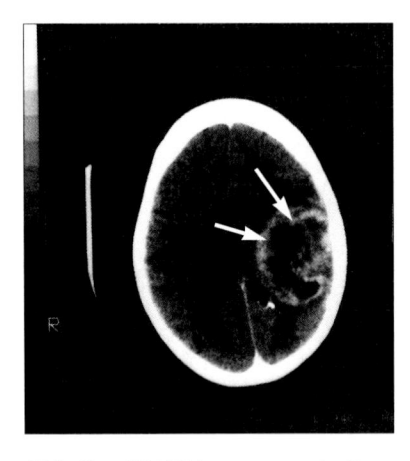

125 Pre-ABMT (pre-surgery). Contrast-enhanced CAT scan shows a large enhancing left parieto-occipital mass with oedema (arrows).

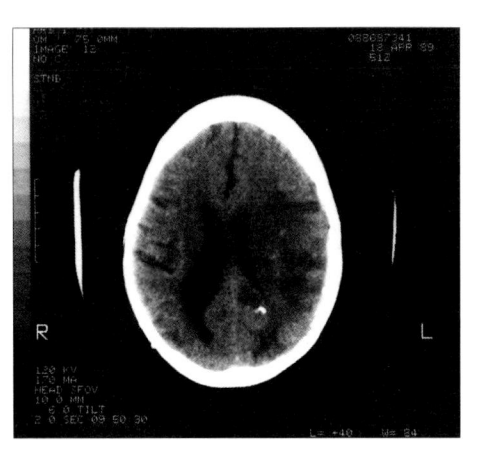

126 Pre-ABMT/post-surgery. Non-contrast scan before chemotherapy reveals partial resolution of mass following debulking. A densely calcified area is seen.

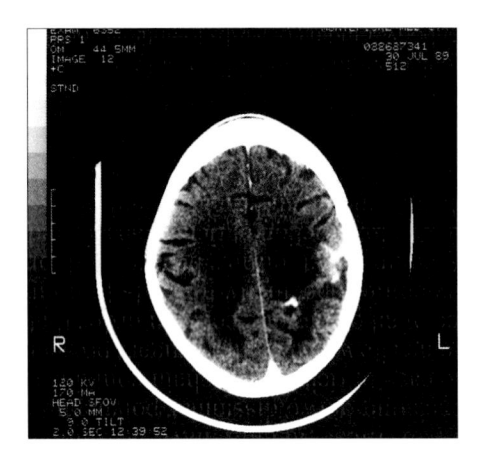

127 Three months after ABMT the area of enhancement was smaller. Ventriculoperitoneal shunting was done because of a trapped expanding lateral ventricle.

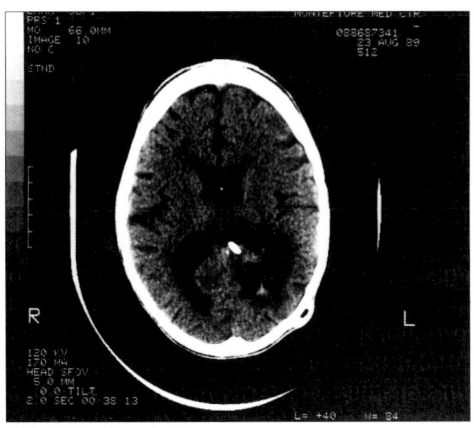

128 Four months after ABMT the ventricles were returning to normal. A shunt tube is seen in place within the lateral ventricle.

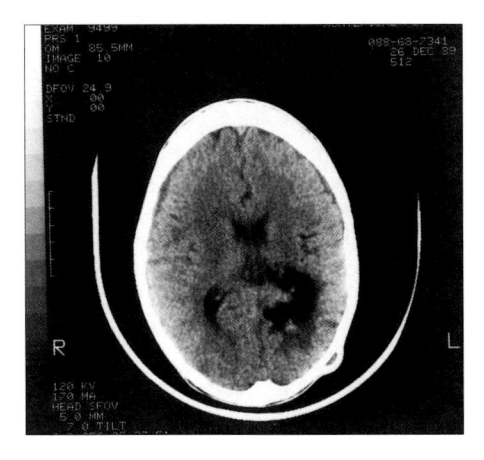

Solid Tumours

129 Eight months later the scan shows that the left ventricle has returned to normal. The left atrium is porencephalic. A small asymptomatic right frontoparietal chronic subdural is present.

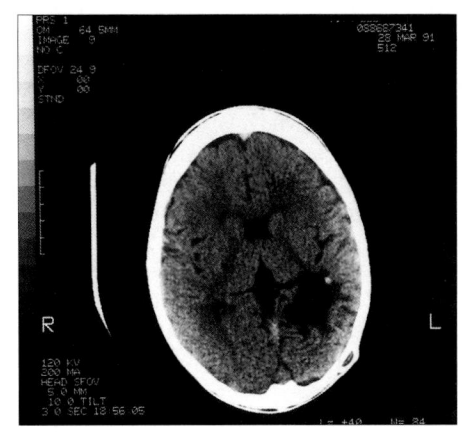

130 Twenty months later the scan is unchanged from that carried out at eight months.

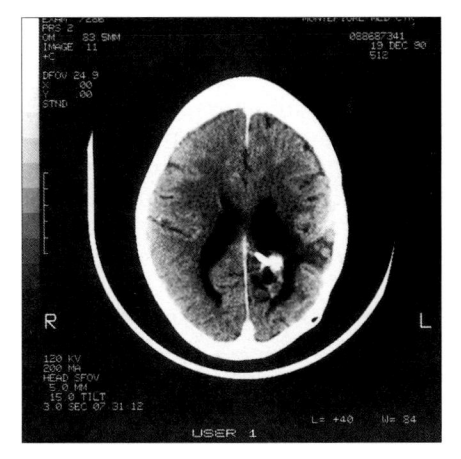

131 Two years post surgery and ABMT the scan shows unchanged ventricular size. A new small dense area along the lateral wall of the left atrium was proven on biopsy to be haemorrhage. No evidence of tumour was seen. One year later a scan with and without contrast was unchanged and the patient has now remained disease-free for five years.

Limited studies have been performed employing agents other than carmustine. Twenty-one patients with previously untreated Grade III or IV astrocytoma which was unresectable, > 5 cm in diameter and/or involving both cerebral hemispheres received thiotepa (750–900 mg/m^2) plus ABMT followed by whole brain radiation therapy (60 Gy) 2–4 weeks after bone marrow re-infusion. Six patients had non-maintained CRs, but further study will be required in order to establish the durability of the responses. In another study, 61 patients received one of three preparative regimens which included: (1) thiotepa (900 mg/m^2) and etoposide (1500 mg/m^2) (n = 33), (2) thiotepa, etoposide plus carmustine (600 mg/m^2) (n = 20), or (3) thiotepa, etoposide, plus carboplatin (1500 mg/m^2) (n = 8) (Finlay *et al.*, 1991). All but five patients were less than 21 years of age, and the majority had progressed after prior therapy. Thirteen patients (21%) died due to treatment-related complications. Six patients (10%) had a CR as evidenced by magnetic resonance imaging of the brain.

In summary, HDC/ABMT combined with whole-brain irradiation appears to be capable of producing sustained progression-free survival in patients with malignant gliomas and other cerebral tumours which have progressed after primary therapy—an unusual occurrence in such patients. Preliminary studies also suggest that this approach is feasible for some patients as primary therapy, particularly patients less than 50 years who have a good performance status. Prospective, randomized trials will be required, however, in order to determine whether this approach can improve the survival for patients with malignant glioma, and in order to determine the long-term effects of this treatment approach on neurological function.

Solid tumours of childhood

The most common solid tumours of childhood in order of decreasing frequency include brain and nervous system tumours, neuroblastoma, Wilms' tumour, rhabdomyosarcoma, retinoblastoma, osteosarcoma and Ewing's sarcoma (Crist and Kun, 1991). Most of the literature regarding HDC/ABMT has focused on the treatment of central nervous system tumours, which have been discussed previously, and neuroblastoma. Only occasional cases of other childhood solid tumours treated with HDC/ABMT have been reported in Phase I trials, limiting any conclusions which can be drawn regarding its efficacy in those settings.

Despite advances in the treatment of neuroblastoma which have led to a doubling of the cure rate, over 80% of children greater than one year of age die due to progressive disease. Most clinical trials, therefore, have focused on this poor prognosis group (**Table 23**). Thirty-three children older than one year of age responding to standard induction chemotherapy received high-dose carmustine, teniposide and melphalan plus autologous marrow purged *in vitro* with Asta-Z7557, a cyclophosphamide derivative (Hartmann *et al.*, 1987). Sixteen patients were alive and progression-free with a median follow-up of 28 months (range 8–50 months). Likewise, 56 children more than one year of age received intensive induction chemotherapy followed by treatment in the 37 responding patients with high-dose melphalan, vincristine and total body irradiation plus re-infusion of autologous bone marrow purged using an immunomagnetic procedure in the majority of cases (Philip *et al.*, 1987). The progression-free survival was 44% at 32 months for the 14 children treated in CR or very good partial remission, but only 13% at 32 months for 23 children treated in partial remission. The overall survival for all 56 patients treated was 39%, compared with 12% for a historical control group. Finally, in another trial, 81 children received high-dose melphalan plus total body irradiation and infusion of allogeneic (n = 7) or autologous (n = 54) bone marrow purged immunomagnetically after achieving a first (n = 54) or second (n = 27) complete or partial remission (Graham Pole *et al.*, 1991). The two year actuarial event-free survival for patients in first CR, first PR, second CR, and second PR were 32, 43, 23, and 5%, respectively. The toxic death rate associated with each of the aforementioned trials were 12, 19, and 12%, respectively.

Therefore, while these studies suggest that high-dose chemotherapy or radiotherapy plus ABMT may produce sustained disease control in select children with poor-prognosis neuroblastoma, further follow-up will be required in order to

Table 23. Selected clinical trials of high-dose chemotherpay and/or radiation therapy in children with neuroblastoma.

Treatment (mg/m²)	Patients (n) *	Results **	Reference
Teniposide (1000) Carmustine (300) Melphalan (180) Purging agent: Asta-Z	62/33	16 patients. alive and in CR at median follow-up of 28 months. (range 8–50 months)	Hartmann *et al.* 1987
Melphalan (180) Vincristine (2.0) TBI (12 Gy) Purging agent: immunomagnetic procedure	56/35	Progression-free survival at 24 months. 39% for study group compared with 12% for historical control group (P < 0.005)	Philip *et al.* 1987
Melphalan (180) TBI (9 or 12 Gy) Purging agent: immunomagnetic procedure	81	23 children continue in CR with a minimum follow-up of 32 months. The two-year actuarial event-free survival for patients. transplanted in first CR, first PR, second CR and second PR were 32%, 43%, 33% and 5%	Graham Pole *et al.* 1991

* Number of children enrolled in trial/number who responded to therapy and received HDC / BMT.
** CR = Complete remission; PR = partial remission.

determine whether relapse is being prevented rather than delayed. The demonstration of improved disease-free survival and survival for children who received high-dose melphalan plus ABMT as consolidation in a randomized trial, however, provides support for continued research in this area (Pinkerton, 1991). The high propensity to relapse may be attributable not only to drug resistance, but perhaps also to occult tumour contamination of the bone marrow and even the blood in such patients, prompting the investigation of novel purging techniques (Moss and Sanders, 1990).

Conclusions

After nearly one decade of clinical investigation examining the feasibility of HDC/ABMT for patients with solid tumours, this treatment modality as yet has no proven therapeutic role in such patients. However, prospective, randomized clinical trials are now in progress comparing standard chemotherapy with HDC/ABMT in specific diseases, such as high-risk operable and advanced breast cancer, high-risk germ cell tumours and neuroblastoma. Furthermore, a substantial amount has been learned about which patients are unlikely to benefit from this approach. Selection of patients with good performance status, minimal tumour burden, and chemotherapy-responsive relapses or poor-prognosis primary responses have resulted in substantially less treatment-related mortality and improved therapeutic outcome. Additional investigation is required in order to further reduce treatment-related morbidity and improve the antineoplastic activity of the treatment regimens. Substantial gains for the former have been accomplished with the development of novel multilineage haematopoietic growth factors, improved methods for stem cell collection and expansion, and investigation of agents which may reduce non-haematopoietic toxicity. For the latter, however, it has become apparent that drug intensification alone may not be sufficient to overcome drug resistance, prompting continued investigation of new drugs and the study of mechanisms whereby drug resistance can be circumvented.

References

Ahmed T, Cook P, Helson L et al. High-dose thiotepa with autologous bone marrow transplant in patients with astrocytoma Grade III–IV. *Eighth Mediterranean Congress of Chemotherapy, Athens, Greece, May 24–29 1992*.

Antman K. The current status of dose intensive therapy with autologous stem cell support in breast cancer. *Ninth Annual Symposium in Autologous Bone Marrow Transplantation, New York, N Y, March 1991*.

Antman K, Ayash L, Elias A et al. A Phase II study of high-dose cyclophosphamide, thiotepa, and carboplatin with autologous marrow support in women with measurable advanced breast cancer responding to standard-dose chemotherapy. *J Clin Oncol* 1992; **10**: 102–110.

Baume D, Pico JL, Droz JP et al. Value of high-dose chemotherapy followed by bone marrow autograft in non-seminomatous germinal tumor with poor prognosis. Results of the combination of cisplatinum, etoposide and cyclophosphamide. *Bull Cancer* 1990; **77**: 169–180.

Biron P, Vial C, Chauvin F et al. Strategy including surgery, high dose BCNU followed by ABMT and radiotherapy in supratentorial high grade astrocytomas: a report of 98 patients. *Autologous Bone Marrow Transplantation. Proceedings of the Fifth International Conference, 1991*, pp. 637–646.

Bensinger WI, Buckner CD, Clift RA et al. Phase I study of busulfan and cyclophosphamide for allogeneic transplantation for patients with multiple myeloma. *J Clin Oncol* 1992; **10**: 1492–1497.

Berman E, Little C, Gee T et al. Reasons that patients with acute myelogenous leukemia do not undergo allogeneic bone marrow transplantation. *New Engl J Med* 1992; **326**: 156–160.

Bianco JA, Appelbaum FR, Nemunaitis J et al. Phase I–II trial of pentoxifylline for the prevention of transplant-related toxicities following bone marrow transplantation. *Blood* 1991; **78**: 1205–1211.

Black PM. Brain tumours I and II. *N Engl J Med* 1991; **324**: 1471–1476 and 1555–1564.

Bodey GP, Buckley M, Sathe YS, Freireich EJ. Quantitative relationships between circulating leukocytes and infection in patients with acute leukemia. *Ann Intern Med* 1966; **64**: 328–340.

Broun ER, Nichols CR, Kneebone P et al. Long-term outcome of patients with relapsed and refractory germ cell tumors treated with high-dose chemotherapy and autologous bone marrow rescue. *Ann Intern Med* 1992; **117**: 124–128.

Budman DR, Wood W, Henderson IC *et al*. Initial findings of CALGB8541: a dose and dose intensity trial of cyclophosphamide, doxorubicin, and 5-fluorouracil as adjuvant treatment of Stage II, node + female breast cancer. *Proc Am Soc Clin Oncol* 1992; **11**: 51 (Abstract 29).

Chapra R, Goldstone AH, Pearc R *et al*. Autologous versus allogeneic bone marrow transplantation for non-Hodgkin's lymphoma: a case-controlled analysis of the European Bone Marrow Transplant group registry data. *J Clin Oncol* 1992; **10**: 1690–1695.

Cheson BD, Lacerna L, Leyland-Jones B *et al*. Autologous bone marrow transplantation. Current status and future directions. *Ann Intern Med* 1989; **110**: 51–65.

Ciobanu N, Runowicz C, Gucalp R *et al*. Reversible central nervous system toxicity associated with high-dose chlorambucil in autologous bone marrow transplantation for ovarian carcinoma. *Cancer Treat Rep* 1987; **71**: 1324–1325.

Ciobanu N, Dutcher J, Gucalp, R *et al*. High dose chemotherapy with autologous bone marrow transplantation (ABMT) for malignant melanoma after failure of interleukin-2 (IL2) and lymphokine activated killer (LAK) cells. *Proc Am Soc Clin Oncol* 1988; **8**: 281 (#1096).

Crist WM, Kun LE. Common solid tumors of childhood. *New Engl J Med* 1991; **324**: 461–471.

Dauplat J, Legros, M, Condat P *et al*. High-dose melphalan and autologous bone marrow support for treatment of ovarian carcinoma with positive second look operation. *Gynecol Oncol* 1989; **34**: 294–298.

Dufour P, Bergerat JP, Liu KL *et al*. High dose melphalan and ABMT with or without abdominal radiotherapy as consolidation treatment for ovarian carcinoma in complete remission or with microscopic residual disease. *Eur J Gynecol Oncol* 1991; **12**: 457–461.

Eddy DM. High-dose chemotherapy with autologous bone marrow transplantation for the treatment of metastatic breast cancer. *J Clin Oncol* 1992; **10**: 657–670.

Eder JP, Elias A, Shea TC *et al*. A Phase I–II study of cyclophosphamide, thiotepa, and carboplatin with autologous bone marrow transplantation in solid tumor patients. *J Clin Oncol* 1990; **8**: 1239–1245.

Elias AD, Eder JP, Shea T *et al*. High-dose ifosfamide with mesna uroprotection: a Phase I study. *J Clin Oncol* 1990; **8**: 170–178.

Finlay J, Packer R, Nachman J *et al*. High-dose chemotherapy with bone marrow rescue in children and young adults with recurrent high-grade brain tumors. *Autologous Bone Marrow Transplantation. Proceedings of the Fifth International Conference*, 1991, pp. 599–605.

Frei E, Antman K, Teicher B *et al*. Bone marrow autotransplantation. *J Clin Oncol* 1989; **7**: 515–526.

Graham Pole J, Casper J, Elfenbein G *et al*. High-dose chemotherapy supported by marrow infusion for advanced neuroblastoma: a Pediatric Oncology Group study. *J Clin Oncol* 1991; **9**: 152–158.

Groopman JE, Molina J, Scadden DT. Hematopoietic growth factors: biology and clinical applications. *N Engl J Med* 1989; **321**: 1449–1457.

Hartmann O, Benhamou E, Beaujean F *et al*. Repeated high-dose chemotherapy followed by purged autologous bone marrow transplantation as consolidation therapy in metastatic neuroblastoma. *J Clin Oncol* 1987; **5**: 1205–1211.

Herzig R, Fay J, Herzig G *et al*. Phase I–II studies with high dose thiotepa and autologous marrow transplantation in patients with refractory malignancies. *Proc Am Soc Clin Oncol* 1988; **7**: 74 (Abstract 285).

Hillner BE, Smith TJ, Desch CE. Efficacy and cost-effectiveness of autologous bone marrow transplantation in metastatic breast cancer. Estimates using decision analysis while awaiting clinical trial results. *J Am Med Assoc* 1992; **267**: 2055–2061.

Hortobagyi GN, Buzdar AU, Bodey GP *et al*. High-dose induction chemotherapy of metastatic breast cancer in protected environment: a prospective randomized study. *J Clin Oncol* 1987; **5**: 178–184.

Hoskins PJ, O'Reilly SE, Swenerton KD *et al*. Ten-year outcome of patients with advanced epithelial ovarian carcinoma treated with cisplatin-based multimodality therapy. *J Clin Oncol* 1992; **10**: 1561–1568.

Hryniuk W, Bush H. The importance of dose intensity in chemotherapy of metastatic breast cancer. *J Clin Oncol* 1984; **2**: 1281–1288.

Huan SD, Hester J, Spitzer G *et al*. Influence of mobilized peripheral blood cells on the hematopoietic recovery by autologous marrow and recombinant human granulocyte–macrophage colony-stimulating factor after high-dose cyclophosphamide, etoposide, and cisplatin. *Blood* 1992; **79**: 3388–3393.

Johnson DB, Thompson JM, Corwin JA *et al*. Prolongation of survival for high-grade malignant gliomas with adjuvant high-dose BCNU and autologous bone marrow transplantation. *J Clin Oncol* 1987; **5**: 783–789.

Lazarus H, Herzig, R, Wolff S *et al*. Treatment of metastatic melanoma with intensive melphalan and autologous bone marrow transplantation. *Cancer Treat Rep* 1985; **69**: 473–477.

Lazarus HM, Crilley P, Ciobanu N *et al*. High-dose carmustine, etoposide, and cisplatin and autologous bone marrow transplantation for relapsed and refractory lymphoma. *J Clin Oncol* 1992; **10**: 1682–1689.

Levin L, Hryniuk WM. Dose intensity analysis of chemotherapy regimens in ovarian carcinoma. *J Clin Oncol* 1987; **5**: 756–767.

Lotz JP, Machover D, Malassagne B *et al*. Phase I–II study of two consecutive courses of high dose epipodophyllotoxin, ifosfamide, and carboplatin with autologous bone marrow transplantation for treatment of adult patients with solid tumors. *J Clin Oncol* 1991; **9**: 1860–1870.

McKenzie RS, Alberts DS, Bishop MR *et al*. Phase I trial of high-dose cyclophosphamide, mitoxantrone, and carboplatin with autologous bone marrow transplantation in female malignancies: pharmacologic levels of mitoxantrone and high response rate in refractory ovarian cancer. *Proc Am Soc Clin Oncol* 1991; **10**: 186. (Abstract 605).

Moss TJ, Sanders DG. Detection of neuroblastoma cells in the blood. *J Clin Oncol* 1990; **8**: 736–740.

Motzer RJ, Bosl G. High-dose chemotherapy for resistant germ cell tumors: recent advanced and future directions. *J Natl Cancer Inst* 1992; **84**: 1703–1709.

Mulder PO, Sleijfer DT, Willemse PH et al. High-dose cyclophosphamide or melphalan with escalating doses of mitoxantrone and autologous bone marrow transplantation for refractory solid tumors. *Cancer Res* 1989a; **9**: 4654–4658.

Mulder PO, Willemse PH, Aalders JG et al. High-dose chemotherapy with autologous bone marrow transplantation in patients with refractory ovarian cancer. *Eur J Cancer Clin Oncol* 1989b; **25**: 645–649.

Naparstek E, Hardan Y, Ben-Shahar M et al. Enhanced marrow recovery by short preincubation of marrow allografts with human recombinant interleukin-3 and granulocyte–macrophage colony stimulating factor. *Blood* 1992; **80**: 1673–1678.

Nemunaitis J, Rabinowe S, Singer JW et al. Recombinant human granulocyte-macrophage colony-stimulating factor after autologous bone marrow transplantation for lymphoid cancer. *N Engl J Med* 1991; **324**: 1773–1778.

Nichols CR, Williams SD, Loehrer PJ et al. Randomized study of cisplatin dose intensity in poor-risk germ cell tumors: a Southeastern Cancer Study Group and Southwest Oncology Group protocol. *J Clin Oncol* 1991; **9**: 1163–1172.

Nichols CR, Andersen J, Lazarus HM et al. High-dose carboplatin and etoposide with autologous bone marrow transplantation in refractory germ cell cancer: an Eastern Cooperative Oncology Group protocol. *J Clin Oncol* 1992; **10**: 558–563.

Ozols R. Intraperitoneal therapy in ovarian cancer: time's up. *J Clin Oncol* 1991; **9**: 197–199.

Ozols R, Corden B, Jacob J et al. High dose cisplatin in hypertonic saline. *Ann Intern Med* 1984; **100**: 19–24.

Peters WP, Eder JP, Henner WD et al. High-dose combination alkylating agents with autologous bone marrow support: a Phase I trial. *J Clin Oncol* 1986; **4**: 646–654.

Peters WP, Ross M, Vredenburgh JJ et al. High-dose chemotherapy and autologous bone marrow support as consolidation after standard-dose adjuvant therapy for high-risk breast cancer. *J Clin Oncol* 1993; **11**: 1132–1143.

Philip T, Bernard JL, Zucker JM et al. High-dose chemoradiotherapy with bone marrow transplantation as consolidation treatment in neuroblastoma: an unselected group of Stage IV patients over 1 year of age. *J Clin Oncol* 1987; **5**: 266–271.

Philips GL, Fay JW, Herzig GP et al. Intensive 1,3-bis(2-choroethyl)-1-nitrosourea (BCNU), NSC #4366650 and cryopreserved autologous marrow transplantation for refractory cancer: a Phase I–II study. *Cancer* 1983; **52**: 1792–1802.

Philips GL, Wolff SN, Fay JW et al. Intensive l,3-bis(2-chloroethyl)-1-nitrosourea (BCNU), monotherapy and autologous marrow transplantation for malignant glioma. *J Clin Oncol* 1986; **4**: 639–645.

Pinkerton CR. ENSG1-Randomized study of high-dose melphalan in neuroblastoma. *Bone Marrow Transplant* 1991; (suppl 3) 7112–7113.

Sarna G, Champlin R, Wells J, Gale RP. Phase I study of high dose mitomycin with autologous bone marrow support. *Cancer Treat Rep* 1982; **66**: 277–282.

Schabel FM. Animal models as predictive systems. In: *Cancer Chemotherapy; Fundamental Concepts and Recent Advances*, 1975. Year Book Medical Publisher, Chicago, pp. 323–355.

Shea TC, Antman KH, Eder JP et al. Malignant melanoma treatment with high-dose combination alkylating agent chemotherapy and autologous bone marrow support. *Arch Dermatol* 1988; **124**: 878–884.

Shea TC, Flaherty M, Elias A et al. A Phase I clinical and pharmacokinetic study of carboplatin and autologous bone marrow support. *J Clin Oncol* 1989; **7**: 651–661.

Shea TC, Mason JR, Storniolo AM et al. Sequential cycles of high-dose carboplatin administered with recombinant human granulocyte macrophage colony-stimulating factor and repeated infusions of autologous peripheral-blood progenitor cells: a novel and effective method for delivering multiple courses of dose-intensive therapy. *J Clin Oncol* 1992; **10**: 464–473.

Shpall EJ, Clarke-Pearson D, Soper JT el al. High dose alkylating agent chemotherapy with autologous bone marrow support in patients with Stage III/IV epithelial ovarian cancer. *Gynecol Oncol* 1990; **38**: 386–391.

Smith I, Evans B, Harland S, Miller JL. Autologous bone marrow rescue is unnecessary after very high dose cycles. *Lancet* 1983; **1**: 76–77.

Stoter G, Sleyfer DT, ten Bokkel Huinink WW et al. High-dose versus low-dose vinblastine in cisplatin–vinblastine–bleomycin combination chemotherapy of non-seminomatous testicular cancer: a randomized study of the EORTC Genitourinary Tract Cancer Cooperative Group. *J Clin Oncol* 1986; **4**: 1199–1206.

Sullivan KM, Storb R, Shulman HM et al. Immediate and delayed neurotoxicity after mechlorethamine preparation for bone marrow transplantation. *Ann Intern Med* 1982; **97**: 182–189.

Sullivan KM, Weiden PL, Storb R et al. Influence of acute graft and chronic graft versus host disease on relapse and survival after bone marrow transplantation form HLA identical siblings as treatment of acute and chronic leukemia. *Blood* 1988; **73**: 1720–1728.

Tannock IF, Boyd NF, Deboer G et al. A randomized trial of two dose levels of cyclophosphamide, methotrexate, and fluorouracil chemotherapy for patients with metastatic breast cancer. *J Clin Oncol* 1988; **6**: 1377–1387.

Thatcher N, Lind M, Morgenstern G et al. High-dose double alkylating agent chemotherapy with DTIC, melphalan or ifosfamide and marrow rescue for metastatic malignant melanoma. *Cancer* 1989; **63**: 1296–1302.

Viens P, Maraninchi D, Legros M et al. High dose melphalan and autologous marrow rescue in advance epithelial ovarian carcinomas: a retrospective analysis of 35 patient treated in France. *Bone Marrow Transplant* 1990; **5**: 227–233.

Von Hoff DD, Clark GM, Weiss GR et al. Use of *in vitro* dose response effects to select antineoplastics for high-dose or regional administration regimens. *J Clin Oncol* 1986; **4**: 1827–1834.

Wheeler C, Antin JH, Churchill WH *et al*. Cyclophosphamide, carmustine, and etoposide with autologous bone marrow transplantation in refractory Hodgkin's disease and non-Hodgkin's lymphoma: a dose-finding study. *J Clin Oncol* 1990; **8**: 648–656.

Wiernik PH, Yeap B, Vogl SE *et al*. Hexamethylmelamine and low or moderate dose cisplatin with or without pyridoxine for treatment of advanced ovarian carcinoma: a study of the Eastern Cooperative Oncology Group. *Cancer Invest* 1992; **10**: 1–9.

Williams SF, Bitran JD, Kaminer L *et al*. A Phase I–II study of bialkylator chemotherapy, high-dose thiotepa, and cyclophosphamide with autologous bone marrow reinfusion in patients with advanced cancer. *J Clin Oncol* 1987; **5**: 260–265.

Wilson W, Jain V, Bryant G *et al*. Phase I and II study of high-dose ifosfamide, carboplatin, and etoposide with autologous bone marrow rescue in lymphomas and solid tumors. *J Clin Oncol* 1992; **10**: 1712–1722.

Wolff S, Fer M, McKay C *et al*. High-dose VP16-213 and autologous bone marrow transplantation for refractory malignancies: a Phase I study. *J Clin Oncol* 1983; **1**: 701–705.

Wolff S, Herzig RH, Fay JW *et al*. High dose thiotepa with ABMT for metastatic melanoma: results of Phase I and II studies of the North American Bone Marrow Transplant Group. *J Clin Oncol* 1989; **7**: 245–249.

III Bone Marrow Harvesting
Keith Patterson

Donor preparation

A full explanation of the procedure and its associated side effects must be given to the donor well before the intended harvest date. Particular points to mention are the requirement for general anaesthetic and post-operative blood transfusion. It should be ensured that the donor appreciates that marrow is self-renewing, unlike a kidney, for example.

Initial blood tests will normally have already been performed to establish blood group and tissue type, and to screen for hepatitis B surface antigen, antibody to hepatitis C, HIV and syphilis. Positive results of these screening tests normally bar the donor from marrow donation. Even in the case of an autograft there is a risk of hepatitis reactivation during the associated chemo/radiotherapy and a risk to operators performing the marrow harvest and processing the marrow.

Autograft candidates should undergo bone marrow examination a week or so before the main procedure to confirm cellularity, ease of aspiration and absence of malignant infiltration.

A standard adult bone marrow harvest contains a red cell concentration equivalent to whole blood. As a litre of marrow is often harvested, blood transfusion is usually required. This is most sensibly and safely provided by autologous transfusion (**132**) in the case of healthy donors or non-anaemic autograft recipients, but homologous blood may be required for patients who are anaemic after previous chemotherapy. The advantages of autologous donation include no risk of sensitization to white cell, red cell or platelet antigens. There is no risk of viral transmission, and stimulation of erythroid hyperplasia in the marrow may allow quicker haemoglobin recovery after harvest. It also provides a suitable opportunity to prepare psychologically for the forthcoming harvest. At least one unit (450 ml of blood in 63 ml of CPD-A1 anticoagulant) is collected between 1 and 4 weeks

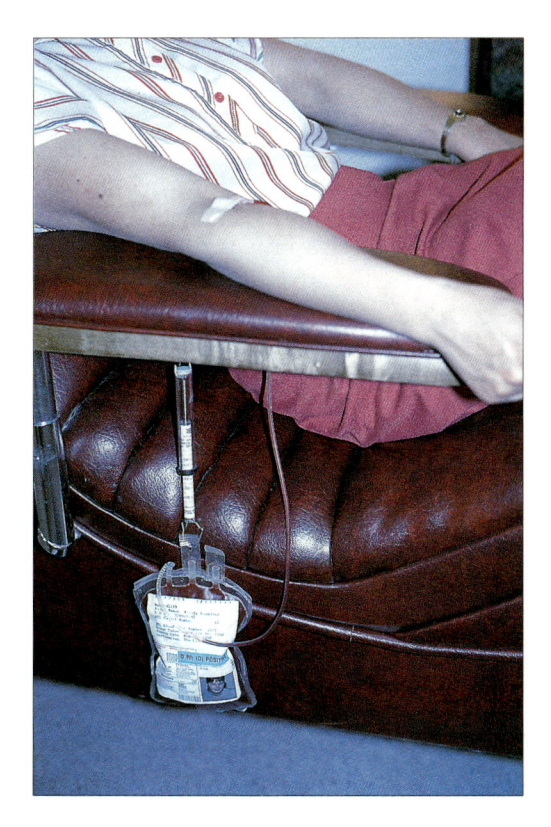

132 Autologous blood donation from bone marrow harvest donor. This is normally performed 1–4 weeks before the planned harvest.

before the harvest procedure. This has a shelf life at 4°C of 5 weeks. Iron supplements (e.g. ferrous sulphate 200 mg b.i.d.) should be administered from the time of blood donation to at least the time of harvest. Collection of blood too close to the harvest date does not allow sufficient time for the haemoglobin to be made up. Stringent safety requirements for autologous blood donation should be observed, particularly as regards identification of the donor unit and check cross-match before transfusion. Such autologous units may be identified by a Polaroid passport-type photograph of the donor, and by having donors sign their autologous blood unit when it is taken, so that they can check their signature prior to return of the unit. The British Society of Haematology has published guidelines for autologous transfusion (1988).

Blood transfusion is usually performed after the harvest procedure, with volume replacement by crystalloid solution during the harvest. This is because of the possibility of blood transfusion reactions occurring under anaesthesia which can be better observed and managed when the patient is awake. If homologous blood is used for transfusion in the case of an autograft it should be irradiated to at least 15 cGy (**133**) to prevent the theoretical possibility of graft contamination with third party viable lymphocytes which may cause later graft-versus-host disease (Graw *et al.*, 1970; Schecter *et al.*, 1977).

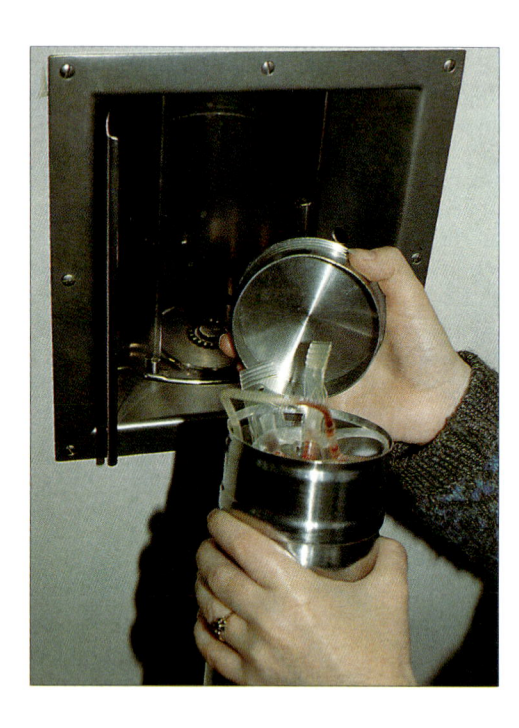

133 Blood irradiator. Blood products for irradiation are inserted into the stainless-steel canister which is then placed on the recessed turntable. The door is then closed and a system of interlocking safety shields internalizes the canister, opens it, and exposes the blood products to a caesium-137 source.

Harvest procedure

Preoperatively, an assistant lays up a sterile trolley with the requirements for the operation (**134**). Many hospitals with a central sterile supplies department (CSSD) may find it convenient to have a pre-autoclaved pack made up, the contents of which are listed in **135**. A 1-litre transfer pack is filled with 150 ml ACD (acid citrate dextrose) solution and the syringes and aspirating needles are flushed through with heparinized saline (**136**).

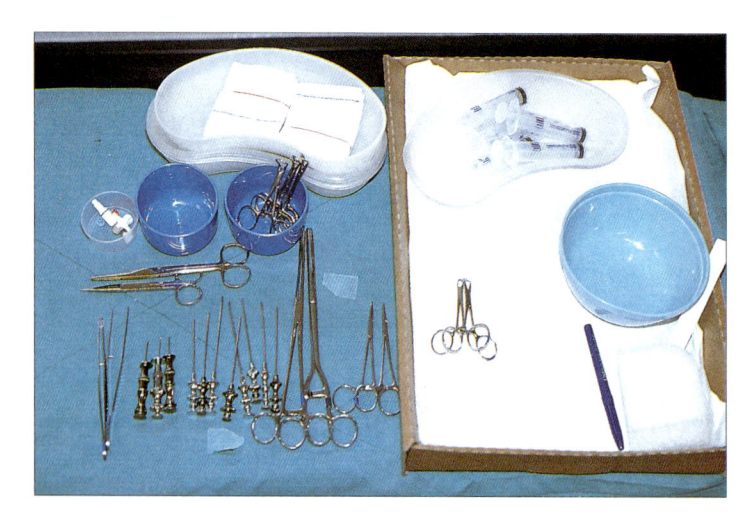

134 Bone-marrow harvest pack showing iliac and sternal aspirate needles in the left foreground. Additional items are the 20-ml disposable syringes and disposable sterile pen.

UNIVERSITY COLLEGE LONDON HOSPITALS CSSD PACK SLIP

BONE MARROW HARVEST 065

TRAY 45 x 30 x 5 cm lined with 50 x 50 cm crepe paper

8	Resenthal needles G14 x 8 cm	) numbers)	join 2 trays no.
		) must)	73 lined with a
3	Child Klima needles G16 x 2.5 cm	) match)	handtowel. Thread
		))	needles individually
		))	onto piece
		))	of paper – stilette
		))	separated from
		))	needle

4	Spongeholding forceps 23 cm	)	Top left-hand corner
6	Bachaus towel clips	)	
2	Mosquito forceps str. 11.5 cm	)	All instruments
2	Gillies dissecting forceps 15 cm	)	marked with blue
1	Mayo scissors str. 17 cm	)	

1   Receiver – top right-hand corner

10   X-Ray detectable swabs 10 x 7.5 cm 32 ply
8   Surgical Skin Prep polyester sponges 5 x 3.6 x 3.6 cm

3   Large sheets

8   Large green towels

2   Paper towels 60 x 60 cm with a hole

3   Surgical sheets 90 x 90 cm – green non-woven

1   Used instrument bag

ASSEMBLED BY ....
CHECKED BY ....
PLEASE COMPLETE FORM AND RETURN WITH INSTRUMENTS TO CSSD

PATIENT'S NAME..
CASE NOTES NO. ....
HOSPITAL ....
OPERATING DEPT...
SURGEON...
DATE OF USE..
SCRUBBED NURSE – initial instrument check ....
SCRUBBED NURSE – final instrument check ....
SUPPLEMENTARY INSTRUMENTS USED...

                                                                                                DATE

135 Contents of CSSD pack used for bone marrow harvesting. This slip also provides quality control information to the CSSD department.

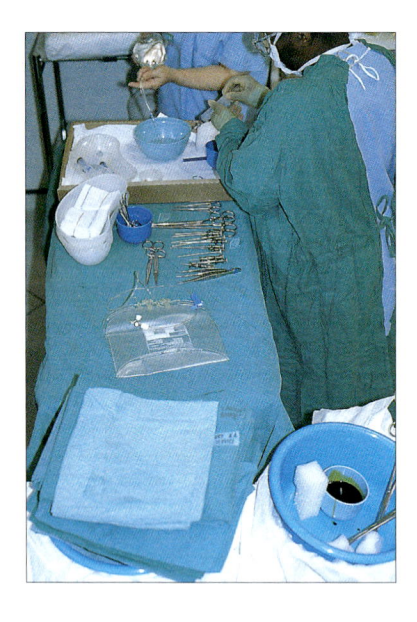

Bone Marrow Transplantation

136 Trolley laid-up for harvest procedure. In the foreground are the swabs for skin-cleansing and towels for draping. On the main trolley is a 1-litre transfer pack containing 150 ml of ACD solution. The operating assistant is flushing syringes and needles with heparinized saline.

Bone marrow may be harvested from anterior and posterior iliac crests and sternum. Care should be taken to identify any sites of previous radiotherapy treatment (e.g. mantle radiotherapy for previously localized Hodgkin's disease) as these generally remain hypocellular and are unsuitable sites for harvesting. Some centres heparinize the donor prior to harvest to prevent occurrence of clots in the marrow harvest. However, this is not strictly necessary providing that there is no delay between aspirating the marrow and mixing it with anticoagulant. Heparinization of the donor may, however, mitigate against lipid embolism (Markwardt, 1984; Shier and Wilson, 1980).

After induction of general or spinal anaesthesia (Filshie *et al.*, 1984) the patient is initially laid prone so that marrow can be aspirated from the posterior iliac crests. In some healthy donors this site provides enough nucleated marrow cells for the total harvest so that the patient need not be turned whilst under the anaesthetic. Normally two operators work on opposite sides of the donor (**137**) and an assistant collects the aspirated marrow.

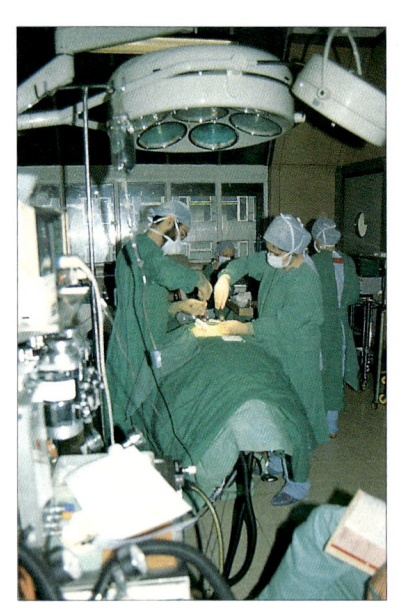

After cleaning the operative field the patient is towelled up to expose the posterior iliac spines and lateral part of the iliac crest (**138**). Bone marrow is aspirated simultaneously from both posterior iliac spines. Several penetrations of the bony cortex may be made through one needle hole in the skin by stretching the skin to one side or the other, thus minimizing trauma and scar formation. The richest site of marrow is the posterior superior spine itself; aspiration is increasingly harder and produces less marrow as the operator moves laterally. Normally at least two-thirds of the marrow harvest can be obtained from the iliac crests.

137 Bone marrow harvest in progress. Two operators work on opposite sides of the patient.

The volumes of marrow aspirated at each site should not generally exceed 10 ml. In general, the smaller the volume aspirated at each site the richer the count of colony forming cells, with less haemodilution (Batinic *et al.*, 1990; Bacipalugo *et al.*, 1992).

After the posterior iliac crests have been exhausted the patient is turned and aspiration from the anterior iliac crests and sternum is performed. Needles with guards should be used for the sternal aspirations (**139**) to prevent sternal perforation. In the case of autograft patients, care should be taken not to

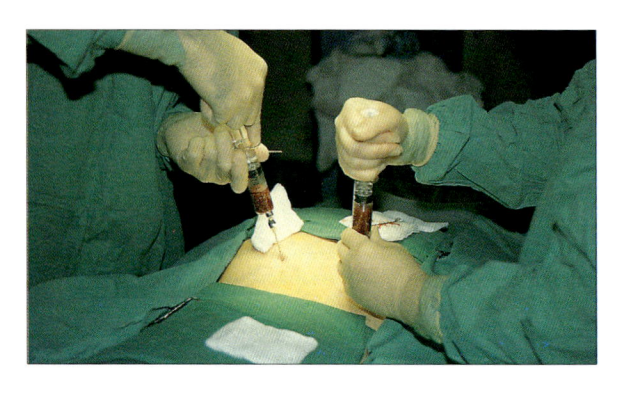

138 Bone marrow is aspirated simultaneously from both sides of the iliac crests. Several cortical penetrations are made through one skin hole.

damage Hickman lines which may have been placed close to the midline. The sternum usually provides a good source of small volumes of rich marrow.

As each aliquot of marrow is aspirated the syringe is passed to the assistant who empties it into the transfer bag through a three-way tap (**140**). Periodically the bag is squeezed to ensure marrow is mixed with anticoagulant. A running total of aspirated marrow volume may be kept if the operators call out the volume of each marrow aspirate as it is completed. Alternatively, the transfer pack can be placed on an electric balance, set at zero after the addition of anticoagulant. One gram of marrow is equivalent to one millilitre. The balance is not sterile, so it should be on a separate trolley, with the transfer pack tube extending to the assistant's sterile trolley. Filtration of harvested marrow is unnecessary, though simple filtration methods are available (Neudorf *et al.*, 1984). The dose of harvested marrow is usually expressed as number of nucleated cells per kilogram of recipient body weight. In practice, this equates to a volume of 10–15 ml/kg of recipient body weight. Some centres correct the nucleated cell count by subtracting the donor's peripheral blood white cell count. For autologous transplantation a total nucleated cell count of 1×10^8/kg of *recipient* weight is needed. For allografting a total nucleated cell count of 2×10^8/kg of *recipient* weight is the minimum required. In the event of donor–recipient HLA mismatch, or if laboratory processing of the marrow is required, then larger numbers of donor cells must be harvested. *Ex vivo* purging will usually more than double the required number of harvested cells. The relationship between number of donor cells harvested and recipient speed of engraftment is poor (Atkinson *et al.*, 1985). Although a more logical approach to measuring the number of cells required for successful engraftment would be to measure the number of colony forming units (CFU_{GM}) in the harvested marrow, the culture process takes more than 1 week, so that data on harvest quality are usually only available retrospectively. The number of CD34-positive mononuclear cells may provide a more useful indicator.

Normally, interim samples of the well-mixed harvested marrow are sent to the laboratory after

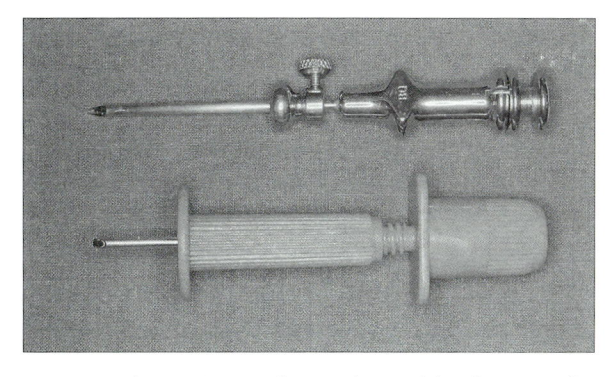

139 Sternal aspirate needles. A disposable Klima needle and re-usable Salah needle. Both have adjustable guards.

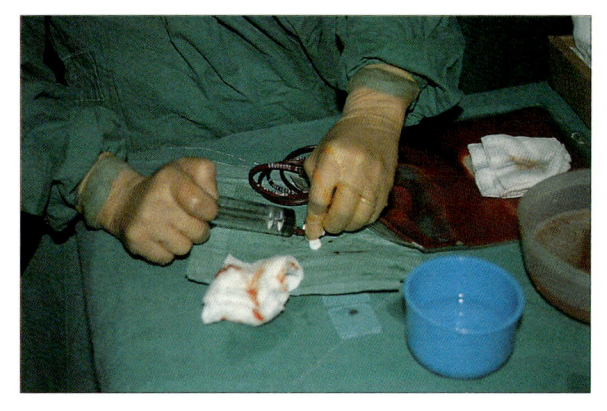

140 Syringes of aspirated bone marrow are handed to the assistant, who injects the marrow into the transfer pack containing ACD solution through a disposable three-way tap.

approximately 500 ml, 800 ml, and 1 litre of marrow has been aspirated to ensure an adequate harvest. For donors of small body weight relative to the recipient it may be necessary to perform two harvests, the first of which is cryopreserved. At the end of the procedure, samples are taken for assessment of colony forming units if required. The marrow bag is labelled with the date, donor's name, recipient's name (where appropriate), volume of harvested marrow and cell count (when known). The marrow may be transferred to the laboratory for further processing, or transfused into the recipient in the case of an ABO-matched allograft.

Donor morbidity from the harvesting procedure is very small and is usually limited to temporary discomfort at the aspiration sites. (Buckner *et al.*, 1984; Cairo *et al.*, 1989) This is important since in the allograft setting donors come from the non-patient population. However, occasional problems have been encountered, and these are listed in **Table 24**.

Table 24. Complications of bone marrow harvesting.

Problems of anaesthesia	Fat embolism
Puncture of vital organs	Air embolism
Bruising	Transient neuropathies
Anaemia	Unexplained postoperative fever
Infection	
Hypovolaemia	Broken needles left at aspiration site
Deep venous thrombosis	
	Pain at puncture sites

Bone marrow reinfusion

This technique of infusion applies equally well to bone marrow or peripheral blood stem cells (PBSC). The recipient should be demonstrated to have immediate venous access (a free-running saline drip into a central venous catheter), before marrow infusion is undertaken.

Frozen marrow should be transported to the patient's bedside in a portable Dewar of liquid nitrogen. This is placed in a secure place. It is important to infuse marrow/PBSC as quickly as possible after thawing to minimize stem cell death.

Because of haemoglobinaemia (Burger et al., 1991) and haemoglobinuria resulting from the lysis of red cells contaminating the marrow or PBSC, prehydration of the recipient with dextrose or normal saline to ensure a high urine flow is advisable. Prophylactic chlorpheniramine and hydrocortisone are usually given 30 min before marrow re-infusion to attenuate allergic-type reactions. The recipient should be warned about the unpleasant smell of dimethylsulphoxide (DMSO) if this has been used as a cryoprotectant, and also about the fact that red cell lysis during thawing will result in a red coloration of the urine. It is advisable to confirm that conditioning chemotherapy has been given as scheduled, to ensure that cytotoxic drugs are not still present in the recipient circulation, which may delay or inhibit engraftment. Normally at least a 24-hour safety margin is required between agents such as melphalan or cyclophosphamide and marrow/PBSC infusion.

A large capacity water bath (or, if unavailable, a ward basin) is filled with clean water at approximately 40°C. Individual marrow/PBSC bags are taken straight from liquid nitrogen and, after checking the donor identity, are plunged into the warm water with continued agitation. When thawed each bag is then rapidly infused into the recipient via a standard blood administration set with integral 170 µm clot filter. Bags are thawed and infused individually. An interval of 1 or 2 hours can be left between infusion of each bag if the recipient is of low body weight and over-hydration is to be avoided.

When marrow/PBSC have been stored in liquid phase nitrogen, this may occasionally have leaked into the bag through an access port or imperfect thermal seal. This may be seen when the marrow is removed from the portable Dewar, or the first indication may be the rapid swelling of a bag when it is thawed. To prevent the bag bursting it may be punctured through

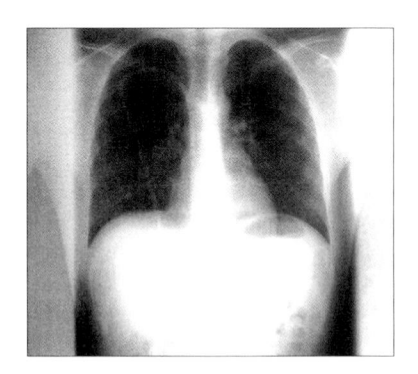

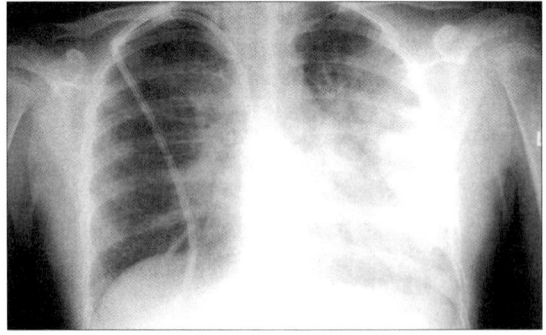

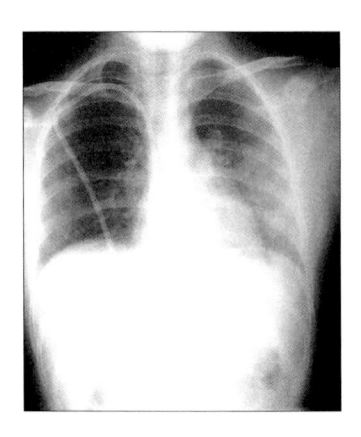

141–143 Pulmonary toxicity of cryopreserved autologous bone marrow. This 10-year-old patient developed cough, haemoptysis and shortness of breath associated with hypoxaemia and bilateral crepitations within 6 hours of an infusion of 800 ml of autologous cryopreserved bone marrow in 5% DMSO. Treatment with oxygen, antibiotics, hydrocortisone and diuretics produced a marked improvement in a few hours. Shown are the chest X-ray films at day −5 before marrow infusion (**141**, above left), 6 hours (**142**, above right), and 24 hours (**143**, left) after infusion. Engraftment on day +16 was followed by complete recovery.

one of the access ports with a sterile hypodermic needle in order to release the nitrogen gas. The puncture hole should then be sealed to prevent extraneous air entry. Whilst this procedure cannot be considered microbiologically safe it is clearly of overriding importance to infuse the marrow/PBSC to ensure engraftment. Marrow harvests may in any case be contaminated with bacteria as a result of the harvesting procedure involving multiple skin punctures (Rowley et al., 1988).

Morbidity associated with marrow infusion may be due to microbial contamination, infusion of particulate material, toxicity of DMSO, or other adverse effects. DMSO infusion may result in nausea, flushing and abdominal pain (Davis et al., 1990). Adult respiratory distress syndrome has also been reported after the infusion of cryopreserved marrow (Roy et al., 1989). Such a case of acute pulmonary toxicity is shown in **141–143**.

References

Atkinson K, Norrie S, Chan P et al. Lack of correlation between nucleated bone marrow cell dose, marrow CFU-GM dose or marrow CFU-E dose and the rate of HLA-identical sibling bone marrow engraftment. *Br J Haematol* 1985; **60**: 245–251.

Bacipalugo A, Tong J, Podesta M et al. Bone marrow harvest for marrow transplantation: effect of multiple small (2 ml) or large (20 ml) aspirates. *Bone Marrow Transplant* 1992; **9**: 467–470.

Batinic D, Marusic M, Pavletic Z et al. Relationship between differing volumes of bone marrow aspirates and their cellular composition *Bone marrow Transplant* 1990; **6**: 103–107.

British Society for Haematology and the British Blood Transfusion Society. Prepared by the British Committee for Standardisation in Haematology Blood Transfusion Task Force. *Clin Lab Haematol* 1988; **10**: 193–201.

Buckner CD, Clift RA, Sanders JE et al. Marrow harvesting from normal donors. *Blood* 1984; **64**: 630.

Burger J, Gilmore MJ, Jackson B, Prentice HG. Acute haemoglobinaemia associated with the reinfusion of bone marrow buffy coat for autologous bone marrow transplantation. *Bone Marrow Transplant* 1991; **7**: 322–324.

Cairo MS, Van de Ven C, Toy C, Sender L. Clinical and laboratory experience in bone marrow harvesting in children for autologous bone marrow transplantation. *Bone Marrow Transplant* 1989; **4**: 305.

Davis J, Rowley SF, Braine HG et al. Clinical toxicity of cryopreserved bone marrow graft infusion. *Blood* 1990; **75**: 781–786.

Filshie J, Pollock AN, Hughes RG, Omar YA. The anaesthetic management of bone marrow harvests for transplantation. *Anaesthesia* 1984; **39**: 480–484.

Graw RG, Buckner CD, Whang-Peng J et al. Complications of bone marrow transplantation: graft-versus-host disease resulting from chronic myelogenous leukaemia leucocyte transfusions. *Lancet* 1970; **2**: 338–340.

Markwardt F. Antilipemic action of heparin. *Thromb Diathesis Haemorrhagica* 1984; **33**: 73.

Neudorf S, Henrixson M, Hammond J et al. A modified method for human bone marrow filtration prior to bone marrow transplantation. *Bone Marrow Transplant* 1984; **4**: 97–100.

Rowley SD, Davis J, Dick J et al. Bacterial contamination of bone marrow grafts intended for autologous and allogeneic bone marrow transplantation: Incidence and clinical significance. *Transfusion* 1988; **28**: 109–112.

Roy V, Veys P, Jackson F et al. Adult respiratory distress syndrome following autologous bone marrow transfusion. *Bone Marrow Transplant* 1989; **4**: 711–712.

Schecter GP, Whang-Peng J, McFarland W. Circulation of donor lymphocytes after blood transfusion in man. *Blood* 1977; **49**: 651–656.

Shier MR, Wilson RF. Fat embolism syndrome: traumatic coagulopathy with respiratory distress. *Surg Annu* 1980; **12**: 139.

IV Bone Marrow Processing

Keith Patterson

Red cell, plasma and T-cell depletion

ABO blood group compatible allografts can be administered without manipulation in the laboratory. In other situations some marrow processing is required, and the most common is red cell depletion. Such depletions are indicated prior to transfusion of fresh ABO incompatible allograft bone marrow, and prior to autologous bone marrow cryopreservation. Small amounts of red cell stroma and haemoglobin contaminating autografted bone marrow do no harm and may have a protective effect during cryopreservation. A large amount of red cells may be associated with an increased possibility of autograft recipient reaction. In ABO-incompatible allografts the infusion of fresh harvested marrow containing incompatible red cells may result in haemolytic transfusion reaction. Donor–recipient incompatibility does not materially affect the rate or nature of engraftment as stem cells lack ABO antigens (Sieff et al., 1982) and therefore cannot be destroyed by anti-A or anti-B in the recipient. However, delayed red cell engraftment may be encountered, lengthening the spell of transfusion dependency after engraftment.

Methods of red cell depletion and concentration of mononuclear cells have been described for a number of centrifugal cell separator machines, including the COBE 2991 (Gilmore et al., 1983), the Fenwal CS 3000 (Dragani et al., 1990) and Haemonetics 30 (**144**) (Linch et al., 1982). In principle, the bag of harvested anticoagulated marrow (usually 0.75–1.25 litres) is attached to the input line of the separator and the buffy coat/mononuclear fraction is collected, leaving the plasma and red cells.

The efficiency of removal of red cells and recovery of stem cells varies between separators and operators. Dragani et al. found the COBE 2991 with a Ficoll–Hypaque gradient to be the most efficient of 5 methods of stem cell concentration, achieving recovery of 89% of mononuclear cells and a volume reduction of 98%; the final product was contaminated with less than 2% of the original red cells.

The deliberate transfusion of cross-match-incompatible red cells into the marrow recipient is an effective way of reducing the titre of anti-A and anti-B, although this is generally employed with preliminary plasmapheresis because of the risk of haemolytic transfusion reaction. Hershko et al. (1980) transfused 1.4 donor group units after a preliminary 20-litre plasma exchange and found no significant haemolytic reactions. The procedures for preventing the transfusion of cross-match-incomp-

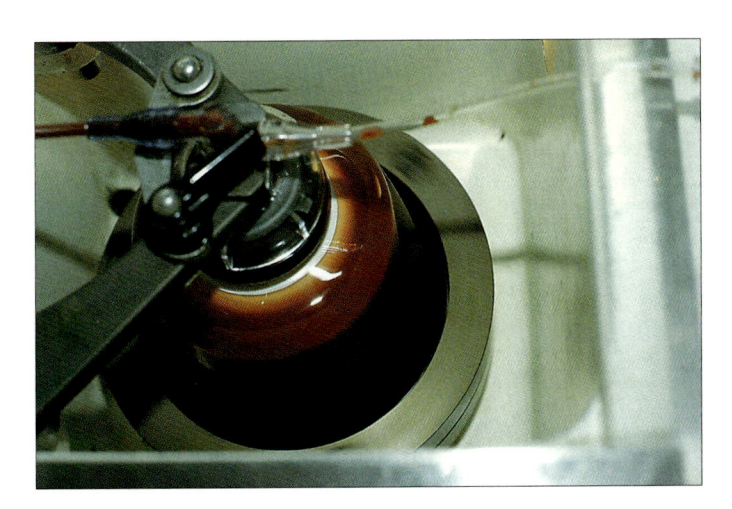

144 Haemonetics model 30 cell separator being used for buffy coat separation from harvested marrow. The red cells are at the bottom of the Lathan-type separation bowl. The supernatant plasma is stained with haemoglobin because of haemolysis, which is not uncommon in harvested marrows. The buffy coat to be collected lies between the red cells and plasma.

atible units in some institutions are so rigorous as to make such procedures difficult to contemplate!

Falkenberg *et al.* (1985) use an ingenious method for enhancing red cell depletion from separated buffy coat. They add recipient-compatible irradiated packed red cells and then repeat the separation procedure.

Plasma depletion of harvested bone marrow to remove anti-A and anti-B is relatively easy to accomplish by a variety of centrifugal and sedimentation methods. The separation of red cells from stem cells is more difficult. Removal of the buffy coat from whole marrow may be accomplished by manual sedimentation using an agent that promotes red cell rouleaux formation or the use of a centrifugal cell separator (**144**). Dinsmore *et al.* (1983) describe a manual method using 6% hydroxyethyl starch (HES) solution. Marrow is mixed with HES (8:1) and the red cells drained off the bottom of the bag after 90 min of sedimentation. This method may still leave enough red cells to cause a haemolytic reaction, however, unless other strategies are employed additionally. Plasmapheresis may be employed to reduce the anti-A and anti-B titres in the recipient circulation prior to infusion of ABO incompatible marrow. In our unit we aim to reduce the anti-A and/or anti-B titre to less than 1 in 16 (measured at 4°C) by 3-litre plasmaphereses on two to four occasions prior to marrow infusion.

Stem cell cryopreservation

The stem cells in harvested bone marrow or peripheral blood remain viable for only 2–3 days at temperatures above freezing. Very few marrow-ablative chemoradiotherapy regimens can be completed in this time, so stem cells are commonly cryopreserved.

Mammalian cells vary in their resistance to cryopreservation. Spermatozoa have been successfully frozen in glycerol since 1948; however, reliable techniques for the cryopreservation of ova have still not been perfected. Stem cells are intermediate in their resistance to cryopreservation.

Cyopreservation damages cells in at least four ways:
1 The formation of intracellular ice crystals damages intracellular organelles.
2 Extracellular ice crystal formation dehydrates the cells by removing pure water from the system.
3 Thawing may also cause damage as the cells rehydrate and expand.
4 At low temperatures some cellular enzyme systems continue to function, but some do not, depending on the characteristics of each particular enzyme. This results in a dislocation of cell metabolism and the accumulation of toxic intermediate metabolites.

Three cryoprotective substances have been extensively investigated for stem cell cryopreservation: glycerol, dimethyl sulphoxide (DMSO) and HES. Glycerol is widely used in the preservation of red cells but is too toxic to be re-infused into the recipient without washing the cryopreserved cells. DMSO is an effective cryoprotectant when used in a concentration of

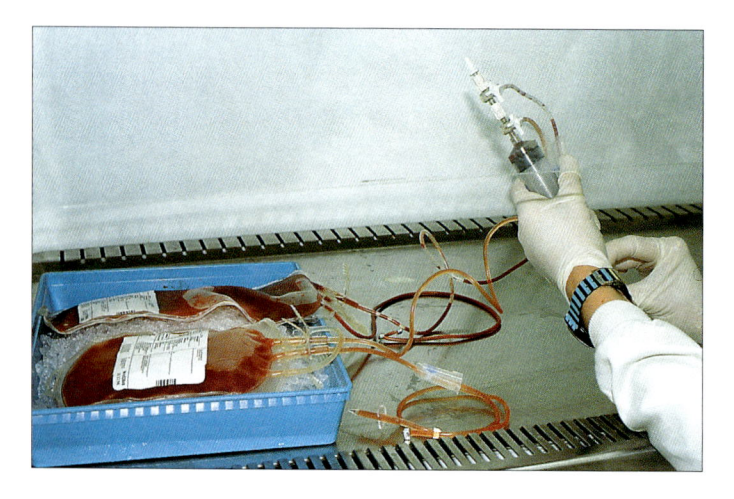

145 Preparation for cryopreservation: a pre-cooled mixture of DMSO and citrated plasma is added a few millilitres at a time to the buffy coat removed from harvested marrow. The marrow is mixed after each addition, the procedure being performed on ice in a sterile cabinet.

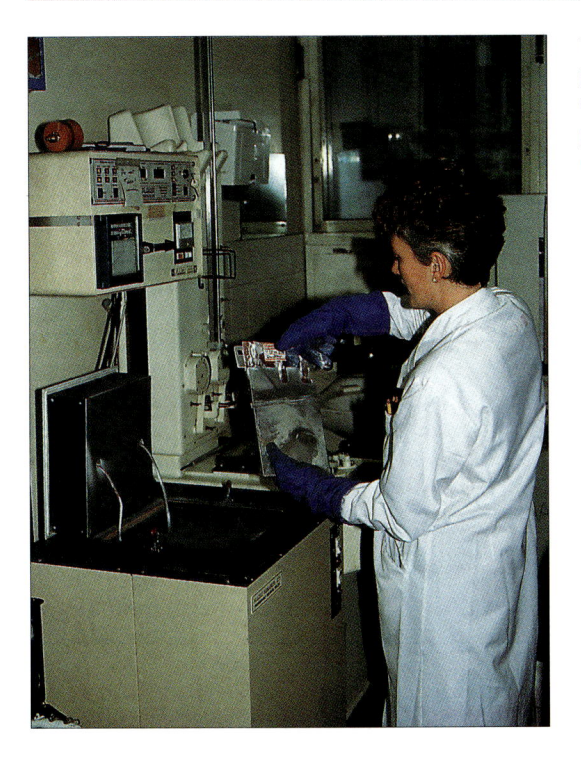

146 Removing cryopreserved bone marrow from the programmed freezer. The frozen marrow in an orange Gambro bag is clamped between two stainless-steel plates which assist heat transfer and ensure the marrow is in a uniform layer 2.3-mm thick.

147 Simplified diagram of programmed freezer. Liquid nitrogen in the storage Dewar on the right of the figure is vaporized by means of an electric heater. The cold vapour passes through a controlling valve (V) via an insulated pipe to the freezer container. Temperature-sensing thermocouples are monitored by the controlling computer and the temperature profile of the material to be frozen is recorded on a chart recorder or similar device. Automatic weighing scales or level sensor ensure that sufficient liquid nitrogen is present to conduct the freezing cycle. The computer controls the freezing cycle by varying the amount of nitrogen vapour entering the freezing chamber.

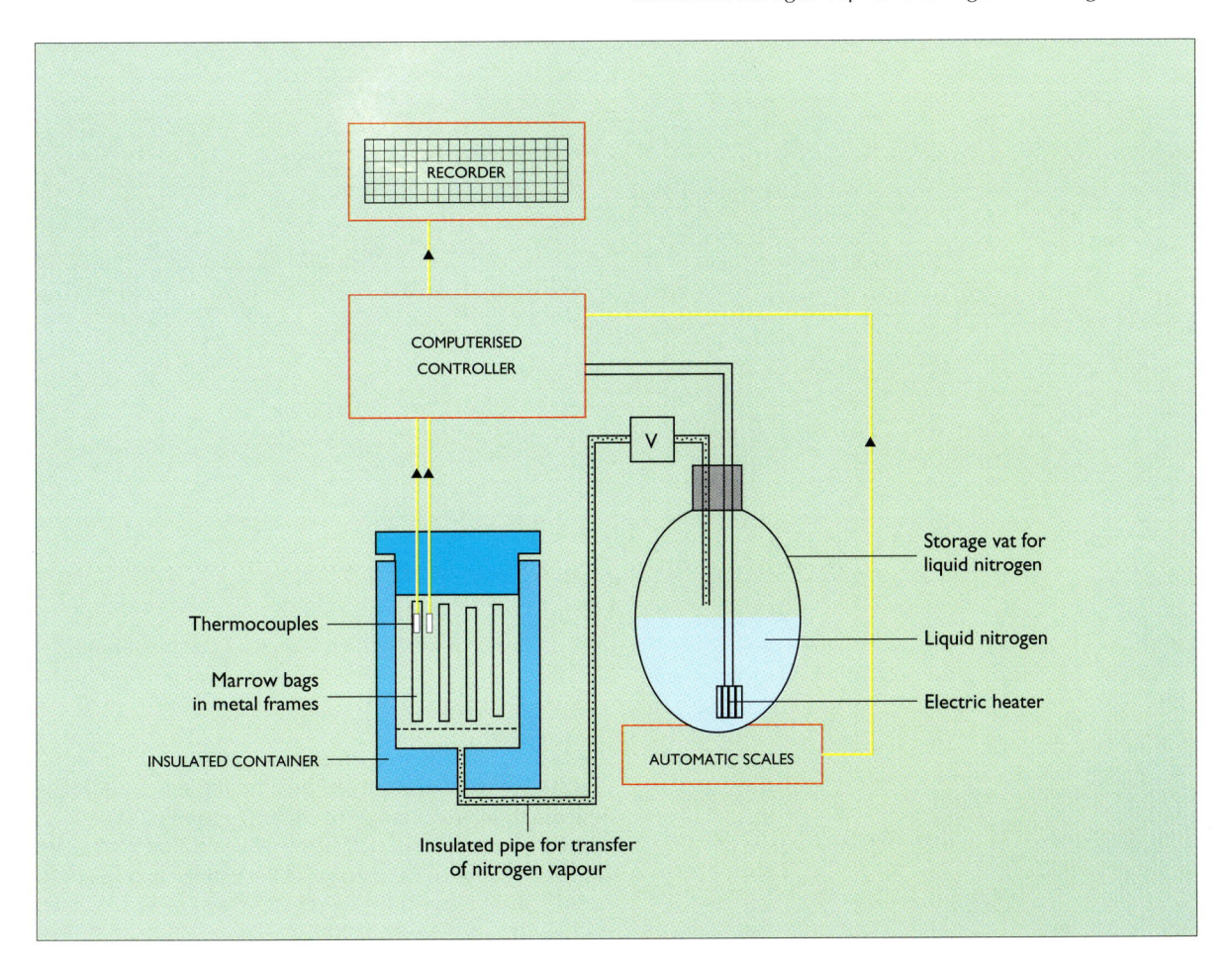

5–10%. It does not need to be washed off the cells but its foul smell, similar to garlic and onions, is noticed by the recipient and his carers for 12–24 hours after administration, since it is excreted through the lungs. Addition of DMSO to water produces an exothermic reaction, which may damage cells. Because of this, DMSO is added to autologous plasma a few millilitres at a time whilst being cooled on ice (**145**). This cold DMSO–plasma mixture is then added to the marrow cells. There is still much that is not understood about the physics of cryopreservation, but some general principles applicable to marrow cryopreservation are clear:

- All parts of the mixture for cryopreservation should follow the same temperature profile at the same time. In practice this is achieved by putting a volume of marrow in a relatively large bag and clamping it between two stainless-steel or aluminium plates (**146**) so that the maximum thickness of marrow exposed to the thawing medium is only 1–2 mm. The metal plates conduct the heat away in uniform way.
- The rate of freezing is controlled, ideally using a programmable freezer (**146, 147**). The initial rate of freezing (area A in **148**) is sufficiently rapid to prevent the disruption of metabolic processes mentioned above. When the liquid starts to freeze solid, heat is released (area B in **148**)—the latent heat of freezing. To minimize cell damage during this period, rapid cooling is essential, effectively smoothing out the plateau. After solidification, a cooling rate of 1–2°C/min (area C) is optimum (Makino *et al.*, 1991)
- Long-term storage may be in the liquid phase of nitrogen at minus 196°C or vapour phase of liquid nitrogen at −140°C. Storage in mechanical freezers at −80°C is acceptable for short periods of time but has been reported to reduce CFU-GM recovery post-thaw (Allieri *et al.*, 1991). Stem cells in nitrogen vapour or liquid remain viable for at least 3 years. After this time it is advisable to check the viability by clonogenic culture of CFU-GM (**149, 150**). Even if this is performed on pilot vials cryopreserved at the same time as the main bags, there is no guarantee that the vial results will reflect those that would be found in the bags. Many institutions save marrow for up to 5 years only, although successful engraftment has been reported up to eight years after cryopreservation (Areman *et al.*, 1990). Our institution prefers storage in the liquid phase of nitrogen (**151–153**) as there are less temperature fluctuations when the storage container is opened.

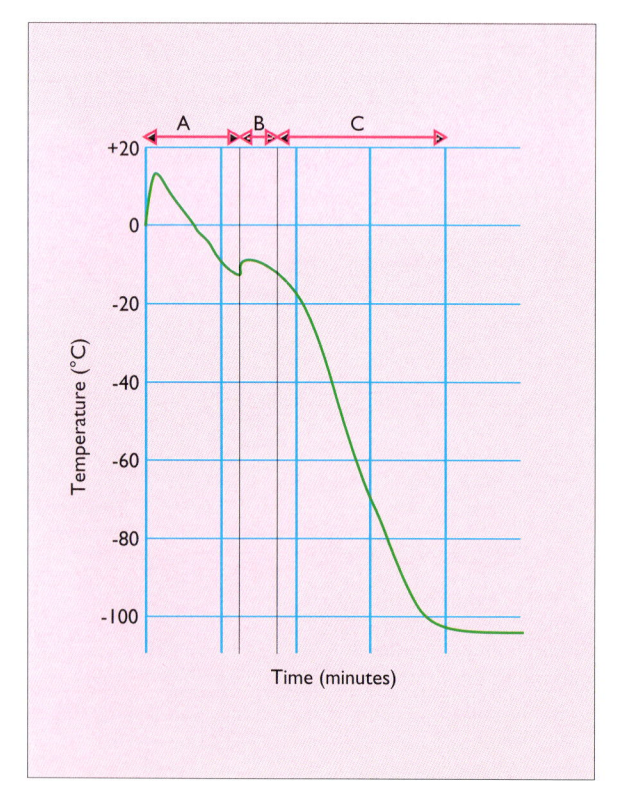

148 Chart recorder record of stem cell freeze. The initial cooling slope is interrupted by a hump representing the release of latent heat by the marrow changing state from liquid to solid. It is during this period that increased cooling is applied to smooth out the plateau and lessen its duration. This period is followed by a slow (1–2°C/min) continuous cooling to −100°C.

Bone Marrow Processing

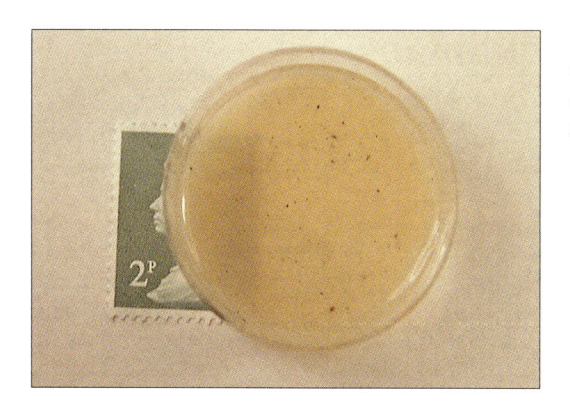

149 Bone marrow/stem cell clonogenic assay. This agar culture plate has been stained with peroxidase to assist in colony counting. Individual colonies stain as black specks.

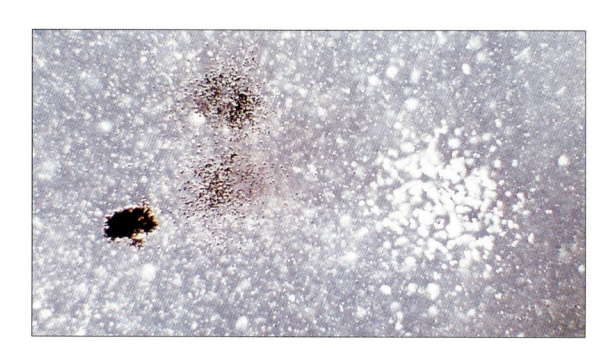

150 Bone marrow/stem cell clonogenic assay. A high power view of the agar plate shown in **149**. Peroxidase-containing myeloid cells stain grey/black and the nature of the colonies can be determined from their morphology and staining characteristics. Four colonies are shown: a diffuse monocyte colony with large unstained cells, two neutrophil colonies staining grey/black, and a tightly clustered eosinophil colony staining black.

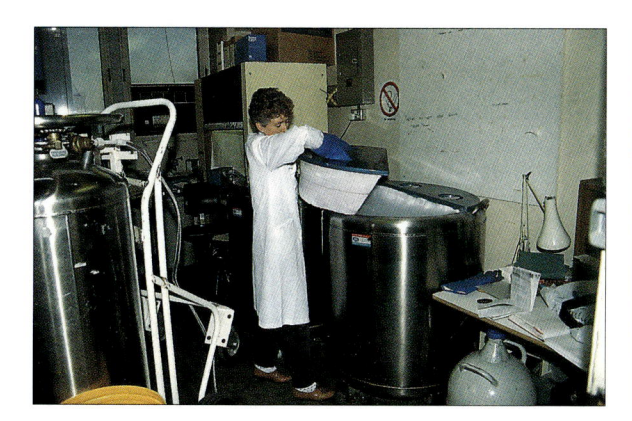

151 Liquid nitrogen freezer being opened prior to insertion of frozen marrow bags.

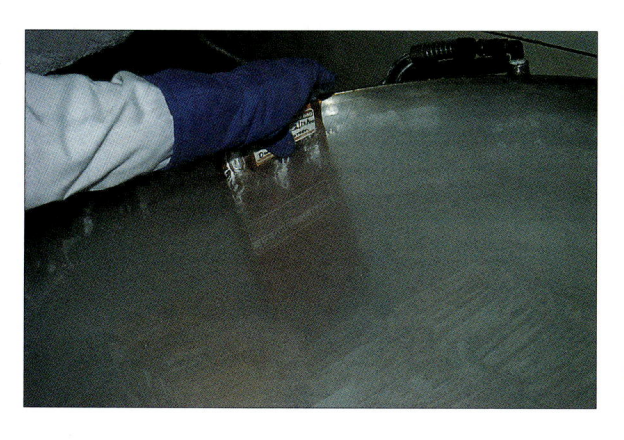

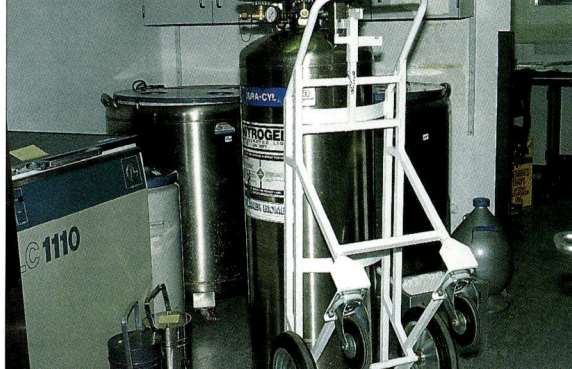

152 Marrow/stem cell storage area. Various types of liquid nitrogen containers are shown. In the foreground are portable Dewars for the transfer of marrow/stem cells in liquid nitrogen to the ward. The tall stainless steel Dewar attached to a white transportation trolley contains the stock supplies of liquid nitrogen. The other tanks contain cryopreserved marrow and stem cells.

153 A bag of frozen marrow being placed in a rack in the liquid phase of nitrogen. The operator is wearing protective gloves.

Cryopreservation without a programmable freezer

Both bone marrow and peripheral blood stem cells can be cryopreserved successfully without the use of a programmed freezer, though this usually involves sacrificing some marrow repopulating capacity. Stiff *et al.* (1987) used a combination of 5% DMSO, 6% HES and 4% human albumin as a cryopreserving solution and froze bone marrow in a standard −80°C laboratory freezer. Their method may also preserve granulocytes in the frozen material. Normally such mature cells are disrupted by the freezing process and their content of nucleic acid may contribute to the formation of a sticky gel likely to block infusion sets and trap stem cells, preventing re-infusion and reducing the efficiency of marrow reconstitution.

Makino *et al.* used a similar mixture for the cryopreservation of peripheral blood stem cells in 50-ml aliquots contained in 100-ml polyolefin freezing bags. They found the duration of the plateau phase (**148**) when frozen at −80°C to be 4 min, with a post-plateau cooling rate of 4.4°C/min. There is thus a necessary compromise in this method between a rapid transition through plateau phase and a slow post-plateau cooling phase.

Quality control of stem cell cryopreservation

The final quality control of stem cell cryopreservation is the haematological reconstitution of the recipient. Before stem cells are infused it is advisable to confirm that reconstitution is likely to happen. The most reliable method of confirming this is the clonogenic culture of CFU-GM (**149, 150**). It is generally accepted that stem cell doses in excess of 13×10^4/kg body weight are satisfactory, and will ensure haemopoietic reconstitution (Bell *et al.*, 1986). The disadvantage of cell culture techniques in assessing graft quality is that the cultures take approximately 2 weeks, and the marrow may well be required in advance of these being ready.

An alternative is the quantitation of CD34-positive cells in the cryopreserved product. CD34 is a primitive antigen present on the surface of stem cells, which may be detected by fluorescent flow cytometry or APAP (alkaline phosphatase anti-alkaline phosphatase) techniques. This must be combined with measurement of viability using trypan blue or eosin exclusion. Dead cells are permeable and take up the dye; living cells exclude it (**154**). Methods for laboratory processing and cryopreservation of stem cells should be clearly documented in standard operating procedures. Liquid nitrogen is potentially dangerous and laboratory, medical and nursing staff must be familiar with the precautions to be taken when handling it, some of which are detailed in **Table 25**.

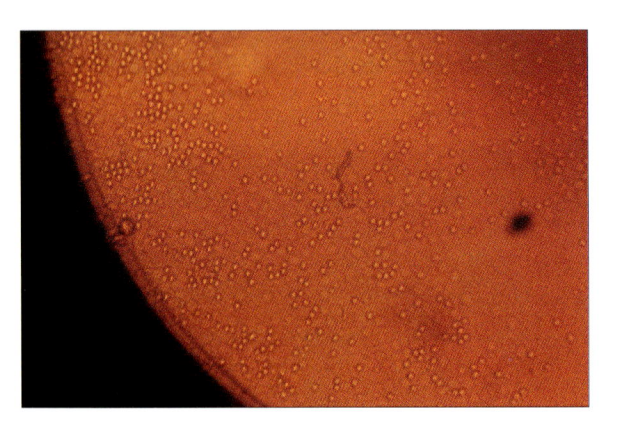

154 This well of a tissue culture plate has been stained with eosin. Viable cells exclude this red dye and show as bubble-like pale areas. Swollen dead cells take up the dye and appear as ghosts in the background.

Table 25. Safe handling of liquid nitrogen.

- Liquid nitrogen causes burns if allowed contact with skin for more than an instant. Initially these burns may be painless and unrecognized because of the numbing effect of intense cold. *Protective gloves should be worn, and manipulations within liquid phase performed using forceps or remote manipulators.*

- Cryogenic mist generated when storage vats are opened can cause a sterile conjunctivitis. *Wear eye protection and trickle liquid nitrogen into the vat to clear mist and improve visibility.*

- *Dispose of unwanted liquid nitrogen by returning it to the storage vat or allowing evaporation to air. If it is essential to pour it away use an outside drain. Do not pour it down basin, sluice or lavatory,* since the ceramic may split because of the intense temperature fluctuations.

- Because of the risk of hypoxia, *rooms containing storage Dewars or programmed freezers should have their doors open at all times* (preferably removed). Where architecture makes continuous ventilation impossible hypoxia alarms should be installed.

- Evacuated storage containers may demonstrate loss of vacuum by a film of frozen condensation on the external surface of the tank. If such a sign becomes apparent, *marrows therein should be moved to another container. Any remaining nitrogen should not be removed until the manufacturers have been contacted as there is a risk of explosion if liquid nitrogen has leaked into the void between the inner and outer layers of the vacuum vessel and evaporates suddenly.*

Marrow purging

The removal of selective populations of cells is required in two situations: T-cell depletion and purging of malignant cells. The most common application is removal of T lymphocytes from harvested marrow prior to transfusion into an allograft recipient. This lessens the possibility of graft-versus-host disease in the post-transplant period. However it should be emphasized that it also decreases the immunological graft-versus-leukaemia effect associated with allografting. Hence, T-cell depletion is usually applied to allograft situations with a high risk of graft-versus-host disease such as matched unrelated donor and single-locus sibling mismatch transplants. T-cell depletion is most commonly accomplished by the addition of complement-fixing monoclonal antibodies directed against T-cell antigens such as CD2, CD3, CD4, CD5, CD6 and CD7. **Table 26** lists other methods of removing selected populations of cells from bone marrow.

Table 26. Methods for the selective removal of populations of cells from bone marrow.

Physical	*Pharmacological*	*Application*
Polystyrene-coated magnetic microspheres	Incubation with complement and monoclonal antibody	T-cell depletion and malignant cell purging
Monoclonal antibody–biotin–avidin–polyacrylamide bead column	Incubation with ricin–monoclonal antibody	T-cell depletion and malignant cell purging
Sedimentation after soya bean agglutinin treatment	Incubation with cytotoxic drugs (e.g. mafosfamide)	T-cell depletion
Sedimentation after sheep erythrocyte rosetting		T-cell depletion and malignant cell purging

The other application of marrow purging is the removal of malignant cells from bone marrow prior to autologous bone marrow transplantation.

Bone marrow purging, positive selection and retention of selected cell populations from the marrow are more fully discussed in Section V.

References

Allieri MA, Lopez M, Douay L *et al*. Clonogenic leukaemic progenitor cells in acute myelocytic leukaemia are highly sensitive to cryopreservation: possible purging effect for autologous bone marrow transplantation. *Bone Marrow Transplant* 1991; **7**: 101–107.

Areman EM, Sacher RA, Deeg HG. Cryopreservation and storage of human bone marrow: A survey of current practices. *Prog Clin Biol Res* 1990; **333**: 523–529.

Bell AJ, Hamblin TJ, Oscier DG. Circulating stem cell autograft. *Bone Marrow Transplant* 1986; **1**: 103–110.

Dinsmore RE, Reich LM, Kapoor N *et al*. ABO incompatible bone marrow transplantion: removal of erythrocytes by starch sedimentation. *B J Haematol* 1983; **54**: 441–449.

Dragani A, Angelini A, Lacone A *et al*. Comparison of five methods for concentrating progenitor cells in human bone marrow transplantation. *Blut* 1990; **60**: 278–281.

Falkenberg JHF, Schaafsma MR, Jansen J *et al*. Recovery of haematopoiesis after blood-group-incompatible bone marrow transplantation with red-blood-cell-depleted grafts. *Transplantation* 1985; **39**: 514–520.

Gilmore MJML, Prentice HG, Corringham RE. Technique for the concentration of nucleated bone marrow cells for *in-vitro* manipulation or cryopreservation using the COBE 2991 blood cell processor. *Vox Sang* 1983; **45**: 294–302.

Hershko C, Gale RP, Ho W, Fitchen J. ABH antigens and bone marrow transplantation. *Br J Haematol* 1980; **44**: 65–73.

Linch DC, Knott LJ, Patterson KG, Cowan DA. Bone marrow processing and cryopreservation. *J Clin Pathol* 1982; **35**: 186–190.

Makino S, Harada M, Akashi K *et al*. A simplified method for cryopreservation of peripheral blood stem cells at –80°C without rate controlled freezing. *Bone Marrow Transplant* 1991; **8**: 239–244.

Sieff C, Bicknell D, Caine G *et al*. Changes in cell surface antigen expression during haemopoietic differentiation. *Blood* 1982; **60**: 703–706.

Stiff PJ, Koester AR, Weidner MK *et al*. Autologous bone marrow transplantation using unfractionated cells cryopreserved in dimethylsulfoxide and hydroxyethyl starch without controlled-rate freezing. *Blood* 1987; **70**: 974–978.

V Bone Marrow Purging

John Kemshead and Adrian Gee

Autologous bone marrow transplantation (ABMT) has found increasing use in the therapy of a number malignant diseases. A potential drawback has been the concern that the transplanted marrow may contain viable occult tumour cells which may contribute to disease relapse. This chapter reviews some of the more widely used approaches to overcome the problems both of detecting and eliminating tumour cells within marrow that is to be used for ABMT.

Detection

Marrow to be used for ABMT is normally harvested when the patient is in clinical remission. Low-level infiltration by leukaemic cells is difficult to detect, as the morphology of the neoplastic cells resembles that of their normal counterparts. However, some solid tumours, such as the small round cell tumours of childhood, and small cell lung carcinoma (SCLC), may also be difficult to differentiate from normal marrow cells (**155, 156**). Detection has, however, been facilitated by the development of monoclonal antibody (MAb) technology.

Immunofluorescent staining using MAbs has also greatly improved the sensitivity of detection of non-haematological malignant cells. Levels of detection

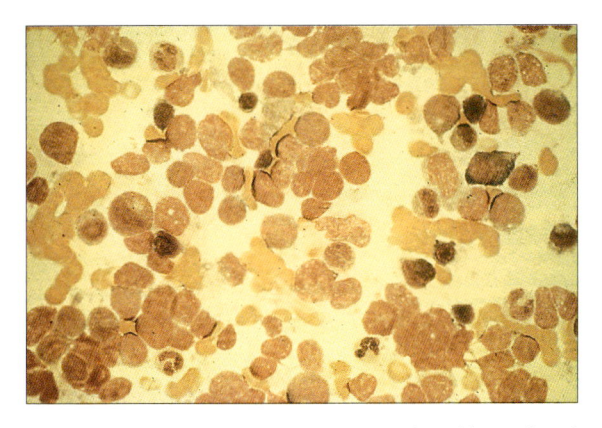

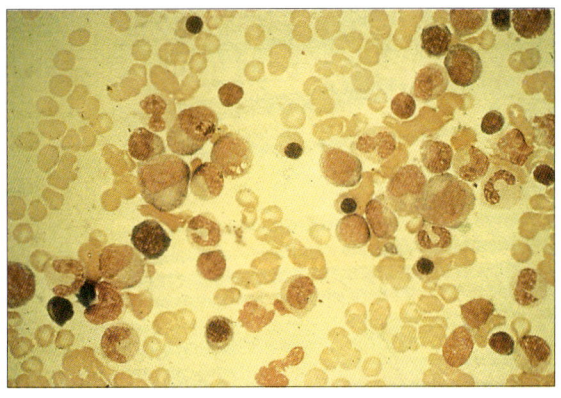

155, 156 Bone marrow aspirate heavily infiltrated with neuroblastoma cells. (H & E staining.) Although it is easy to detect the tumour cells when they are present in large numbers, identification at low levels of infiltration is difficult as the neuroblastoma can appear morphologically identical to normal marrow elements. **155** Heavy infiltration of neuroblastoma cells in bone marrow. **156** Normal bone marrow.

of one malignant cell in 1000–10 000 normal cells are possible (**157**) (Kemshead *et al.*, 1983). Staining with multiple MAbs and fluorochromes, and use of automated flow cytometric analysis, may add an additional log of detection sensitivity. The disadvantage of these techniques is that they do not permit easy examination of the morphology of the labelled cells. This can be achieved by use of immunocytochemical staining (**158, 159**), which, under optimal conditions, may detect 1 cell in 100 000 (Moss *et al.*, 1991). Molecular techniques, such the polymerase chain reaction (PCR) may further enhance tumour cell detection sensitivity in certain instances, where it is possible to define clearly oligonucleotides which only bind to mRNA within the tumour population (**160**). In theory, this approach could also be used to detect leukaemic progenitor cells if the sequence of either rearranged B-cell immunoglobulin genes or T-cell receptor genes is known.

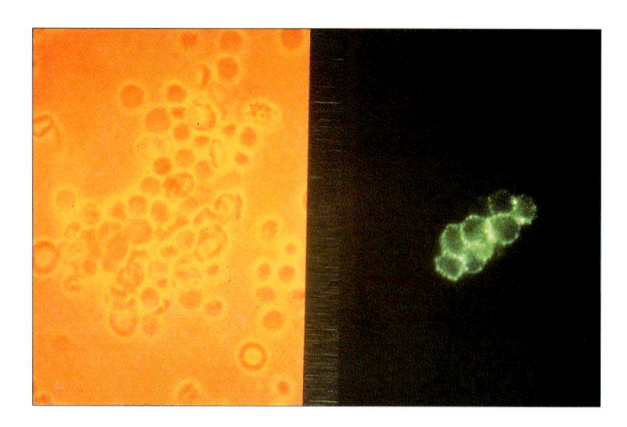

157 Bone marrow aspirate containing a low number of neuroblasts detected by indirect immunofluorescence. Bone marrow was incubated with a monoclonal antibody that binds to neuroblastoma cells, but not to normal haemopoietic cells within the aspirate. Binding of the MAb was visualized using a fluorescently labelled rabbit anti-mouse immunoglobin. Extending the technology to its highest sensitivity, it is possible to detect 1 tumour cell in 10 000 normal progenitors.

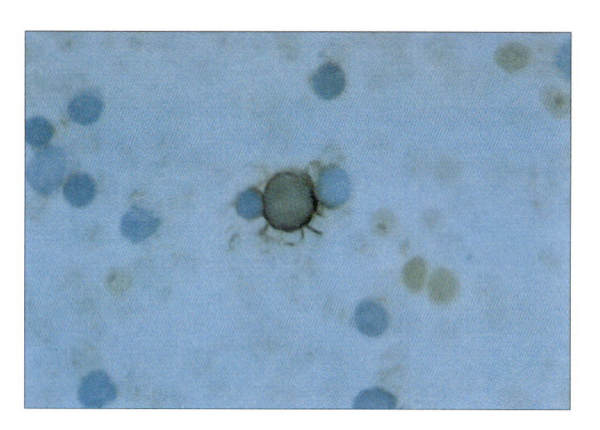

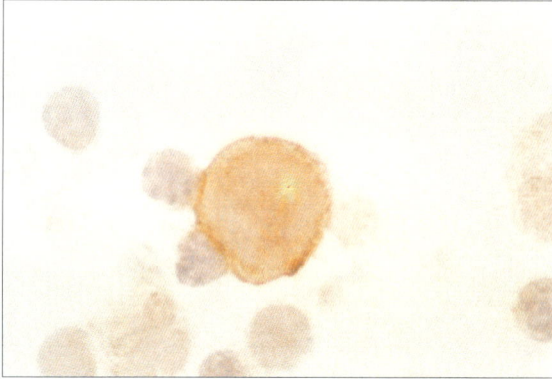

158, 159 Immunoperoxidase staining of bone marrow taken from patients with neuroblastoma at diagnosis. Specimens were judged to be tumour-free by routine histopathological analysis. **158** Positive tumour cell in a patient with Stage IV disease (× 400). **159** Neuroblastoma cell identified in a patient with Stage III disease (× 600).

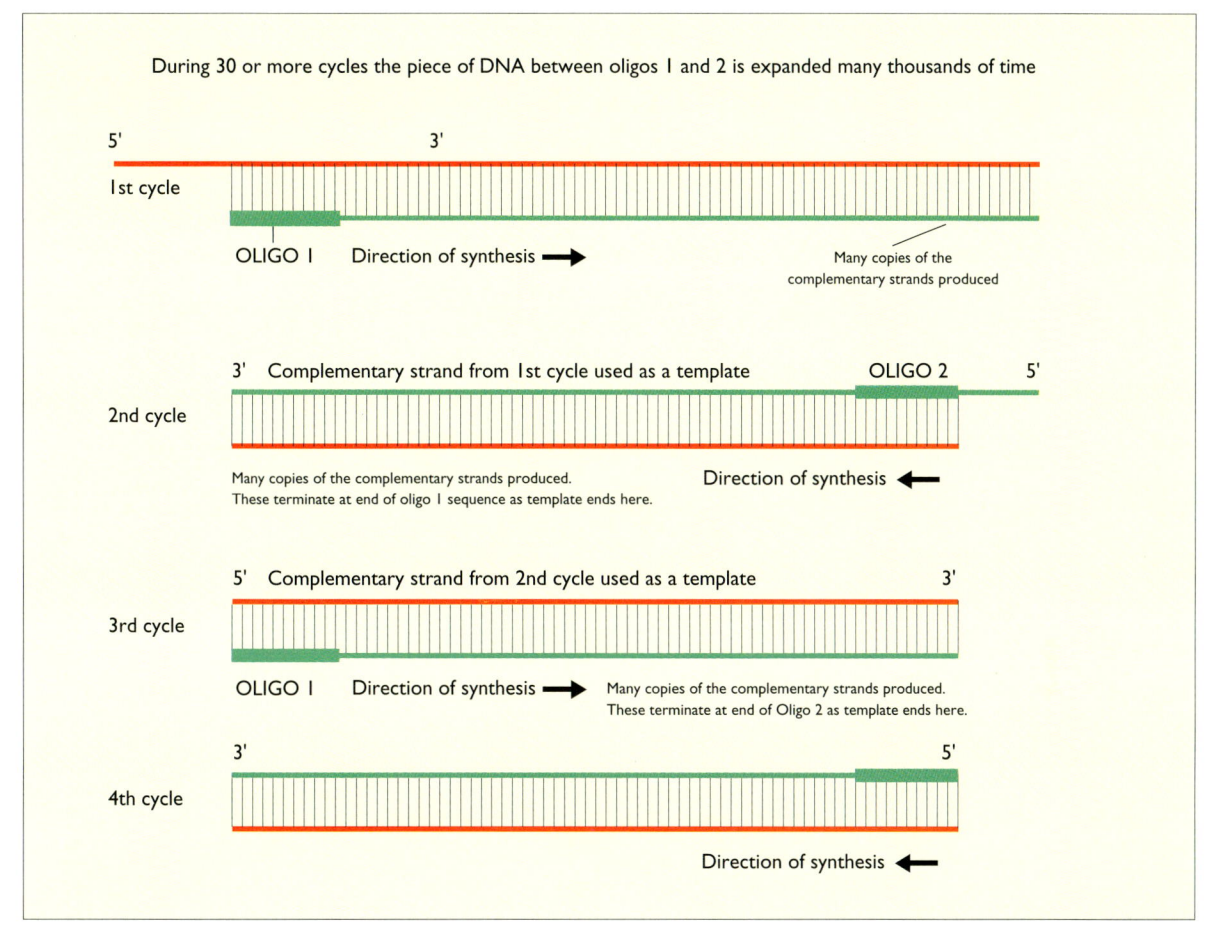

During 30 or more cycles the piece of DNA between oligos 1 and 2 is expanded many thousands of time

1st cycle
5' — 3'
OLIGO 1   Direction of synthesis →   Many copies of the complementary strands produced

2nd cycle
3' Complementary strand from 1st cycle used as a template   OLIGO 2   5'
Many copies of the complementary strands produced. These terminate at end of oligo 1 sequence as template ends here.   Direction of synthesis ←

3rd cycle
5' Complementary strand from 2nd cycle used as a template   3'
OLIGO 1   Direction of synthesis →   Many copies of the complementary strands produced. These terminate at end of Oligo 2 as template ends here.

4th cycle
3'   5'
Direction of synthesis ←

160 The polymerase chain reaction (PCR) allows the amplification of specific pieces of DNA. The sequence must be known so that oligonucleotides can be designed to span the area of interest. Binding of the first oligonucleotide allows the synthesis of a complementary strand of DNA. This is produced in excess and then serves as a template for the second oligonucleotide. Once this binds it allows synthesis of the original DNA strand, as far as the area where the first oligonucleotide binds. The majority of the DNA strands present in the incubation mix now span the area between (and including) oligonucleotides 1 and 2. Further cycles expand this region hundreds of thousands of times.

It is important to note that the sensitivity of all of these approaches is further limited by the number of diagnostic aspirates that are taken from the patient. Even using the most sensitive of the currently available techniques, in a harvest of 1×10^{10} nucleated cells, up to 1×10^5 tumour cells may be returned to a patient (Favrot et al., 1986). A variety of methods have, therefore, been developed to achieve maximal removal of tumour cells from marrow that is harvested for ABMT. These can be conveniently grouped into physical, chemical and immunological techniques (**Table 27**).

Table 27. Methods of separating tumour cells from bone marrow.

Method	Efficacy of depletion ($\times \log$)	In clinical use
Physical		
Gravity sedimentation	1	No
Centrifugal elutriation	1–2	Minimal
Density centrifugation	1–2	No
Hyperthermia	1–3	No
Chemical		
Photoactivators	1–3	Minimal
Alkyl lysophospholipids	1–3	No
Antisense Oligonucleotides	1–3	No
Radiopharmaceuticals	1–3	No
Cytotoxic drugs	1–5	Yes
Immunological		
LAK cells	1–2	No
Antibody complement	1–3	Yes
Immunotoxins	1–4	Yes
Solid-phase capture:		
Magnetic microspheres	1–4	Yes
Panning	1–4	Yes
Columns	1–3	Yes

Physical techniques

Physical methods, including gravity sedimentation, centrifugal elutriation and hyperthermia, generally achieve only 1–2 logarithms of tumour depletion and have not, therefore, found widespread clinical use except as an adjunct to other separation techniques. Chemical methods for purging are highly diverse and are at various stages of development. Less frequently used methods include selective uptake of photoactive agents (merocyanine 450 and photofrin) by tumour cells and the use of alkyl lysophospholipids, which induce the production of free radicals (Sieber *et al.*, 1987).

Antisense oligonucleotides have been proposed as effective purging agents and have shown promise in preclinical experiments.

Targeting of the agent to the tumour cell can be improved by exploiting biochemical pathways that are only expressed in the malignant cell population. An example of this type of reagent is the radiopharmaceutical *m*-iodobenzylguanidine (*m*-IBG), which is an analogue of adrenalin (epinephrine) (Wieland *et al.*, 1980). This is selectively taken up into the cytoplasm of neuroblastoma cells (**161**) and into dense core granules in phaeochromocytoma.

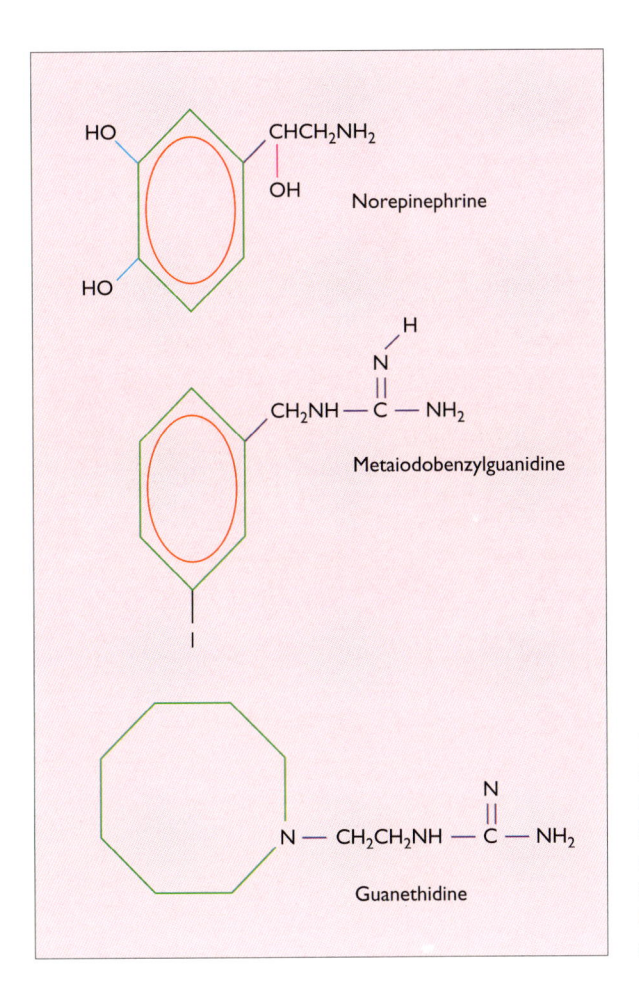

161 Metaiodobenzylguanidine (m-IBG) structure as compared to adrenalin (norepinephrine) and guanethidine. m-IBG has structural similarity to both adrenalin and the hypotensive drug guanethidine. It is actively taken up into either the cytoplasm of neuroblastoma cells or neurosecretory granules within phaeochromocytoma cells. Incorporation of isotopes of iodine (^{131}I/^{125}I) can lead to the selective destruction of the malignant cells

Bone Marrow Transplantation

Chemical techniques

The most widely used chemical agent has been 4-hydroperoxycyclophosphamide (4-HC), a cyclophosphamide derivative which does not require activation in the liver (**162**). This has been used extensively for purging in AML (acute myeloblastic leukaemia) and, more recently, in breast cancer either alone or in combination with other agents such as VP-16 (Yeager *et al.*, 1986). Uniquely, among purging agents, the clinical efficacy of 4-HC can be predicted using *in vitro* assays. Initial problems of delayed engraftment can be overcome by use of carefully optimised treatment conditions.

162 Metabolism of 4-hydropeoxycyclophosphamide (4-HC). 4-HC has a short half-life in solution and degrades to the active compounds 4-hydroxycyclophosphamide and phophoramide mustard. Unlike cyclophosphamide it does not require internal metabolism by the liver to generate these cytotoxic intermediates. 4-HC has been used successfully as a pharmacological approach to eliminating tumour cells contaminating bone marrow.

Immunological techniques

Immunological approaches to tumour 'purging' can be subdivided on the basis of whether they employ MAbs. Non-antibody-mediated methods, such as the LAK cell purging, are still in the experimental stages, whereas MAb-based techniques have found extensive clinical application. Initially, a single MAb was used to sensitize the tumour cells, which were subsequently eliminated by incubation with animal complement (**163, 164**). Heterogeneity of antigen expression by malignant cells has led to the use of panels of MAbs to achieve maximal tumour kill (Bast *et al.*, 1983). However, this technique has been limited by;
- The requirement to use antibodies of particular isotypes.
- Lack of a standardized high titre complement sources.
- Concerns regarding the use of unfractionated animal sera in clinical treatments.
- The resistance of low target antigen cells to complement-mediated lysis by IgG MAbs.

MAbs can be used to target highly potent toxins obtained from bacteria, plants or fungi. The most widely used of these is ricin isolated from the castor bean plant (*Ricinus communis*) (**165**) (Jansen *et al.*, 1982). Many of these agents have a similar structure, consisting of two dissimilar polypeptide chains. In the case of ricin, the B chain contains a galactose binding site which binds to sugars present on the surface of all eukaryotic cells. In order that the MAb may confer specificity towards tumour cells, the B chain must either be blocked or removed. The cytotoxic action of ricin is associated with the A chain, which is internalized and blocks

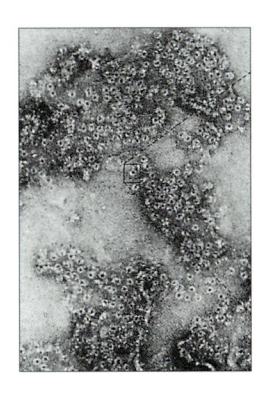

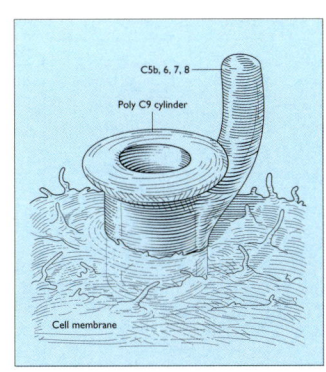

163, 164 Complement-mediated killing of tumour cells coated with antibody. Binding of MAbs to antigens on the target cell activates the complement cascade resulting in lysis of the cells. MAbs of the appropriate isotype must be used and, in the case of IgG MAbs, they must bind to the tumour cells at a high enough density to activate the complement system. **163** (left) Electron micrograph of a membrane lysed by complement ($\times$ 130 000). **164** (right) Schematic drawing of complement components inserted into the cell membrane.

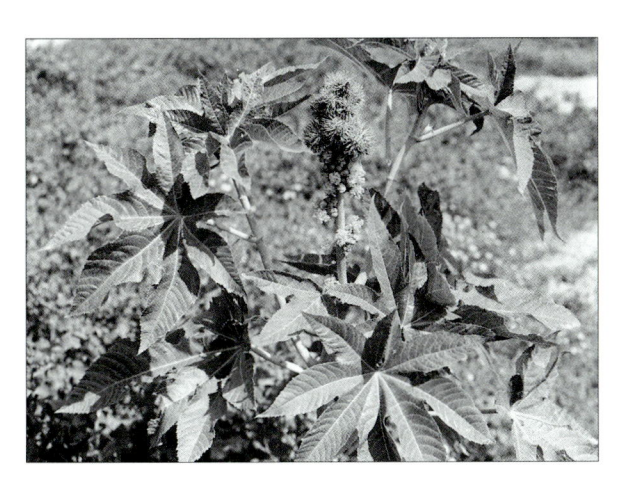

165 Castor bean plant (*Ricinus communis*), cultivated in Egypt. (Courtesy of Dr Robin Mattocks, Tadworth, Surrey.)

protein synthesis by binding to the ribosomes (**166**). Unlike complement-mediated purging, it is necessary to conjugate each MAb in a panel of reagents to the toxin molecule prior to addition to the bone marrow. Conjugate preparation must be performed under strictly controlled conditions as these compounds are highly toxic. Effective cytotoxic activity will depend on internalization of the antigen to which the immunotoxin conjugate is directed. Immunotoxin efficiency is also highly dependent on the correct combination of MAb and toxin molecules. These agents have been most widely used for T-cell leukaemia purging, *in vivo* immunotherapy for B-cell leukaemia/lymphoma, and for the elimination of T-cell subsets in allogeneic transplantation as prophylaxis of graft-versus-host disease.

These methods eliminate the tumour cells within the marrow. It is possible, however, to remove the malignant cell population using a variety of solid phase capture techniques. Either the MAb can be conjugated to a solid phase, e.g. columns, plates or

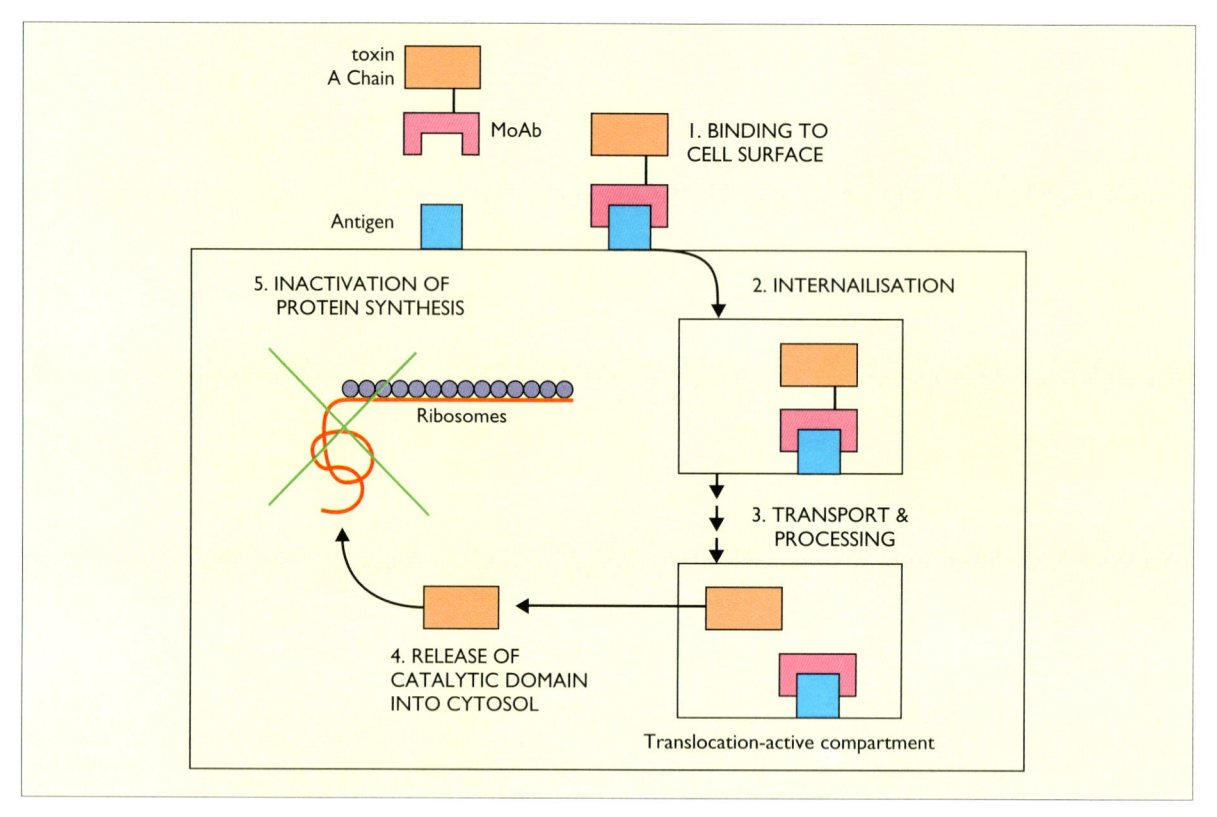

166 Mode of action of ricin A chain in blocking protein synthesis. MAbs conjugated to the A chain of ricin bind to antigens on the surface of the cell. Following internalization, the A chain must be released into the cytoplasm to inactivate ribosomal protein synthesis.

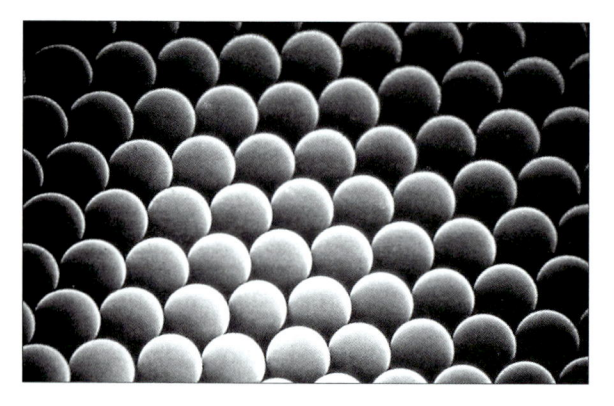

167 Monodispersed magnetic microspheres used for the removal of tumour cells from bone marrow. These are produced by polymerization of styrene. The microspheres are identical in size and contain ferromagnetic iron uniformly distributed throughout their core. They are coated with methacrylate to reduce any non-specific sticking to cells. Proteins can be linked to the surface either by passive adsorption or by covalent linkage. The diameter of the microspheres is 4.5 μm.

beads (direct method), or the tumour cells can be presensitized with the MAb and collected onto an antimouse immunoglobulin-coated support matrix (indirect method) (Treleaven *et al.*, 1984). Monodispersed polystyrene microspheres containing ferromagnetic material are the most commonly used solid phase (**167**). To compensate for antigenic heterogeneity, the indirect method employing panels of MAbs is most widely used for tumour purging (**168–171**). For example, in neuroblastoma, marrow to be purged is incubated with a cocktail of 5 tumour-directed IgG MAbs, and

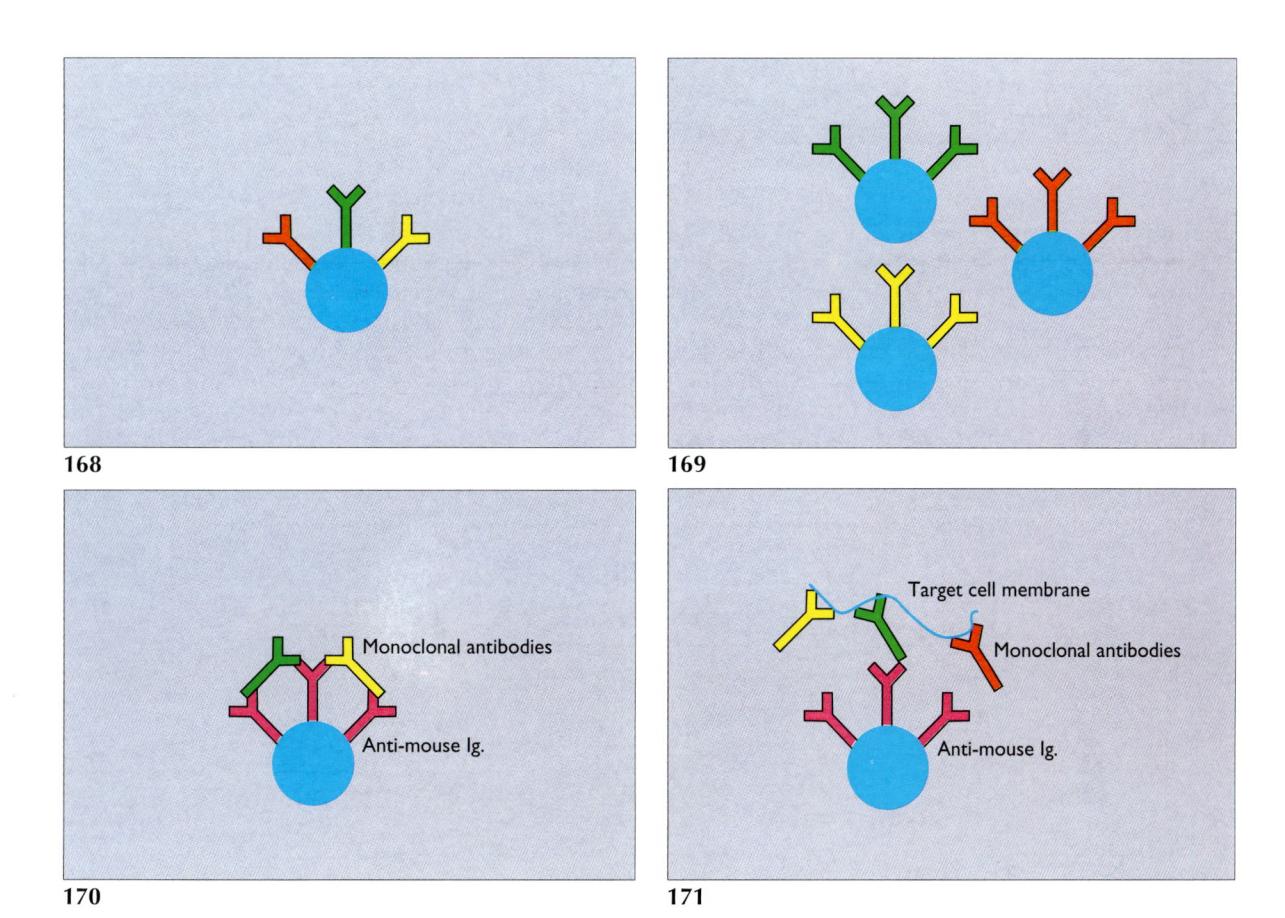

168–171 Four different approaches to the attachment of MAbs to a solid-phase matrix. In this example, the use of magnetic microspheres is illustrated. The capture of tumour cells in bone marrow is best achieved using a panel of MAbs. All four methods for attaching the monoclonal antibody panel to microspheres were investigated to maximize the capture of the malignant population. In most instances the indirect approach gave the best results. **168** One bead coated with several monoclonal antibodies. **169** A cocktail of MAbs are attached to each preparation of microspheres. **170** Antimouse immunoglobulin coated heads premixed with MAbs. **171** Two step targeting: (i) Monoclonal antibodies bound to tumour cells. (ii) Microspheres bound to normal antibodies.

Bone Marrow Transplantation

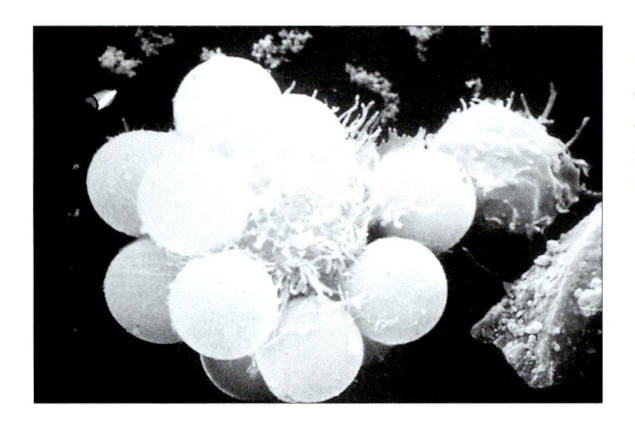

172 Scanning electromicrograph showing the targeting of magnetic microspheres to tumour cells in bone marrow. Contaminated bone marrow was initially incubated with a cocktail of MAbs. After washing, microspheres coated with sheep antimouse immunoglobulin were added, and these bind to the antibodies on the malignant cell population.

then washed and mixed with an excess of sheep antimouse Ig-coated microspheres which rosette with the tumour cells (**172**) (Kemshead *et al.*, 1986).

The immunomagnetic method is readily adaptable for use with a variety of tumours for which suitable MAbs are available and the tumour cells may be recovered from the beads for further study. One disadvantage of this method is the relatively high cost of microspheres.

The ability to recover cells from the beads has opened up the possibility of using this approach for the positive selection of haematopoietic stem cells using an anti-CD34 MAb (**173, 174**) (Lansdorp and Thomas, 1991). However, it has proven difficult to recover the cells from the beads with consistent high yields and purities. Two techniques have been developed: the first uses digestion of an epitope on the CD34 antigen using the enzyme chymopapain, and the second employs an antibody to the Fab region of the MAb (**175**). Under optimal conditions release using chymopapain results in >50% yields of

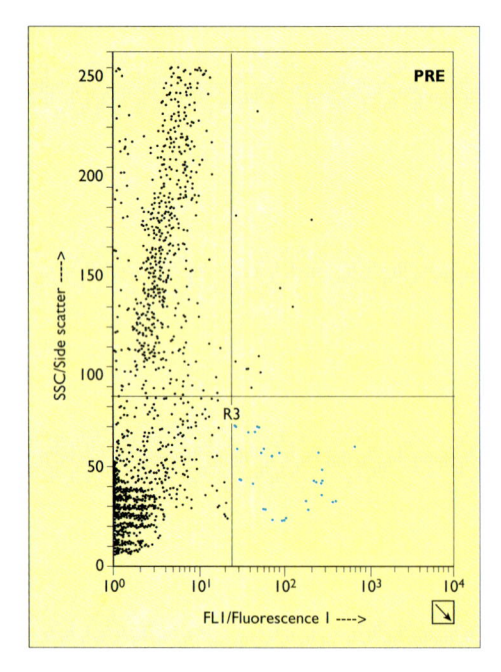

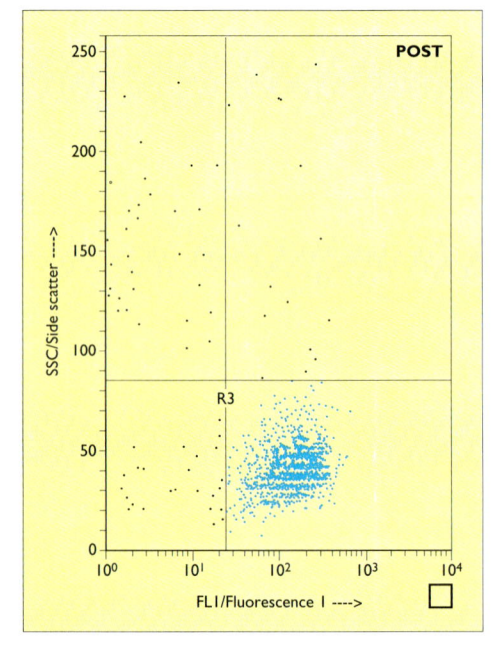

173, 174 Flow cytometric analysis of CD34+ cells in bone marrow. **173** (left) Prior to positive immunomagnetic selection, the CD34+ subpopulation represents 1–3% of the total nucleated cells (bottom left rectangle contains CD34+β cells). **174** (right) Following selective collection of the CD34+ cells onto immunomagnetic beads and release by incubation with chymopapain, the cells can be enriched to purities of >90% with yields in excess of 50% (bottom right rectangle).

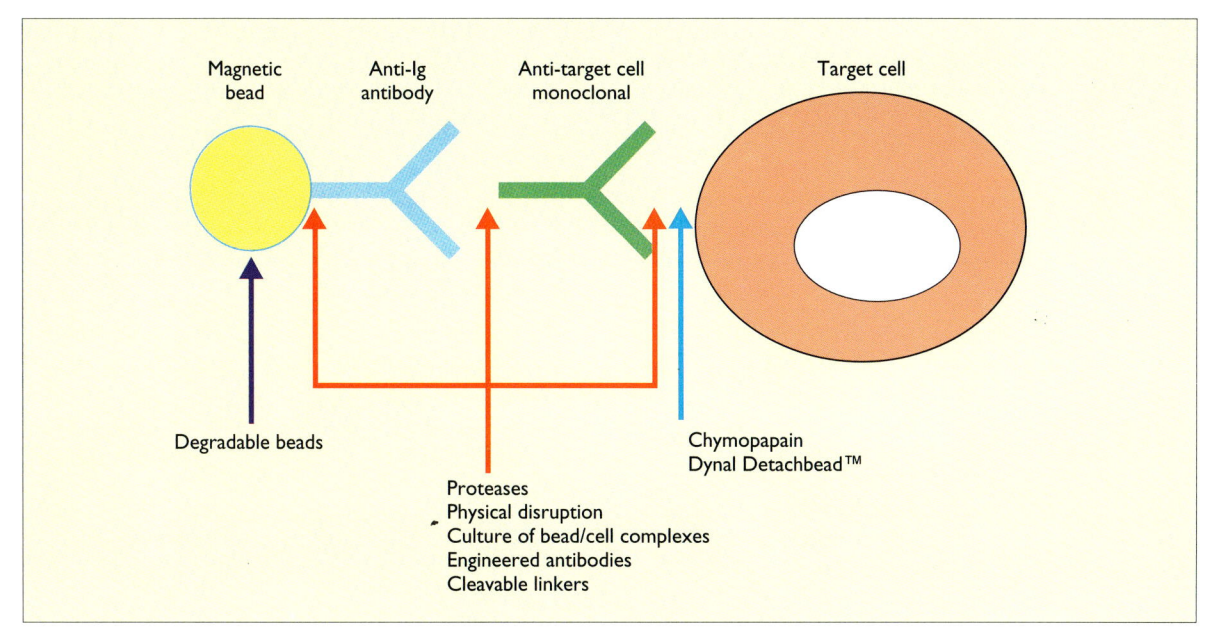

175 Different possibilities for the removal of tumour cells attached to solid supports. Several different approaches to the removal of magnetic microspheres from CD34+ cells have been developed. The bond between the MAb and antigen on the cell membrane of the target cell can be destroyed by either chymopapain or the Dynal Detachbead™ system. Alternatively, methods can disrupt either the bonds between the MAb and antimouse immunoglobulin or the bonds holding the antimouse immunoglobulin to the magnetic bead. Finally, biodegradable beads may be available in the future.

CD34+ cells, with purities in excess of 90%. Alternative technologies for selection of CD34+ cells include the use of panning on MAb-coated polystyrene plates and the collection of stem cells sensitized with biotinylated MAb onto streptavidin columns (**176**). In both cases, the cells are released from the solid phase by physical disruption.

All of the techniques for purging that have found widespread clinical use achieve a 3–4 logarithmic depletion of tumour cells from marrow. No randomized trial has yet been undertaken to demonstrate definitively the benefit of purging to the patient, since such a trial would require large numbers of patients and prolonged follow-up. It is important to appreciate that use of stem cell preparations does not solve the problem of tumour removal since even those methods which achieve

176 The selection of CD34+ cells using MAbs and a commercially available column device. Haemopoietic cells are coated with biotin-linked anti-CD34 and captured by passage down an avidin column. The captured population can be removed from the column by gentle stirring of the avidin matrix (using an integral impellor). (Courtesy of CellPro Inc.)

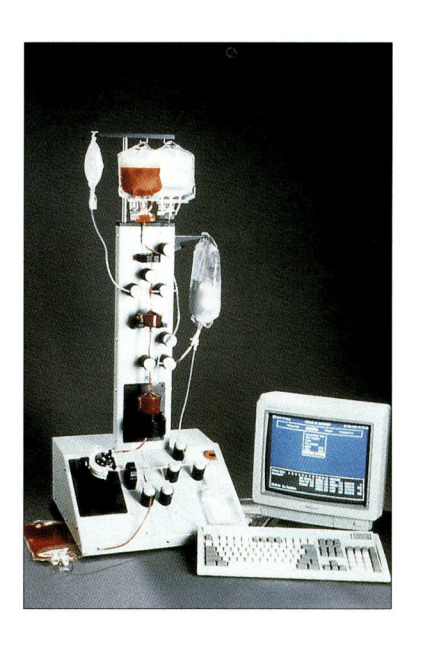

high purities will only result in a 1–2 logarithmic depletion of tumour cells (**Table 28**). The development of efficient pluripotent progenitor cell selection techniques have, however, facilitated *ex vivo* cell expansion for supportive infusions, allogeneic stem cell transplants and gene therapy.

Table 28. Enrichment of CD34+ progenitor cells does not resolve the problem of tumour cell contamination of marrow harvested for autologous transplantation.

Efficiency of CD34+ cell enrichment	Starting population		
	CD34+ cells 5×10^7 *(1%)*	*Bone marrow* 5×10^9	*Tumour cells* 5×10^7 *(1%)*
	CD34+ recovered cells	Contaminated with	
		Bone marrow	Tumour
50%	2.5×10^7	2.5×10^7	2.5×10^5
60%	3.0×10^7	2.0×10^7	2.0×10^5
70%	3.8×10^7	1.5×10^7	1.5×10^5
80%	4.0×10^7	1×10^7	1×10^5
90%	4.5×10^7	0.5×10^7	5×10^4
99%	4.95×10^7	0.05×10^7	5×10^3

The assumption has been made that 5×10^9 nucleated bone marrow cells were harvested and these are contaminated with 5×10^7 tumour cells (1%). Also, the number of CD34+ cells is assumed to be 5×10^7; 1% of the total harvested marrow population

References

Bast RC, Ritz J. Lipton JM *et al*. Elimination of leukaemic cells from human bone marrow using monoclonal antibody and complement. *Cancer Res* 1983; **43**: 1389–1394.

Favrot M, Frappez D, Maritaz O *et al*. Histological, cytological and immunological analysis are complementary for the detection of neuroblastoma cells in bone marrow. *Br J Cancer* 1986; **54**: 637–641.

Jansen FK, Blythman HE, Carriere D. Immunotoxins: Hybrid molecules combining high specificity and potent cytotoxicity. *Immunol Rev* 1982; **62**: 185–216.

Kemshead JT, Goldman A, Fritschy J *et al*. The use of panels of monoclonal antibodies in the differential diagnosis of neuroblastoma and lymphoblastic disorders. *Lancet* 1983; **1**: 12–14.

Kemshead JT. Heath L, Gibson F *et al*. Magnetic microspheres and monoclonal antibodies for the depletion of neuroblastoma cells from bone marrow. Experiences, improvements and observations. *Br J Cancer* 1986; **54**: 771–778.

Lansdorp PM, Thomas TE. Selection of human haemopoietic stem cells. In: *Bone Marrow Processing and Purging*, 1991. Ed: Gee AP. CRC Press, Boca Raton, pp. 351–362.

Moss TJ, Reynolds CP, Sather HN *et al*. Prognostic value of immunocytologic detection of bone marrow metastases in neuroblastoma. *N Engl J Med* 1991; **324**: 219–226.

Sieber F, Stuart RK, Rowley SD, Sieber-Blum M. Dye mediated photolysis of normal and neoplastic haematopoietic cells. *Leuk Res* 1987; **11**: 43–49.

Treleaven J, Gibson F, Ugelstad J *et al*. Removal of neuroblastoma cells from bone marrow with monoclonal antibodies conjugated to magnetic microspheres. *Lancet* 1984; **1**: 70–73.

Wieland DM, Wu J, Brown LE *et al*. Radiolabelled adrenergic neuron blocking agents: adrenomedullary imaging with [^{131}I]iodobenzylguanidine. *J Nucl Med* 1980; **21**: 349–353.

Yeager AM, Kaizer H, Santos GW *et al*. Autologous bone marrow transplantation in patients with acute non-lymphocytic leukaemia: A study of *ex vivo* marrow treatment with 4-hydroperoxycyclophosphamide. *N Engl J Med* 1986; **315**: 141–147.

VI Venous Access

Richard Stacey and Jacqueline Filshie

Successful bone marrow transplantation (BMT) is dependent upon repeated safe venous access for administration of drugs and supportive therapy. Access is also required for monitoring treatment progress. Patients who receive bone marrow transplantation have usually received extensive treatment beforehand and may have few usable peripheral veins (Hickman *et al.*, 1979; Thomas, 1979).

Inadequate venous access has many consequences; as venepuncture becomes more difficult, access becomes less secure, and extravasation becomes a greater risk. When the peripheral veins are exhausted central venous cannulation is attempted in patients who may already be thrombocytopenic. It may be difficult to keep patients adequately hydrated and supported with blood products and parenteral nutrition. Drug treatment may also be compromised by delays in administration (Raaf, 1985).

Initially, venous access is needed for high-dose cytoreductive therapy and for subsequent infusion of the harvested marrow. Mucositis, nausea and taste changes, which commonly occur as complications of the initial high dose cytoreductive treatment, radically interfere with calorie intake during the first month of BMT (Aker *et al.*, 1982). In Seattle, for example, the average oral intake over the first two weeks was only 150 calories per day (Sanders *et al.*, 1982). Gastrointestinal losses of fluid and electrolytes require replacement at an early stage, and total parenteral nutrition is often necessary for at least one month following transplantation (Hickman *et al.*, 1979). Neutropenic patients almost inevitably become febrile and require a variety of antibacterial and antifungal drugs that are continued until patients become apyrexial and their white cell count has recovered. Pancytopenia usually persists for 2–5 weeks after transplantation and the haemoglobin and platelet counts require support with transfusions during this period.

Multiple blood samples are necessary to monitor the progress of therapy. Some blood samples, however, should not be taken from the central venous catheter. Coagulation studies carried out on blood drawn from a Hickman type catheter, for example, are often inaccurate as a result of residual heparinization (Barton and Poon, 1986), and spuriously high aminoglycoside levels have been reported after sampling through central venous lines (Franson *et al.*, 1987). Patients will therefore still require peripheral venepunctures for these investigations as well as for some blood cultures. Finally, when engraftment has occurred, patients may need intravenous support should graft versus host disease develop. **Table 29** summarizes the uses of venous access in BMT.

Table 29. The purposes for which access to the vasculature is needed in patients undergoing bone marrow transplantation.

High-dose chemotherapy.
Marrow transfusion following TBI/high-dose chemotherapy
Blood sampling
Fluids and electrolytes
Nutritional support
Marrow support with red cells and platelet transfusions
Antimicrobial therapy
Support and treatment of graft-versus-host disease

Central venous catheters

Central venous catheters are usually placed in the superior vena cava or right atrium, via the cephalic, subclavian, external or internal jugular veins. The femoral vein has also been used for inferior vena caval access (Lazarus et al., 1990). Lines may be tunnelled if needed for a prolonged period, which enables outpatient use.

A range of lines, from single to triple lumen, is available, and in the transplant population the need for more than one line is usual since there is often a need for simultaneous infusion of incompatible drugs. Parenteral nutrition requires a dedicated line to minimize handling and to avoid frequent interruptions for other supportive therapy. Double or triple lumen lines are preferred.

Non-tunnelled lines

Most non-tunnelled lines are now made from polyurethane which, when compared to silicone, is less vulnerable to damage by most chemotherapeutic agents (Ranchere et al., 1988) but offers no advantage in terms of bacterial adherence to the catheter material (Gilsdorf et al., 1989). The stiffer materials are more likely to cause vessel wall perforation than the softer silicone catheters (Gravenstein and Blackshear, 1991) but there is wide variation in individual catheter performance. The use of non-tunnelled lines has certain disadvantages in patients requiring long-term venous access: these catheters must be removed if patients leave hospital, they are less secure, and multiple subclavian venepunctures are required if access is needed for a prolonged period.

The incidence of infection and thrombosis increases the longer lines are left in place (Gil et al., 1989). It is possible that the stiff materials used to manufacture these lines contribute to thrombus formation by causing intimal damage. Thrombus then produces areas of decreased blood flow which can form a nidus for infection, in much the same way that abnormal heart valves predispose to endocarditis (Lewis et al., 1989). This results in higher infection rates for thrombosed lines (Press et al., 1984). In a randomised prospective study comparing tunnelled and non-tunnelled lines in patients with a variety of solid and haematological tumours, the incidence of sepsis and thrombosis was comparable. Non-tunnelled lines were changed more frequently (Wagman et al., 1984). These lines may become colonized extraluminally, intraluminally or via blood-borne seeding. The use of topical antimicrobial ointments provides an element of protection against catheter-related sepsis (Maki and Band, 1981). Conversely, occlusive dressings that allow build-up of moisture are likely to be associated with an increased incidence of infection (Conly et al., 1989; Toltzis and Goldmann, 1990).

Non-tunnelled lines may be used if a short period of myelosuppression is anticipated. However, repeated subclavian venepuncture in patients who are thrombocytopenic is potentially hazardous. An alternative to contralateral venepuncture is changing the line over a guidewire if the exit site is not inflamed (Michel et al., 1988).

Tunnelled lines

Tunnelled silicone rubber right atrial catheters were first used for parenteral nutrition (Broviac et al., 1973). Special features of these catheters were the inert, antithrombogenic and flexible material. Flexibility was considered important when sclerosant infusions were used, since movement of the catheter with each heartbeat was permitted, thus minimizing contact with any single endothelial area. Recent evidence also suggests that this flexibility makes the catheter less likely to cause vessel perforation (Gravenstein and Blackshear, 1991). A subcutaneous Dacron cuff attached to the catheter was used which secured the line by obliterating part of the subcutaneous tunnel secondary to fibroblastic ingrowth. This feature had been shown to be associated with a decrease in the incidence of peritonitis when used with peritoneal dialysis catheters (**177**).

Central venous catheters are tunnelled to decrease the incidence of catheter-related sepsis by creating a barrier to extraluminal migration of microorganisms (Franceschi and Specht, 1989). There is conflicting evidence over whether or not this is achieved (Kappers-Klunne et al., 1989), presumably because catheters may also be colonized intraluminally or by blood-borne seeding (Root et al., 1988). Tunnelling of lines does not always decrease the rate of sepsis in patients receiving parenteral nutrition because infections often originate from contaminated hubs (Sitges-Serra and Linares, 1984; Linares et al., 1985). In studies comparing microorganisms isolated from

Venous Access

lines with skin exit site and hub cultures, the latter has been implicated as the portal of entry (Sitges-Serra *et al.*, 1985; Weightman *et al.*, 1988). After sufficient fibroblastic ingrowth into the cuff has occurred, extra luminal migration of microorganisms is probably halted. Exit-site infections are usually confined by the cuff (Reed, 1983; Newman *et al.*, 1989), unless they occur within 1 or 2 weeks after placement.

The use of the Broviac catheter in bone marrow transplantation was first reported in Seattle in 1976 (Riella and Scribner, 1976). Further reports soon followed (Blune *et al.*, 1978; Thomas, 1979). The catheter was modified by Hickman and his colleagues, who created a larger lumen of 1.6-mm internal diameter to facilitate blood sampling (Hickman *et al.*, 1979).

There is now a wide variety of catheters available, ranging from single to triple lumen. The catheters are made of polymeric silicone rubber impregnated with barium to make them radio-opaque. The different catheters have many names, although in practice they are all referred to as Hickman lines.

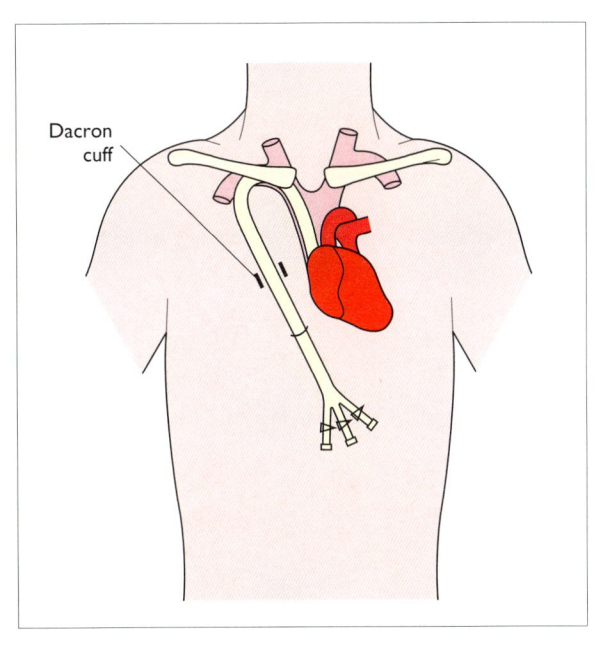

177 Correct placement of Hickman line with Dacron cuff and tip in the mid-atrium.

Preparation

Preoperative identification of lung and mediastinal pathology, cardiac disease, coagulopathy and bacteraemia is necessary to minimize complications. In thrombocytopenic patients, line placement is possible with aggressive platelet support. At the Royal Marsden Hospital, six to eight pools of platelets are given if the platelet count is less than $50 \times 10^9/l$. Catheters should not be inserted if there is uncontrolled bacteraemia, since this predisposes to tunnel infections, although fever, neutropenia, and infection at other sites are not contraindications (Press *et al.*, 1984). Prophylactic antibiotics are commonly administered but may they be unnecessary (Ranson *et al.*, 1990) since the majority of infections occur secondary to contamination at a later stage.

Insertion

The aim at insertion is to place the catheter tip in the right atrium, or if this causes arrhythmias, in the superior vena cava (**178, 179**). Early techniques involved venous cut-down onto the cephalic vein

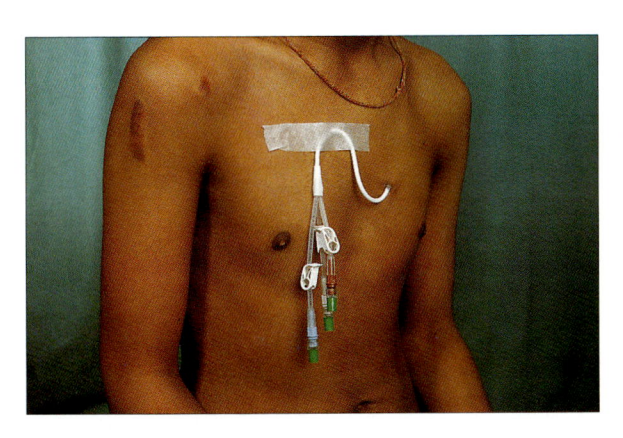

178 Patient with Hickman line *in situ*.

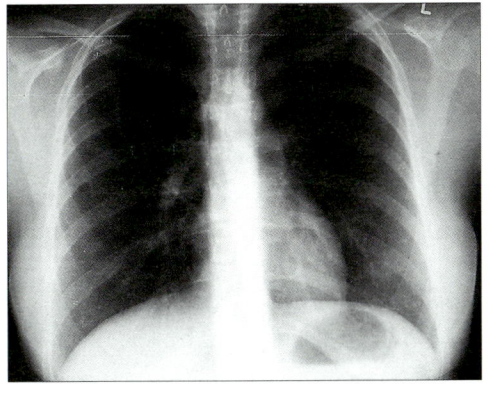

179 X-ray showing correct siting of Hickman line.

Bone Marrow Transplantation

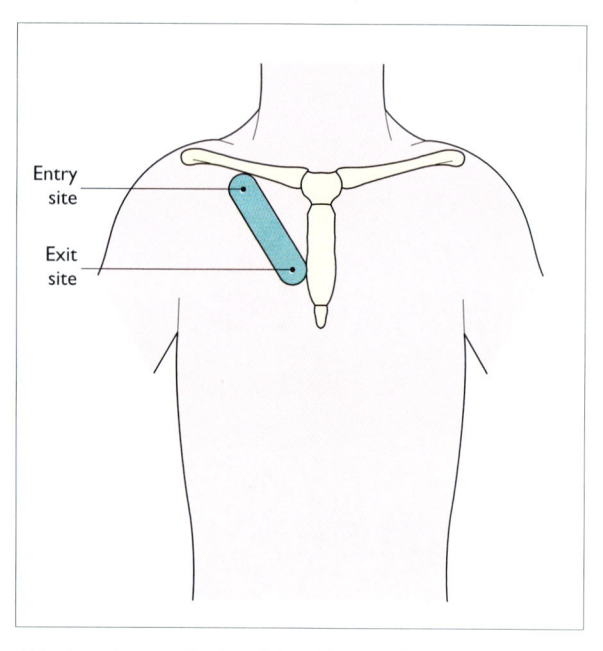

180 Local anaesthetic is liberally introduced into the subcutaneous tissues as illustrated by the shaded area.

(Heimbach and Ivy, 1976), the external jugular vein (Hawkins and Nelson, 1982), or the internal jugular vein (Hickman *et al.*, 1979). The cephalic vein is usually too small for the large multilumen catheters and may have been obliterated by phlebitis in those who have had previous chemotherapy.

When catheters are inserted directly into the vein without a guidewire, the catheter is often difficult to manipulate into the superior vena cava. At the Royal Marsden Hospital (Sutton, Surrey, UK), catheters are inserted percutaneously, using a Seldinger technique, directly into the subclavian vein. A split sheath introducer, adapted from pacemaker insertion sets, is used for placement of the catheter. Considerable savings in theatre time can be made because positioning of the catheter is much easier when introduced into the superior vena cava through a sheath.

Surgical cut down is used in small children below the age of about 6 years as the large stiff dilators used in the percutaneous method are potentially hazardous in this age group.

When superior vena caval obstruction from thrombosis or compression is present, catheters placed in the superior vena cava commonly malfunction (Raaf, 1985). In this situation, inferior vena caval placement, often via the femoral vein, is necessary. Femoral lines have been safely maintained in the groins of marrow recipients without excess infection (Lazarus *et al.*, 1990)

Insertion is carried out in the operating theatre under aseptic conditions with fluoroscopic control and ECG monitoring (Stacey *et al.*, 1991). After preparation of the skin from the chin to below the nipples with antiseptic solution (0.5% chlorhexidine in spirit or povidone-iodine), the skin is anaesthetized. A relatively large volume (30–40 ml) of 0.25% bupivicaine or 0.5% lidocaine with 1 in 200 000 adrenalin is used to distend the tissue planes. Adrenalin is used to minimize capillary bleeding and limit local anaesthetic absorption (**180**).

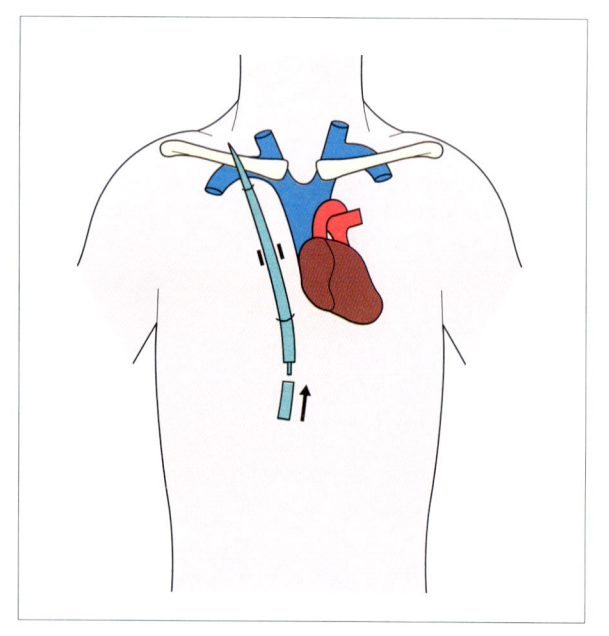

181 The Hickman line is tunnelled subcutaneously using a Redivac introducer.

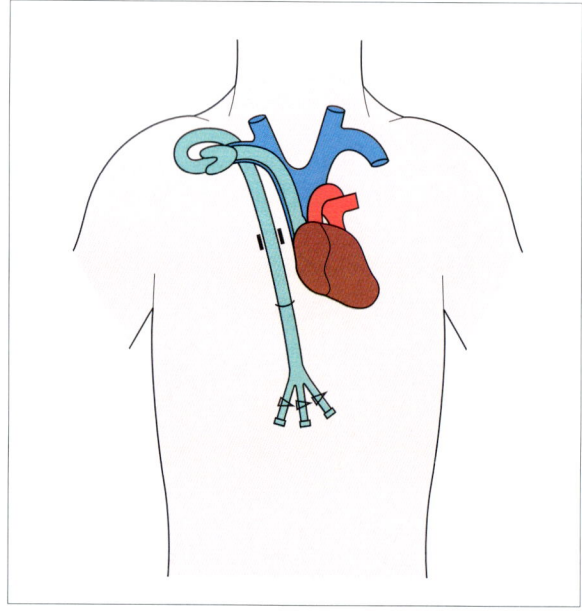

182 The Hickman catheter is quickly and carefully threaded through the lumen of the split-sheath introducer.

Insertion too close to the clavicle can result in damage to the split sheath introducer, leading to difficulty threading the catheter. An approach which is too medial may result in sharp angulation and kinking of the introducer sheath under the clavicle (Robertson *et al.*, 1989). It will also predispose to pinching between the clavicle and the first rib which could result in catheter malfunction or breakage (Reed *et al.*, 1989).

The vein is identified with an 18 gauge needle through which the J-wire is introduced. Correct placement of the wire may be assumed if ectopics beats are seen on the ECG, or the wire vibrates with the heartbeat. An image intensifier is used to confirm that the wire is positioned correctly, and to aid manipulation if it is not.

A variety of forceps may be used to form the tunnel (Cohen and Wood, 1982) or a metal rod may be passed, which is less traumatic (Kirkemo and Johnston, 1982). A Redivac drain introducer may be used to pull the catheter through from a 5-mm incision at the lower end of the tunnel, to a similar one cut down onto the guidewire at the insertion site (**181**). The tunnel should be kept medial, in the immobile tissues near the sternum. This prevents catheter retraction when patients sit up from lying down, a particular problem in women with pendulous breasts (Wagman and Neifield, 1986; Moorman *et al.*, 1987).

The Dacron cuff is placed in a mid-tunnel position at least 3–5 cm from the exit site. There is the danger of cuff extrusion if it is positioned too close to the exit site (Hayward *et al.*, 1990). The catheter is then cut to the desired length over the surface marking of the right atrium, at the third or fourth rib interspace. The tip should not be bevelled as this makes the line more likely to lie against the vessel wall, resulting in positional functioning and possibly perforation. Once cut, the lumens of the catheter are primed with heparinized saline. The tract is dilated over the guidewire using dilators that have been curved to suit the lie of the blood vessel entered. For larger catheters a series of graded dilators is used. After lubrication with liquid paraffin the split sheath is placed in the superior vena cava over the dilator. This can be painful if local anaesthetic has not been used liberally under the clavicle. In small children, the insertion of the dilator may be performed with continuous fluoroscopy. The dilator is advanced no further than the upper superior vena cava, avoiding kinking of the guidewire and distortion of the mediastinum. The sheath is then advanced over the dilator so that its tip lies just beyond that of the dilator.

On removal of the dilator, the catheter is passed through the sheath, using non-toothed forceps (**182**). After correct positioning of the catheter, the sheath is removed by splitting the sides apart. The two incisions are then closed with a stitch to each. The lower stitch is extended to secure the line and should remain in place until there is an adequate fibroblastic response to secure the catheter.

Duration of use

In a series of 357 bone marrow recipients from Seattle (Petersen *et al.*, 1986) the median duration of use was 93 days with a range of 16–209 days. Of the catheters inserted, 40% were kept until the end of treatment and 16% were removed for complications. The decision to remove a catheter depends upon the gravity of the complication, the need for the catheter to remain, the risks of inserting a new one, and the overall life expectancy of the patient.

Complications

Complications associated with right atrial catheters may be divided into those occurring at insertion or soon after, or those occurring late due to the presence of the line (**Tables 30, 31**).

Bone Marrow Transplantation

Table 30. Complications related to insertion.

Venous cutdown	Haemomediastinum	*Dilator and split-sheath insertion*
Inadequate size or sclerosis of vein	Nerve injury	Guidewire displacement
Misplacement of catheter		Damaged or kinked introducing
	Guidewire	sheath
Subclavian venepuncture	Arrhythmias	Perforation of vessel or
Haematoma	Ectopic placement	mediastinum
Venous laceration		
Arterial puncture	*Tunnel*	*Catheter insertion*
Pneumothorax	Bleeding	Arrhythmias
Haemothorax		Air embolus

Table 31. Complications related to the continued presence of the line.

Infection	Superior vena caval perforation
Exit site	Positional functioning
Bacteraemia	Catheter breakage
Tunnel	Catheter embolization
Septic thrombophlebitis	Arrhythmia
Endocarditis	Catheter migration
Thrombosis	Catheter ballooning and rupture
Fibrin sheath	Extravasation
Catheter occlusion	Catheter damage
Large-vessel thrombosis	Cuff extrusion
Right-atrial thrombosis	Accidental removal
Pulmonary thromboembolism	

Insertion-related complications

There is always a risk of pleural injury with subclavian venepuncture. Pneumothorax occurs in 0.7–6% of subclavian lines (Lechner *et al.*, 1989) (**183, 184**).

Varying amounts of bleeding may result from injury to the subclavian vein or artery, or from perforation of the vessel with the dilator. Depending on the extent of the damage, and competence of haemostasis, outcome will vary from haematoma to life-threatening exsanguination. Bleeding may also occur into the tunnel. The perforating branches of the internal mammary artery are at risk from the tunnelling device if the tunnel is not kept in the superficial tissues.

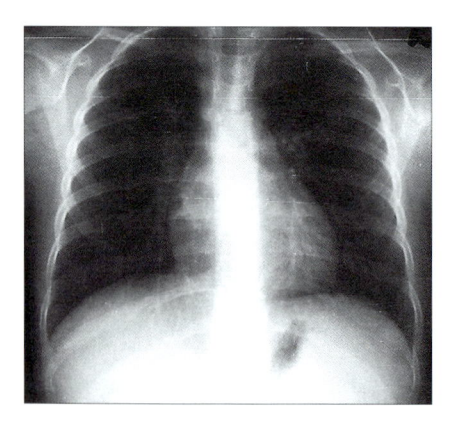

183 PA X-ray of the chest of a child prior to insertion of Hickman line.

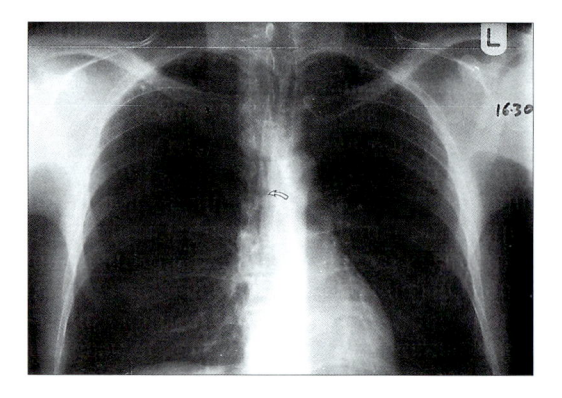

184 X-ray showing pneumothorax which occurred after insertion of a Hickman line.

Haematomas increase infection risk (Reed *et al.*, 1983; Robertson *et al.*, l989) and may also allow seeding of tumour cells (Amiraian *et al.*, 1988; Davidson, 1990).

Arrhythmias may be precipitated by the guidewire (Stuart *et al.*, 1990) or catheter. These are rarely dangerous but if they occur it is prudent to leave the tip of the catheter in the superior vena cava rather than the right atrium.

The guidewire does not always travel down to the heart and may require screening into the correct position. If the dilator is not curved to suite the lie of the blood vessel entered it may displace the guidewire into the opposite subclavian vein.

The introducing sheath may be damaged on the under surface of the clavicle and may kink when the dilator is removed. Either may result in difficulty passing the catheter, with the concomitant risk of air embolus or haemorrhage.

Infection

There is much confusion when talking about infected lines because of imprecise definition of infection (Kropek and Daschner, 1990), difficulty in making an exact diagnosis unless the line is removed (Maki *et al.*, 1977), and a tendency to attribute any episode of bacteraemia to the line. Bacteraemia with no obvious source is extremely common in neutropenic patients, and the majority of these bacteraemias are not catheter-related (Newman *et al.*, 1989). However, infection is, without doubt, a troublesome complication of long-term right atrial catheters (Guenier *et al.*, 1989). In a review of 1088 catheters in an unselected oncology population there were 0.14 catheter infections per 100 catheter-days. Of these, 45% were exit site, 20% tunnel and 31% bacteraemic, with a 3.5% incidence of septic thrombophlebitis (Press *et al.*, 1984). Chances of infection increase the more a line is handled, and poor catheter care is the most important preventable factor. It is possible to reduce infection rate by implementing a meticulous handling technique, and possibly by less frequent flushing and changing of giving sets. Microbiological evidence from exit site and hub culture (Sitges-Serra and Linares, 1984; Linares *et al.*, 1985; Sitges-Serra and Linares, 1985) suggests that hubs are usually the source of microorganisms when bacteraemia is associated with tunnelled lines. Production of haematomas at insertion, and insertion of lines into bacteraemic patients both predispose to tunnel infections. Thrombosis is strongly associated with bacteraemic infections and infections are commoner in neutropenic patients (Press *et al.*, 1984). Patients with haematological malignancies tend to have higher rates of infection than those with solid tumours (Landay *et al.*, 1984). Catheter damage may also lead to bacterial inoculation and subsequent sepsis (Schuman *et al.*, 1985).

The organisms implicated in line sepsis are the coagulase-negative staphylococci (Schuman *et al.*, 1985; Kappers-Klunne *et al.*, 1989). The success of this organism is due to its prevalence on the skin (Rotstein *et al.*, 1988), its ability to adhere to and degrade catheter materials (Gilsdorf *et al.*, 1989), and the production of a protective slime. However, it should not be assumed that all bacteraemias due to this organism originate from the line as it is often isolated from the gut (Rotstein *et al.*, 1988) and respiratory tract (Press *et al.*, 1984) in the neutropenic population (**Table 32**). It is often stressed that when neutropenic patients develop fever or bacteraemia, the right atrial catheter should not be removed immediately even if it is thought to be the source of infection (Raaf, 1985). Aggressive treatment with broad-spectrum antibiotics given through the catheter will often salvage the line (Newman *et al.*, 1989). *Staphylococcus aureus* (Dugdale and Ramsey, 1990) and fungal infections (Hendrick and Wilkinson, 1985) may be resistant to treatment. Exit site infections are well localized by the Dacron cuff and will often resolve with a combination of antibiotics, daily cleaning and povidone-iodine ointment (Newman *et al.*, 1989). Tunnel infections are difficult to treat and usually require catheter removal. Osteomyelitis of the clavicle has been reported in one patient with a tunnel infection (Kravitz, 1989).

It is often recommended that the catheter be removed if bacteraemia or fever persists despite treatment, if there is associated thrombus, or fungal infection (Abrahm and Mullen, 1982; Hendrick and Wilkinson, 1985). Some such situations may respond to treatment. Persistent bacteraemia may be due to infected catheter-associated thrombus. This has been successfully treated without removing the catheter with a combination of antibiotic and fibrinolytic therapy (Schuman *et al.*, 1985; Lewis *et al.*, 1989). If

Table 32. Microorganisms involved in catheter related infections from a study of over one million catheter-days (Press *et al.*,1984).

Staphylococcus epidermidis	54%
Staphylococcus aureus	20%
Candida spp.	7%
Pseudomonas spp.	6%
Corynebacterium	5%
Klebsiella spp.	4%
Enterococcus spp.	4%

this therapy is used, it is important to establish therapeutic antibiotic levels before fibrinolytic therapy is started, which may prevent seeding of microorganisms throughout the circulation.

Fungal infections may also be the cause of persistent fever, and amphotericin B has been used with good effect in febrile neutropenic patients who failed to improve after 5 days broad spectrum antibiotics (Lazarus *et al.*, 1984). Endocarditis is an occasional complication (Quinn *et al.*, 1986) but it occurred in only 5% of bone marrow recipients in a recent prospective study (Martino *et al.*, 1990).

Thrombosis

Intravascular fibrin formation occurs at an early stage and is often present by 48 hours. It was noted in 78% of patients when random venograms were performed on removal of the catheter (Wagman *et al.*, 1984). Fibrin may form a sleeve around the catheter causing infused fluids to track up alongside it and exit from the vessel alongside the catheter (Lewis *et al.*, 1989). This association with extravasation has been noted by others (Gemlo *et al.*, 1988; Anderson *et al.*, 1989) (**185–187**).

Catheter occlusion occurs at a rate of about 0.6 per 1000 catheter days (Bagnall *et al.*, 1989) although it varies with the size of the catheter. Similar incidences occur whether or not routine flushing is performed. Clots may be aspirated from the catheter in 30% of samples taken from heparinized lines (Anderson *et al.*, 1987), and it is possible that disodium EDTA (20mg/ml) may become an alternative to flushing the line. This has the advantage of having bactericidal properties against *Staphylococcus epidermidis*, the most common infecting organism (Root *et al.*, 1988). It has been suggested that measurement of catheter resistance can be used to detect partial occlusion (Stokes *et al.*, 1989). When faced with an occluded catheter, forceful injection with a small syringe may result in catheter rupture (Wagman *et al.*, 1989). An effective treatment is to instil either streptokinase (250 U/ml) or urokinase (5000 U/ml) in a volume equal to the catheter dead space (Lawson *et al.*, 1982). If this fails, a low dose infusion is usually effective (Bagnall *et al.*, 1989).

Large-vessel thrombosis is a very common complication in marrow transplantation recipients (Haire

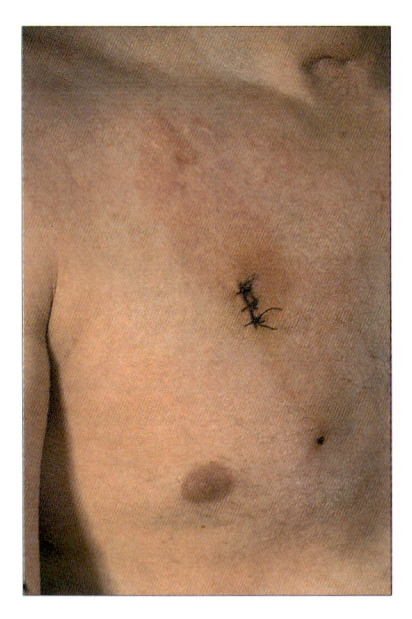

185 Inflamed skin around an area where chemotherapy has extravasated into the subcutaneous tissue of a Hickman catheter track.

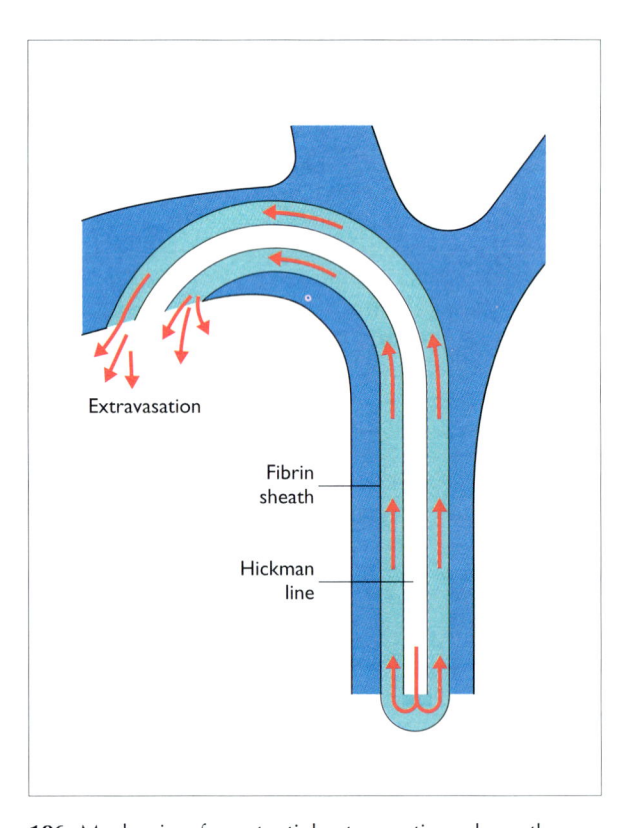

186 Mechanism for potential extravasation: chemotherapy injected down a Hickman line may track back along fibrin sheath and spill into tissues where the line leaves the vein.

et al., 1990). Venograms performed on all patients identified 62% with intravascular thrombus, and only one-third of patients with totally occluded subclavian veins were symptomatic (Haire *et al.*, 1991). Superior vena caval obstruction and lesser degrees of thrombosis have been treated with urokinase while the right atrial catheter was retained (Lewis *et al.*, 1989; Meister *et al.*, 1989; Moss *et al.*, 1989). Therapy is more effective if instituted early and if the central venous catheter is retained (Gray *et al.*, 1991). High-dose fibrinolytic therapy is used. An example of an effective regimen is streptokinase (250 000 U) to load followed by 100 000 U/hour for 24–48 hours.

Right-atrial thrombi have been described (Blune *et al.*, 1978; Reed *et al.*, 1985; Williams *et al.*, 1988), and can reach dangerously large sizes that obstruct the tricuspid valve (Benbow *et al.*, 1987; Chakravarthy *et al.*, 1987). Pulmonary thromboembolism has been described as a result of Hickman-catheter-associated thrombosis (Leiby *et al.*, 1989). In a population of patients with solid tumours receiving infusion chemotherapy via Hickman catheters, use of a daily dose of 1 mg warfarin was found to significantly reduce the incidence of large-vessel thrombosis without producing any detectable change in coagulation studies (Bern *et al.*, 1990).

Other complications

Superior vena caval perforation into the right mediastinum has occurred with left-sided lines (Russell *et al.*, 1987). All lines were bevelled and it is likely that this, plus intravascular thrombus in 2 of the 3 cases, caused the tip to lie against the vessel wall in an area of decreased blood flow, thus allowing sclerosant infusions to erode the vessel. **188** shows a haemomediastinum, the result of puncture of the vasculature during line insertion.

Catheter function may be dependent on patient position, and this may be due to the catheter tip impinging on the vessel wall, as happens if the tip is bevelled (Thomas and Schnett, 1988). Alternatively, an excessive length of catheter in the right atrium may bend and impinge on the endocardium (Reed *et al.*, 1983). Shoulder girdle movements may result in pinching of the catheter between the first rib and clavicle, which initially causes catheter malfunction and may eventually lead to catheter breakage (Franceschi and Specht, 1989) with possible embolization (**189, 190**). The retrieval of embolized fragments is possible (Mehta *et al.*, 1989) with right-heart catheterization using a snare biopsy forceps or a wire basket that can be closed around the fragment. Broken fragments should be removed as soon as possible since the fragment tends to move through the right heart into the pulmonary circulation.

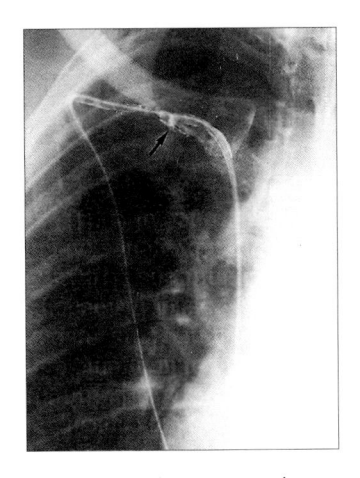

187 X-ray showing Hickman catheter *in situ*. The arrow indicates the point at which extravasation has occurred.

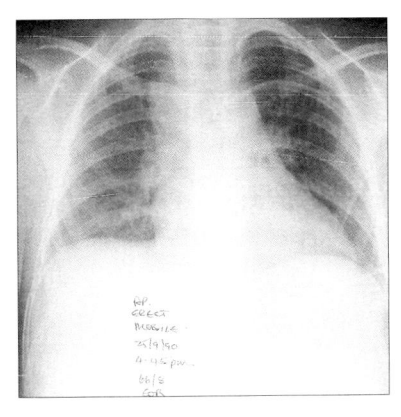

188 This AP chest X-ray taken postoperatively shows a haemomediastinum. The catheter was successfully sited in the left side.

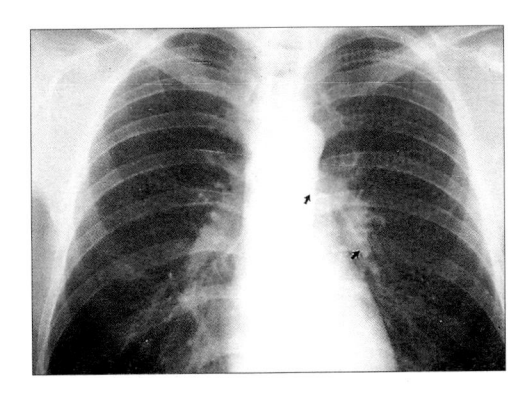

189 X-ray showing the amputated end of a Hickman line (arrows), which has migrated into the descending branch of the left main pulmonary artery.

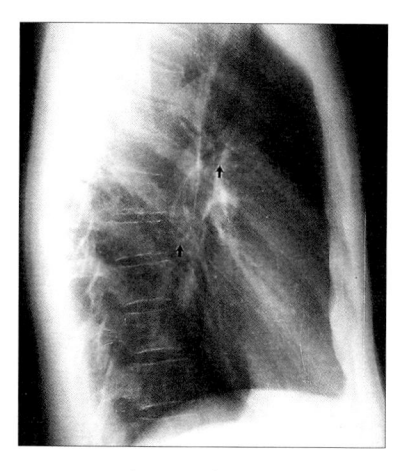

190 Lateral view of amputated Hickman line shown in **189**.

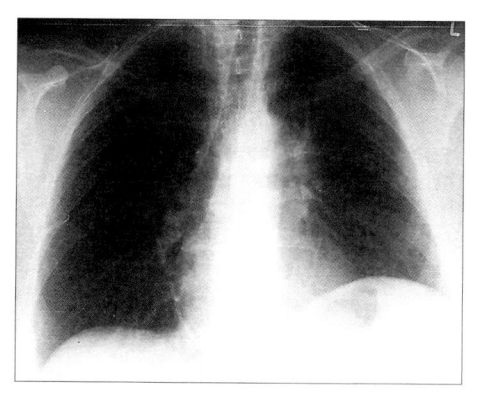

191 The Hickman tip has been directed superiorly into the right internal jugular vein in a patient with consolidation in the right upper lobe.

Arrhythmias have been reported with the tip of the catheter positioned in the right atrium, and pulling the catheter back led to resolution (Spearing et al., 1987). Some authorities recommend that the catheter tip be left just above the right atrium in order to avoid arrhythmias (Reed et al., 1983). Catheter tip migration was noted in 10% of one series (Hendrick and Wilkinson, 1985) (**191**). Lines that have migrated may be hooked back down into the superior vena cava by a pigtail catheter passed up from the femoral vein (Walker et al., 1988). Alternatively, the subclavian puncture site may be re-opened and the catheter pulled back and manipulated with fluoroscopic guidance (Wagman and Neifield, 1986).

Catheter ballooning and rupture (Wagman and Neifield, 1986; Wagman et al., 1989) are associated with forceful injections into an occluded catheter. These may occur externally or beneath the skin, resulting in pain and possibly extravasation.

Extravasation is a serious complication which occurs in association with the split sheath method of insertion (Gemlo et al., 1988). Venous thrombosis (Watterson et al., 1988) or fibrin sheath formation usually precede extravasation which may be caused by excessive bolus flushing of clogged catheters where the path of least resistance is alongside the catheter into the tissues (Gemlo et al., 1988).

Some catheters are damaged by cutting with scissors while removing dressings or broken by traction. These problems occurred in 7% of catheters in one series (Franceschi and Specht, 1989). Repair kits exist for most of the currently marketed catheters.

Cuff extrusion usually occurs in the early stages before the Dacron cuff has been properly anchored (Thomas and Sinnett, 1988). It is more likely to occur if the tunnel is short or the cuff is left close to the exit site. Reported rates vary from 0.9% (Raaf, 1985) to 6% (Wagman et al., 1984).

Accidental removal due to traction accidents is more common in children (Petersen, 1986) and usually occurs shortly after insertion in 1–3% of cases (Raaf, 1985).

Implantable devices

In order to decrease infection risk and minimize the limitation of patient activities, the access point of these devices is buried under the skin. The use of subcutaneous ports was first reported in the early 1980s (Bothe et al., 1984; Gyves et al., 1984). There are various subcutaneous devices available consisting of a reservoir with a silicone rubber diaphragm attached to a Hickman like catheter (Reed et al., 1989). Access is via a Huber needle, which cuts a slit, rather than taking a core, through the skin and silicone diaphragm. Infections are much less common than with Hickman catheters but thrombosis occurs with a similar frequency (Guenier et al., 1989). Skin puncture is necessary, which may cause bleeding in thrombocytopenic patients thus increasing the risk of infection. Needle dislodgement and extravasation may occur, as may a limited fluid infusion rate (Newman et al., 1989). Most of these devices are single lumen only and may be better suited to patients needing limited access for short periods of time (Reed et al., 1989).

References

Abrahm J, Mullen J. A prospective study of prolonged central venous access in leukaemia. *J Am Med Assoc* 1982; **248**: 2868–2873.

Aker SN, Cheney CL, Sanders JE, *et al* Nutritional support in marrow graft recipients with single versus double lumen right atrial catheters. *Exp Hematol* 1982; **10**: 732–737.

Amiraian R, Penn TE, Hamann S *et al*. Leukaemic dermal infiltrates as a complication of central venous catheter placement. *Cancer* 1988; **62**: 2223–2225.

Anderson AJ, Krasnow SH, Boyer MW *et al*. Hickman catheter clots: a common occurrence despite daily heparin flushing. *Cancer Treat Rep* 1987; **71**: 651– 653.

Anderson AJ, Krasnow SH, Boyer MW *et al*. Thrombosis: the major Hickman catheter complication in patients with solid tumours. *Chest* 1989; **95**: 71–75.

Bagnall HA, Gomperts E, Atkinson JB. Continuous infusion of low dose urokinase in the treatment of central venous catheter thrombosis in infants and children. *Paediatrics* 1989; **83**: 963–966.

Barton JC, Poon MC. Coagulation testing of Hickman catheter blood in patients with acute leukaemia. *Arch Intern Med* 1986; **146**: 2165–2169.

Benbow EW, Love EM, Love HG *et al*. Massive right atrial thrombus associated with a Chiari network and a Hickman catheter. *Am J Clin Path* 1987; **88**: 243–248.

Bern M, Lokich J, Wallach S *et al*. Very low doses of warfarin can prevent thrombosis in central venous catheters. *Ann Intern Med* 1990; **112**: 423–428.

Blune KG, Bross KJ, Riihinaki DU *et al*. The use of a right atrial catheter in bone marrow transplantation for acute leukaemia. *Exp Haemat* 1978; **6**: 636–638.

Bothe A, Piccione W, Ambrosino JJ *et al*. Implantable central venous access system. *Am J Surg* 1984; **147**: 565–569.

Broviac JW, Cole JJ, Scribner BH. A silicone rubber atrial catheter for prolonged parenteral nutrition. *Surg Gynecol Obstet* 1973; **136**: 602–606.

Chakravarthy A, Edwards WO, Fleming CR. Fatal tricuspid valve obstruction due to a large infected thrombus attached to a Hickman catheter. *J Am Med Assoc* 1987; **257**: 801–803.

Cohen AM, Wood WC. Simplified technique for placement of long-term central venous silicone catheters. *Surg Gynecol Obstet* 1982; **154**: 721–724.

Conly J, Grieves K, Peters B. A prospective, randomised study comparing transparent and dry gauze dressing for central venous catheters. *J Infect Dis* 1989; **159**: 310–319.

Davidson N. Tumour metastasis from multiple myeloma in Hickman catheter tract. *Eur J Surg Oncol* 1990; **16**: 170–171.

Dugdale D, Ramsey P. *Staphylococcus aureus* bacteraemia in patients with Hickman catheters. *Am J Med* 1990; **89**: 137–141.

Franceschi D, Specht MA. Implantable venous access device. *J Cardiovasc Surg* 1989; **30**: 124–129.

Franson TR, Ritch PS, Quebbenan EJ. Aminoglycoside serum concentration sampling via central venous catheters: potential source of clinical errors. *J Parenter Enter Nutr* 1987; **11**: 77–79.

Gemlo BT, Rayner AA, Swanson RJ *et al*. A serious complication of the split sheath introducer technique for venous access. *Arch Surg* 1988; **123**: 490–492.

Gil RT, Kruse JA, Thill-Baharuzian MC *et al*. Triple versus single lumen central venous catheters. A prospective study in a critically ill population. *Arch Intern Med* 1989; **149**: 1139–1143.

Gilsdorf JR, Wilson K, Beals TF. Bacterial colonisation of intravenous catheter materials *in vitro* and *in vivo*. *Surgery* 1989; **106**: 37–44.

Gravenstein N, Blackshear R. *In vitro* evaluation of relative perforating potential of central venous catheters: comparison of materials, selected models, number of lumens, and angles of incidence to simulated membrane. *J Clin Monit* 1991; **7**: 1–6.

Gray BH, Olin JW, Graor RA *et al*. Safety and efficacy of thrombolytic therapy for superior vena cava syndrome. *Chest* 1991; **99**: 54–59.

Guenier C, Ferreira J, Pector JC. Prolonged venous access in cancer patients. *Eur J Surg Oncol* 1989; **15**: 553–555.

Gyves JW, Ensminger WD, Niederhuber JE. A totally implanted injection port system for blood sampling and chemotherapy administration. *J Am Med Assoc* 1984; **251**: 2538–2541.

Haire W, Lieberman R, Edney J *et al*. Hickman catheter-induced thoracic vein thrombosis. Frequency and long-term sequelae in patients receiving high-dose chemotherapy and marrow transplantation. *Cancer* 1990; **66**: 900–908.

Haire W, Lieberman R, Lund G *et al*. Thrombotic complications of silicone rubber catheters during autologous marrow and peripheral stem cell transplantation: prospective comparison of Hickman and Groshong catheters. *Bone Marrow Transplant* 1991; **7**: 57–59.

Hawkins J, Nelson EW. Percutaneous placement of Hickman catheters for prolonged venous access. *Am J Surg* 1982; **144**: 624–626.

Hayward S, Ledgerwood A, Lucas C. The fate of 100 prolonged venous access devices. *Am Surg* 1990; **56**: 515–519.

Heimbach OM, Ivey TD. Technique for placement of a permanent home hyperalimentation catheter. *Surg Gynecol Obstet* 1976; **143**: 635–636.

Hendrick AM, Wilkinson A. Infective complications of prolonged central venous (Hickman) catheterisation., *South Med J* 1985; **78**: 639–642.

Hickman RO, Buckner CD, Clift RA *et al*. A modified right atrial catheter for access to the venous system in marrow transplant recipients. *Surg Gynaecol Obstet* 1979; **148**: 871–875.

Kappers-Klunne MC, Degenerb JE, Stijnen T *et al*. Complications from long-term indwelling central venous catheters in haematologic patients with special reference to infection. *Cancer* 1989; **64**: 1747–l752.

Kirkemo A, Johnston MR. Percutaneous subclavian vein placement of the Hickman catheter. *Surgery* 1982; **91**: 349–351.

Kravitz AB. Osteomyelitis of the clavicle secondary to infected Hickman catheter. *J Parenter Enter Nutr* 1989; **13**: 426–427.

Kropek A, Daschner F. Intravascular device related infections. In: *Ballières Clinical Anaesthesiology*, 1990. Eds: Stoutenbeck C, VanSaene H. Infection and the Anaesthetist pp. 108–122.

Landay Z, Rotstein C, Lucey J et al. Hickman-Broviac catheter use in cancer patients. *J Surg Oncol* 1984; **26**: 215–218.

Lawson M, Bottino JC, Hurtubise MR et al. The use of urokinase to restore the patency of occluded central venous catheters. *Am J Intravenous Ther Clin Nutr* 1982; **9**: 29–32.

Lazarus H, Creger R, Bloom A et al. Percutaneous placement of femoral central venous catheter in patients undergoing transplantation of bone marrow. *Surg Gynecol Obstet* 1990; **170**: 403–6.

Lazarus HM, Lowder JN, Anderson JM et al. A prospective randomised trial of central venous catheter removal versus intravenous Amphotericin B in febrile neutropenic patients. *J Parenter Enter Nutr* 1984; **8**: 501–505.

Lechner P, Anderhuber F, Tesch NP. Anatomical basis for a safe method of subclavian venipuncture. *Surg Radiol Anat* 1989; **11**: 91–95.

Leiby J, Purcell H, DeMaria J et al. Pulmonary embolism as a result of Hickman catheter related thrombosis. *Am J Med* 1989; **86**: 228–231.

Lewis JA, LaFrance R, Bower-RH. Treatment of an infected silicone right atrial catheter with combined fibrinolytic and antibiotic therapy. *J Parenter Enter Nutr* 1989; **13**: 92–98.

Linares-J, SitgesSerra A, Garau J et al. Pathogenesis of catheter sepsis: a prospective study with quantitative and semiquantitative cultures of catheter hub and segments. *J Clin Microbiol* 1985; **21**: 357–360.

Maki D, Weise C, Sarafin H. A semiquantitive culture method for identifying intravenous catheter related infection. *N Eng J Med* 1977; **296**: 1305–1309.

Maki D, Band J. A comparitive study of polyantibiotic and iodophor ointments in prevention of vascular catheter-related infection. *Am J Med* 1981; **70**: 739–744.

Martino P, Micozzi A, Venditti M, et al. Catheter-related right-sided endocarditis in bone marrow transplant recipients. *Rev Infect Dis* 1990; **12**: 250–257.

Mehta J, Archie D, Kincaid W et al. Percutaneous retrieval of a Hickman catheter fragment. *J Tenn Med Assoc* 1989; **82**: 129–130.

Meister FL, Mclavglin TF, Tenney RD et al. Urokinase. A cost effective alternative treatment of superior vena caval thrombosis and obstruction. *Arch Inter Med* 1989; **149**: 1209–1210.

Michel LA, Bradpiece HA, Randour P et al. Safety of central venous catheter change over guidewire for suspected catheter-related sepsis. A prospective randomised trial. *Int Surg* 1988; **73**: 180–186.

Moorman DW, Horattas MC, Wright D et al. Hickman catheter dislodgement due to pendulous breasts. *J Parenter Enter Nutrition* 1987; **11**: 502–504.

Moss JF, Wagman LD, Riihimaki DU et al. Central venous thrombosis related to the silastic Hickman Broviac catheter in an oncologic population *J Parenter Enter Nutr* 1989; **13**: 397–400.

Newman KA, Reed WP, Biustanante CI et al. Venous access devices utilised in association with intensive cancer chemotherapy. *Eur J Cancer Clin Oncol* 1989; **25**: 1375–1378.

Petersen FB, Clift R, Hickman RO et al. Hickman catheter complications in marrow transplant recipients. *J Parenter Enter Nutr* 1986; **10**: 58–62.

Press OW, Ramsey PG, Larson EB et al. Hickman catheter infections in patients with malignancies. *Medicine (Baltimore)* 1984; **63**: 189–200.

Quinn JP, Counts GW, Meyers JD. Intracardiac infections due to coagulase negative staphylococcus associated with Hickman catheters. *Cancer* 1986; **57**: 1079–1082.

Raaf JH. Results from use of 826 vascular access devices in cancer patients. *Cancer* 1985; **55**: 1312–1321.

Ranchere JY, Tabone E, Latour JF. Polyurethene catheters and antineoplastic chemotherapy. An experimental study. *Ann Fr Anesth Reanim* 1988; **7**: 517–519.

Ranson M, Oppenheim B, Jackson A et al. Double-blind placebo controlled study of vancomycin prophylaxis for central venous catheter insertion in cancer patients. *J Hosp Infect* 1990; **15**: 95–102.

Reed WP, Newman KA, DeJongh CA et al. Prolonged venous access for chemotherapy by means of the Hickman catheter. *Cancer* 1983; **52**:185–192.

Reed WP, Newman KA, Tenney J. Autopsy findings after prolonged catheterisation of the right atrium for chemotherapy in acute leukaemia. *Surg Gynecol Obstet* 1985; **160**: 417–420.

Reed WP, Newman KA, Wade JC. Choosing an appropriate implantable device for long-term venous access. *Euro J Cancer Clin Oncol* 1989; **25**: 1383–1391.

Riella MC, Scribner BH. Five years` experience with a right atrial catheter for prolonged parenteral nutrition at home. *Surg Gynaecol Obstet* 1976; **143**: 205–208.

Robertson LJ, Mauro MA, Jaques-PF. Radiologic placement of Hickman catheters. *Radiology* 1989; **170**: 1007–1009.

Root JL, McIntyre OR, Jacobs NJ, et al. Inhibitory effects of disodium EDTA upon growth of staphylococcus epidermis *in vitro*: Relation to infection prophylaxis of Hickman catheters. *Antimicrob Agents Chemotherapy* 1988; **32**: 1627–1631.

Rotstein C, Higby D, Killion K et al. Relationship of surveillance culture to bacteraemia and fungaemia in bone marrow transplant recipients with Hickman or Broviac catheters. *J Surg Oncol* 1988; **39**: 154–158.

Russell SJ, Giles FJ, Edwards D et al. Perforation of superior vena cava by indwelling central venous catheters. *Lancet* 1987; **i**: 568–569.

Sanders JE, Hickman RO, Aker S et al. Experience with double lumen right atrial catheters. *J Parenter Enter Nutr* 1982; **6**: 95–99.

Schuman ES, Winters V, Gross GF et al. Management of Hickman catheter sepsis. *Am J Surg* 1985; **149**: 627–628.

Sitges-Serra A, Linares-J. Tunnels do not protect against venous catheter related sepsis. *Lancet* 1984; **i**: 459–460.

Sitges-Serra A, Linares-J, Garau-J. Catheter sepsis: The clue is the hub. *Surgery* 1985; **97**: 355–357.

Spearing RL, Mackie EJ, Wright-JG. Ventricular arrythmias despite an apparently correctly placed Hickman-Broviac catheter. *Lancet* 1987; **i**: 924.

Stacey R, Filshie J, Skewes D. Percutaneous insertion of Hickman type catheters. *Br J Hosp Med* 1991; **46**: 396–398.

Stokes DC, Rao BN, Mirro J et al. Early detection and simplified management of obstructed Hickman and Broviac catheters. *J Pediatr Surg* 1989; **24**: 257–262.

Stuart R, Shikora S, Akerman P et al. Incidence of arrhythmia with central venous catheter insertion and exchange *J Parenter Enter Nutr* 1990; **14**: 152–155.

Thomas-M. The use of the Hickman catheter in the management of patients with leukaemia and other malignancies. *Br J Surg* 1979; **66**: 673–674.

Thomas PR, Sinnett HD. An evaluation of prolonged venous access catheters in patients with leukaemia and other malignancies. *Eur J Surg Oncol* 1988; **14**: 63–68.

Toltzis P, Goldmann D. Current issues in central venous catheter infection. *Annu Rev Med* 1990; **41**: 169–76.

Wagman LD, Kirkemo A, Johnston R. Venous access: A prospective, randomised study of the Hickman catheter. *Surgery* 1984; **95**: 303–308.

Wagman LD, Konrad P, Schmit P. Internal fracture of a paediatric Broviac catheter. *J Parenter Enter Nutr* 1989; **13**: 560–561.

Wagman LD, Neifeld JP. Experience with the Hickman catheter: Unusual complications and suggestions for their prevention. *J Parenter Enter Nutr* 1986; **10**: 311–315.

Walker TG, Geller SC, Waltman AC et al. A simple technique for redirection of malpositioned Broviac or Hickman catheters. *Surg Gynecol Obstet* 1988; **167**: 246–248.

Watterson J, Heisel M, Cich JA, et al. Intrathoracic extravasation of sclerosing agents associated with central venous catheters. *Am J Pediatr Haemat Oncol* 1988; **10**: 249–251.

Weightman NC, Simpson EM, Speller DC et al. Bacteraemia related to indwelling central venous catheters: Prevention, diagnosis, and treatment. *Eur J Clin Microbiol Infect Dis* 1988; **7**: 125–129.

Williams D, Silove E, Stevens M. Intracardiac thrombus and tricuspid valve obstruction: a complication of Hickman catheter use. *Pediatr Hematol Oncol* 1988; **5**: 47–52.

VII Graft-Versus-Host Disease

Edward Kanfer

One of the main barriers to curing patients by allogeneic bone marrow transplantation (BMT) is graft-versus-host disease (GvHD). This disorder, a consequence of the recognition by donor immunocompetent cells of antigenic differences on recipient tissues, is responsible for considerable morbidity and mortality following BMT, both by causing direct organ dysfunction and by significantly increasing liability towards serious infection. The major effectors of this phenomenon are donor T lymphocytes, although other cell types and the subsequent amplification of this process by various cytokines are closely involved (see below). An important insight into the mechanisms by which BMT may cure leukaemia has been provided by analysis of the outcome of large numbers of BMTs by the International Bone Marrow Transplant Registry (IBMTR). It was noted that the risk of disease relapse after BMT for leukaemia was significantly greater in patients who had not developed GvHD (either acute or chronic) and, conversely, was smallest in those who had developed both acute and chronic forms of the disease (Horowitz et al., 1990). In support of the concept that GvHD was statistically related to a graft-versus-leukaemia (GvL) effect, it was also evident that recipients of identical twin (syngeneic) BMT (who only rarely develop GvHD—see below) were at high risk of subsequent relapse. This additionally explained the apparent paradox that T-cell depletion, extremely effective at reducing mortality from GvHD, had not benefited overall survival after BMT for leukaemia, primarily due to the increased probability of disease relapse. This GvL effect was not equally obvious in all types of leukaemia, but was most significant following BMT for chronic myeloid leukaemia (CML) (Goldman et al., 1988). For the above reasons it has become clear that simple reduction in GvHD incidence and severity is not of major influence in the long-term cure of leukaemia patients receiving allogeneic BMT in itself, although it does result in improved short-term survival.

Acute and chronic graft-versus-host disease

Two distinct syndromes are recognisable and are termed acute and chronic GvHD, although they are distinguished by timing of onset (before and after day 100, respectively) and pattern of organ involvement. In practice the two forms often merge into one another. The incidence of acute GvHD in published BMT studies has ranged from 15 to 80% in patients undergoing allogeneic BMT, the major determinants of this great variability being:
1 The relationship between donor and recipient (within family or unrelated, HLA-identical or mismatched, sex-identical or mismatched).
2 The type of GvHD prophylaxis employed.
Donor and recipient ages are also of relevance, although less so than (**1**) and (**2**) (Gale et al., 1987). The effects of these and other parameters on GvHD incidence are shown in **Table 33**. The clinical syndrome of acute GvHD may develop as early as a few days after allogeneic marrow infusion, particularly if there is significant HLA-antigen disparity between donor and recipient or if no immunosuppressive therapy is given. This form of GvHD is often very severe and is termed 'hyperacute GvHD' (Sullivan et al., 1986). In the more common context of HLA-matched sibling BMT, the median day of onset of acute GvHD is day 17 (Bortin et al., 1989). The clinical manifestations centre around the triad of skin rash, diarrhoea and hepatic dysfunction, to which may be added fever and marrow suppression (Peralvo et al., 1987) in a proportion of patients. The majority of marrow recipients do not exhibit clinical features involving all three organs, and there is marked variation in the degree of severity with which individuals are affected. Specifically, the clinical findings may range from a faint skin rash, minimal diarrhoea and minor hepatic enzyme elevation to widespread skin desquamation, profuse diarrhoea (several litres daily) and fulminant hepatic failure. A clinical and pathological grading system for acute GvHD is in common usage and allows comparison between different studies of prophylactic and therapeutic measures (Thomas et al., 1975).

Chronic GvHD has a median day of onset of 111 days post-BMT and usually arises following acute

Table 33. Influences on GvHD incidence.

Degree of significance	Less GvHD	More GvHD
Most significant		
Donor–recipient relationship	Identical twins 'Self' (autologous) Matched sibling	Mismatched relative Unrelated donor
Type of prophylaxis used	T-cell depletion MTX + CSP combined	None MTX alone CSP alone
Donor-recipient sex match	Male to male Male to female Nulliparous female to male	Parous female to male
Less significant		
Age of recipient and donor	Younger	Older
BMT conditioning regimen	Less intensive	More intensive
Post-BMT viral infection (particularly cytomegalovirus)	No	Yes

GvHD, or less frequently it may present *de novo*. Approximately 30% of patients are affected and many of these suffer considerable impairment in their general wellbeing, together with specific organ dysfunction. Chronic GvHD may target the same sites as acute GvHD, but in addition shows many similarities to autoimmune processes such as primary biliary cirrhosis, Sjögren's syndrome and systemic sclerosis (Sullivan et al., 1991). Both forms of GvHD greatly increase the tendency towards infectious complications, due to the immunosuppressive nature of both the disease and its therapy. For this reason infection prophylaxis is an important part of management. While the probability of developing GvHD can be assessed in broad terms using risk factor assignment as outlined above, the advantages of being able to directly predict this likelihood in an individual patient is obvious. Two methods of attempting to do this have been:

1. By using an in vitro skin explant culture model (Vogelsang et al., 1985).
2. By the enumeration of host-reactive donor cytotoxic or helper T-lymphocyte precursors (CTLp or HTLp) in limiting dilution assay (Kaminski et al., 1988; Schwarer et al., 1993). These assays may play a particular role in aiding choice between prospective donors by predicting individual risk for GvHD in specific donor–recipient pairs.

Aetiology

Experimental and clinical evidence strongly supports the idea that GvHD initiation results from T-cell recognition of antigenic differences between donor and recipient. This disparity classically centres around the major histocompatibility complex (MHC) group of antigens (HLA-A, -B and -DR), which are determined by genes on chromosome 6. However, the occurrence of GvHD after fully HLA-matched sibling BMT clearly suggests that minor histocompatibility antigen differences are sufficient stimuli for GvHD. This hypothesis is supported by the increased incidence and severity of GvHD following HLA-matched unrelated donor BMT, a situation in which minor antigen disparity would be expected to be greatest (Martin, 1991). In addition to the above, GvHD following syngeneic and autologous BMT has been described despite lack of obvious immunological disparity between donor and recipient. It should be noted that many such cases of GvHD have been of mild degree, often affecting only the skin, and that the clinical and histological differentiation between Grade I GvHD and other potential aetiological factors (such as drug toxicity or viral infection) may be very difficult to accomplish. Nevertheless, clear cut cases of GvHD in such circumstances have occurred (Hood *et al.*, 1987) and the suggestion that these may be related to 'imbalance' in the reconstituting immune system with consequent autoimmune manifestations is supported by the reproducibility of 'autologous GvHD' with cyclosporin (Jones *et al.*, 1989).

The exact identification of the cell populations responsible for GvHD remains unclear, and there is evidence that both CD4+ and CD8+ T lymphocytes and natural killer (NK) cells may play a role in the disorder (Korngold and Sprent 1987; Ferrara *et al.*, 1989). Cytokines, including interferons, tumour necrosis factor (TNF), granulocyte–macrophage colony-stimulating factor (GM-CSF) and several interleukins may be involved particularly in the amplification of the GvH reaction and subsequent tissue damage (Dickinson *et al.*, 1991; Jadus and Wepsic, 1992). Clinical studies of anticytokine agents in the prevention of GvHD are mentioned below.

Options for prophylaxis

Early studies in BMT (Thomas *et al.*, 1977) established GvHD as one of the three principal causes of treatment failure after BMT for leukaemia (together with leukaemic relapse and interstitial pneumonia). Several approaches to reducing the incidence and severity of GvHD have been tried with varying degrees of success (**Table 34**).

Methotrexate

Methotrexate (MTX) is an N^{10}-methyl derivative of aminopterin, itself a 4-NH$_2$ derivative of folic acid. The cytotoxic effect of MTX is mediated via the inhibition of dihydrofolate reductase, an enzyme which reduces dihydrofolic acid to tetrahydrofolic acid. This latter step is essential for thymidylate and purine nucleotide synthesis. Initial studies in a canine transplant model demonstrated the efficacy of MTX in the prevention of GvHD (Storb *et al.*, 1970), and the early Seattle human BMT series utilised an MTX regimen of 15 mg/m^2 on day 1 followed by 10 mg/m^2 on days 3, 6, 11 and then weekly until day 100 (Thomas *et al*, 1977). Approximately 50% of these 100 patients developed moderate to severe GvHD, an incidence subsequently confirmed in a larger number of patients (Gale *et al.*, 1987). The principal toxicities following BMT associated with MTX at this dosage are marrow suppression and mucositis. Folinic acid 'rescue' has been used for the amelioration of these, and one study has shown positive benefit without compromise of GvHD-preventive efficacy (Nevill *et al.*, 1992). Other complications of MTX used for GvHD prevention are unusual although it may possibly contribute towards the development of interstitial pneumonitis (Weiner

Table 34. Options for GvHD prevention.

Cytotoxic agents

    Methotrexate
    Cyclophosphamide

Immunosuppressive Agents

    Corticosteroids
    Cyclosporin
    FK-506

Ex-vivo T-cell depletion

    Monoclonal anti-T-cell antibody
    Counterflow centrifugation
    Soybean agglutination
    Sheep red cell (E-)rosetting
    Ricin-conjugated anti-T-cell antibody

In-vivo T-cell depletion

    Anti-lymphocyte (anti-thymocyte) globulin
    Monoclonal anti-T-cell antibody

Anticytokine Agents

    Anti-interleukin-2 receptor antibody
    Anti-tumour necrosis factor antibody (and pentoxiphylline)

et al., 1989) and hepatic veno-occlusive disease post-BMT (Dulley *et al.*, 1987; Essel *et al.*, 1992).

An alternative to MTX used in early studies was cyclophosphamide (7.5 mg/kg on days 1, 3, 5, 7, 9 and then weekly to day 100). The incidence of acute GvHD was similar to that seen with MTX although the severity, in terms of GvHD-attributable mortality, may have been somewhat higher (Santos *et al.*, 1983; Geller *et al.*, 1989).

Trimetrexate is a folate analogue closely related to MTX but it is metabolized in the liver rather than excreted in the urine. Studies with trimetrexate in a canine BMT model have shown encouraging activity in the prevention of GvHD (Appelbaum *et al.*, 1989).

Cyclosporin

Cyclosporin (CSP) is a hydrophobic cyclic peptide of fungal origin. Its immunosuppressive properties appear to reside in the ability of helper T lymphocytes to profoundly reduce interleukin-2 (IL-2) production and thus block the amplification of the alloimmune response. Its effect is much greater on primary, as opposed to secondary, immune responses, and the molecular basis for its action is almost certainly related to the observed reduction in IL-2 mRNA generation by CSP-treated cells (Kromke *et al.*, 1984).

The demonstrated efficacy of CSP in both human (Powles *et al.*, 1980; Hows *et al.*, 1982) and canine (Deeg *et al.*, 1981) GvHD prevention led to its increasing use in allogeneic BMT during the 1980s. Randomized trials of CSP versus MTX in patients with leukaemia showed equivalent results (Deeg *et al.*, 1985; Storb *et al.*, 1985) and this was confirmed in an IBMTR study (Gale *et al.*, 1987). However, an analysis of IBMTR data of patients with severe aplastic anaemia receiving BMT concluded that CSP, either alone or in combination with MTX, resulted in a superior overall survival compared with MTX alone (Gluckman *et al.*, 1992).

A common dosage schedule for CSP has been 3 mg/kg/24 hours intravenously (usually given as 1 hour infusions 12 hourly) starting 1–3 days prior to BMT and changing to 12.5 mg/kg/24 hours orally when tolerance to oral medication has become established, continued for 3–6 months.

It has been common practice to monitor whole blood or serum levels of CSP and to alter dosage as necessary. However, although levels correlate well with the toxicities associated with CSP, there have been conflicting reports concerning the relationship between levels and GvHD incidence (Bacigalupo *et al.*, 1984; Yee *et al.*, 1988). An alternative method of controlling CSP dosage is to use the serum creatinine value, which is a sensitive indicator of CSP toxicity. It should also be noted that hepatic dysfunction may increase the incidence of CSP toxicity (Yee *et al.*, 1984).

One of the earliest noted problems associated with CSP GvHD prevention was renal toxicity (Powles *et al.*, 1980; Barrett *et al.*, 1982; Hows *et al.*, 1983). Although mild and reversible in the majority of patients this complication may occasionally be severe and contribute significantly to morbidity, particularly in patients receiving other nephrotoxic agents (such as aminoglycoside antibiotics or amphotericin) or in patients who have coincidental renal impairment from other causes such as sepsis or VOD (veno-occlusive disease) with consequent hepato-renal syndrome. CSP may also be associated with hypertension, liver dysfunction, hypomagnesaemia, neurological toxicity and microangiopathic haemolysis (reviewed by Atkinson, 1987) (**192–194**). However, in comparison with MTX, CSP causes less mucositis and permits speedier marrow engraftment. **195** shows the potential side effects of CSP administration, and **196** and **197** show the hirsutism associated with CSP administration.

As mentioned above, CSP, when given to patients undergoing autologous BMT, may paradoxically induce GvHD, usually limited to the skin. In view of the negative correlation between GvHD and post-BMT leukaemia relapse risk in allogeneic marrow recipients, studies concerning use of CSP in patients with malignancy receiving autologous BMT are in progress (Talbot *et al.*, 1990; Yeager *et al.*, 1992). It is unknown to date whether this strategy will improve the long-term outcome for such patients.

An agent which may provide an alternative to CSP in future studies is FK-506. Limited initial evidence suggests that its efficacy in the prevention of GvHD may be at least as good as CSP but with a more favourable toxicity profile (Hiraoka *et al.*, 1992).

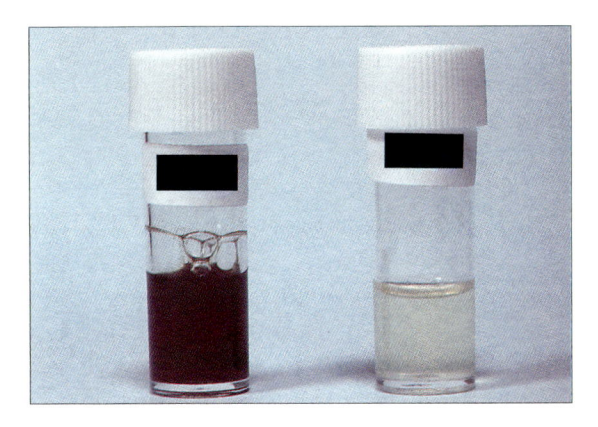

Graft-Versus-Host Disease

192 Cyclosporin-induced haemolysis resulting in red cell debris and free haemoglobin in the patient's plasma.

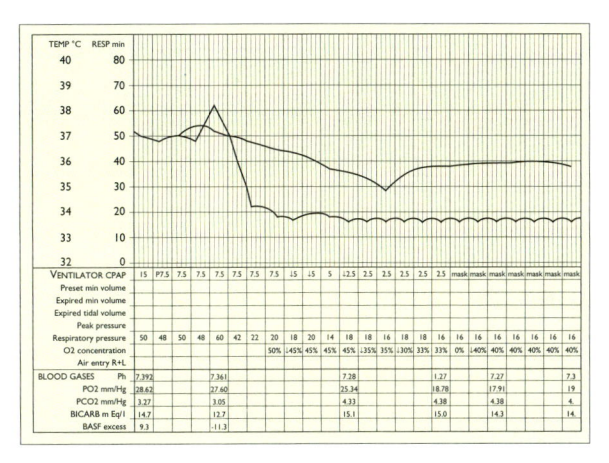

193 Observation chart on patient whose plasma is shown in **192**. Prior to plasmapheresis, respiratory rate is rapid with a high requirement for continuous positive airways pressure (CPAP) and she has a high oxygen requirement. Following plasmapheresis, respiratory rate and blood gases improve with decreased requirement for CPAP.

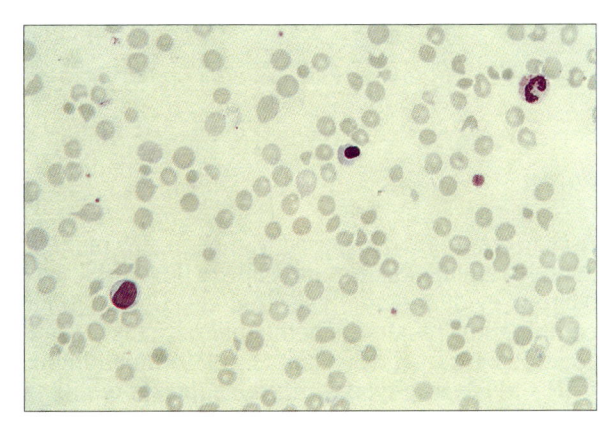

194 Blood film from patient above showing polychromasia, fragments, spheres and a nucleated red cell.

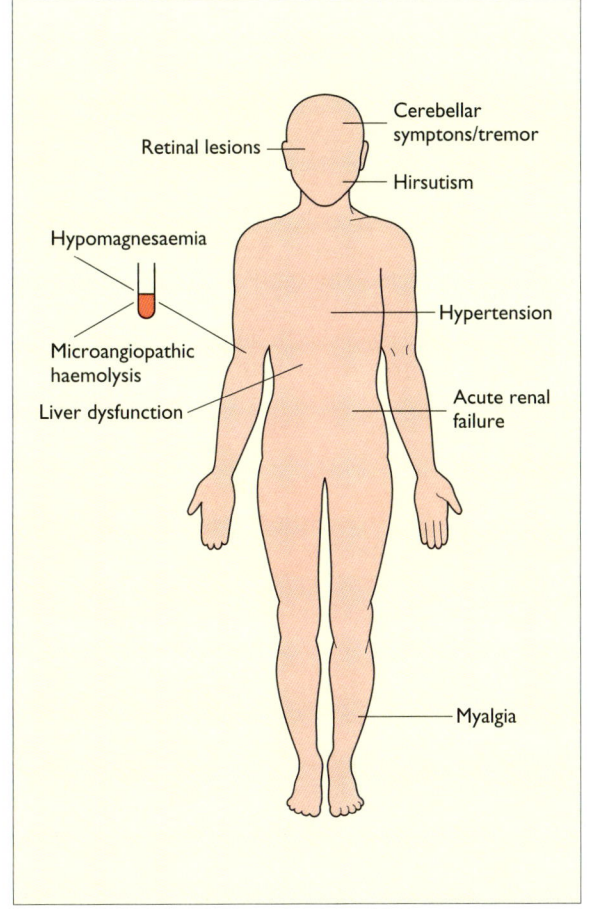

195 Potential complications of cyclosporin therapy.

147

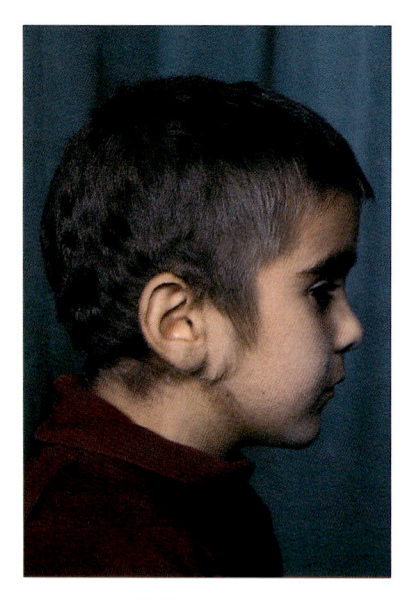

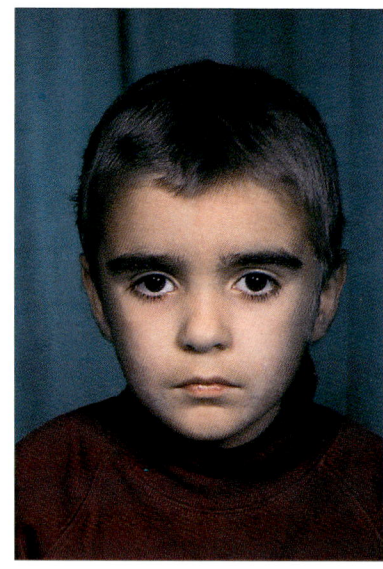

196, 197 Child with hirsutism induced by cyclosporin, three months after bone marrow transplantation.

Combination of methotrexate and cyclosporin

Studies of BMT in canine models demonstrated that the combination of MTX with CSP is more effective for GvHD prophylaxis than either agent alone, and this has subsequently been shown to be the case in human BMT (Storb et al., 1986a, b). The schedule developed in Seattle comprised the standard CSP dosage (see above—starting on the day prior to BMT), together with four doses of MTX (15, 10, 10 and 10 mg/m^2) given on days 1, 3, 6 and 11. However, it soon became apparent that the lower GvHD incidence effected by CSP + MTX immunosuppression was counterbalanced by an increase in leukaemic relapse risk leading in general to equivalent long-term survival (Storb et al., 1989; Aschan et al., 1991). Importantly, though, this may not apply to all leukaemic indications for BMT and current evidence suggests that the CSP + MTX combination results in better overall survival for patients with CML (Storb et al., 1989). In addition, CSP + MTX prophylaxis may be superior to either agent alone in recipients of marrow from donors other than HLA-identical siblings (Ringden et al., 1992).

There is evidence to suggest that reducing the dose of CSP within the combination of MTX + CSP may permit good GvHD prophylaxis without relative increase in relapse probability (Hunter et al., 1992), but this strategy requires testing in a randomized study.

Steroids

Steroids are effective in the therapy of established GvHD and they have been used occasionally in combination with other drugs for prophylaxis (Santos et al., 1987; Yau et al., 1990). However, one randomized study showed that the addition of prednisolone to the combination of CSP and MTX was of no benefit in HLA-identical sibling BMT (Atkinson et al., 1991).

In vitro *T-cell depletion*

Several studies involving the *ex vivo* removal of T lymphocytes from donor marrow prior to infusion have shown that this method of GvHD prevention is by far the most effective currently available (reviewed in Poynton, UK, 1988). Patients with both malignant and non-malignant disease have received T-depleted BMT (Mitsuyasu et al., 1986; Morgan et al., 1986), and these procedures have not been restricted to HLA-matched sibling transplants (O'Reilly et al., 1985a; Trigg et al., 1989; Ash et al., 1991). Several different methods have been used for T-cell depletion including monoclonal antibodies (Prentice et al., 1984; Heit et al., 1986; Herve, 1986), counterflow centrifugation (de Witte et al., 1986), soybean agglutinin and E-rosetting (Reisner et al., 1981), and immunotoxins (Filipovich et al., 1984). It is not clear which method offers the most advantages.

The efficacy of T-cell depletion in the prevention of GvHD has been largely offset by the two major complications of graft rejection (Martin et al., 1985; Patterson et al., 1986) and, as noted above, increased probability of leukaemic relapse (Apperley et al., 1986; Maraninchi et al., 1987).

The increase in host-versus-graft resistance associated with T-cell depletion (O'Reilly et al., 1985a; Bunjes et al., 1987), and the consequent failure to achieve sustained engraftment has been a particular problem with BMT for aplastic anaemia (Hows et al., 1989) and in patients receiving non-HLA identical marrow (Irle and van Rood, 1987). Attempts to overcome this have concentrated on increased immunosuppression, and have included intensified total body irradiation (O'Reilly et al., 1985b), and total lymphoid irradiation (Slavin et al., 1986). Studies involving modifications to T-depletion strategies, for example, by the selective depletion of T-cell subsets (Champlin et al., 1990) or by adding back to the marrow infusion a specified dose of T cells (Potter et al., 1991), are ongoing.

In vivo *antibody therapy*

Anti-lymphocyte globulin

Anti-lymphocyte globulin (ALG) has been used in the therapy of active GvHD, for which it is moderately effective. Two trials have studied whether ALG might be a useful addition to post-BMT MTX for the prevention of GvHD. In one case, ALG was started on day 7 (a total of 6 doses administered on alternate days) and in the other it was started only when engraftment had been established (at a median of 16.5 days post-BMT) (Doney et al., 1981; Weiden et al., 1979). No benefit was demonstrated in either study.

Anti-T-cell monoclonal antibodies

Therapy of acute GvHD with OKT3, an anti-CD3 antibody, has been associated with severe toxicity in some cases. A recent report has described the use of another CD3 antibody, BC3, which shows little interaction with the Fc receptor on monocytes, and which therefore does not lead to T-cell activation and consequent complications (Anasetti et al., 1992). Results in patients with GvHD have been encouraging and studies utilising this approach for the prevention of GvHD can be anticipated.

Anti cytokine agents

Anti-interleukin-2 receptor antibody (aIL-2-ra)

Monoclonal antibodies directed against structures associated with the IL-2 receptor abolish most of the *in vitro* proliferative responses of antigen-stimulated T-cells. Animal studies have shown, for example, that parenteral therapy with rat aIL-2-ra prolonged survival of both heart and skin grafts between H-2-incompatible mice (Kirkman et al., 1985). Investigations in human BMT have demonstrated the efficacy of aIL-2-ra in some patients with steroid-resistant GvHD (Herve et al., 1990; Cuthbert et al., 1992), resulting in trials of this agent for prophylaxis. To date, results are inconclusive in that aIL-2-ra may effectively prevent GvHD (Blaise et al., 1991) or only delay its onset (Anasetti et al., 1991). Further studies are clearly necessary to define a role for this particular strategy.

Anti-TNF agents

TNF is strongly-suspected to participate in the GvHD reaction (see above). In a study of a monoclonal antitumour necrosis factor antibody for the therapy of steroid-resistant GvHD, 14 of 19 patients experienced a partial response but the majority relapsed when treatment was stopped (Herve et al., 1992). Greater efficacy may perhaps be evident if therapy is anticipatory, and a study of prophylactic oral pentoxiphylline (an inhibitor of TNF production) has shown significant reductions in the incidence of acute GvHD as well as VOD (veno-occlusive disease), mucositis and the duration of parenteral nutrition necessary after BMT (Bianco et al., 1991). However, another study failed to confirm these benefits (Kalhs et al., 1992).

Conclusion

GvHD remains one of the most important topics within the field of allogeneic BMT because, although its amelioration is readily achievable, this has not been clearly translated into an improved overall survival for patients with haematological malignancy. A possible way forward may be provided by future research focusing on the separation of GvHD from the anti-neoplastic effect of allogeneic bone marrow (Slavin et al., 1990; Brenner and Heslop, 1991; Jiang et al., 1991). If this proves exploitable in clinical practice, the prevention of GvHD may eventually fulfil its objective of improved safety for patients undergoing allogeneic BMT without compromising the chances of cure.

References

Anasetti C, Martin PJ, Storb R et al. Prophylaxis of graft-versus-host disease by administration of the murine anti-IL-2 receptor antibody 2A3. *Bone Marrow Transplant* 1991; **7**: 375–381.

Anasetti C, Martin PJ, Storb R et al. Treatment of acute graft-versus-host disease with a non-mitogenic anti-CD3 monoclonal antibody. *Transplantation* 1992; **54**: 844–851.

Appelbaum FR, Raff RF, Storb R et al. Use of trimetrexate for the prevention of graft-versus-host disease. *Bone Marrow Transplant* 1989; **4**: 421–424.

Apperley JF, Jones L, Hale G et al. Bone marrow transplantation for patients with chronic myeloid leukaemia: T-cell depletion with Campath-1 reduces the incidence of graft-versus-host disease but may increase the risk of leukaemic relapse. *Bone Marrow Transplant* 1986;; **1**: 53-66.

Aschan J, Ringden O, Sundberg B et al. Methotrexate combined with cyclosporin A decreases graft-versus-host disease, but increases leukemic relapse compared to monotherapy. *Bone Marrow Transplant* 1991; **7**: 113–119.

Ash RC, Horowitz MM, Gale RP et al. Bone marrow transplantation from related donors other than HLA-identical siblings: effect of T-cell depletion. *Bone Marrow Transplant* 1991; **7**: 443–452.

Atkinson K. Cyclosporin in bone marrow transplantation. *Bone Marrow Transplant* 1987; **1**: 265–270.

Atkinson K, Biggs J, Concannon A et al. A prospective randomised trial of cyclosporin and methotrexate versus cyclosporin, methotrexate and prednisolone for prevention of graft-versus-host disease after HLA-identical sibling marrow transplantation for haematological malignancy. *Austr N Z J Med* 1991; **21**: 850-856.

Bacigalupo A, Di Giorgio F, Frassoni et al. Cyclosporin A serum and blood levels in marrow graft recipients: correlation with administered dose, serum creatinine and graft-versus-host disease. *Acta Haematol (Basel)* 1984; **72**: 155–162.

Barrett AJ, Kendra JR, Lucas CF et al. Cyclosporin A as prophylaxis against graft-versus-host disease in 36 patients. *Br Med J* 1982; **285**: 162–166.

Bianco JA, Appelbaum FR, Nemunaitis J et al. Phase I–II trial of pentoxifylline for the prevention of transplant-related toxicities following bone marrow transplantation. *Blood* 1991; **78**:1205–1211.

Blaise D, Olive D, Hirn M et al. Prevention of acute GvHD by *in vivo* use of anti-interleukin-2 receptor monoclonal antibody (33B3.1): a feasibility trial in 15 patients. *Bone Marrow Transplant* 1991; **8**: 105–111.

Bortin MM, Ringden O, Horowitz MM et al. Temporal relationships between the major complications of bone marrow transplantation. *Bone Marrow Transplant* 1989; **4**: 339–344.

Brenner MK, Heslop HE. Graft versus leukaemia effects after marrow transplantation. *Baillière Clin Haematol* 1991; **4**: 727–749.

Bunjes D, Heit W, Arnold R *et al*. Evidence for the involvement of host-derived OKT8-positive T cells in the rejection of T-depleted, HLA-identical bone marrow grafts.*Transplantation* 1987; **43**: 501–505.

Champlin R, Ho W, Gajewski J *et al*. Selective depletion of CD8+ T lymphocytes for prevention of graft-versus-host disease after bone marrow transplantation. *Blood* 1990; **76**: 418–423.

Cuthbert R, Phillips GL. Barnett MJ *et al*. Anti-interleukin-2 receptor monoclonal antibody (BT 563) in the treatment of severe acute GvHD refractory to systemic corticosteroid therapy. *Bone Marrow Transplant* 1992; **10**: 451–455.

de Witte T, Hoogenhout J, de Pauw B *et al*. Depletion of donor lymphocytes by counterflow centrifugation successfully prevents acute graft-versus-host disease in matched allogeneic marrow transplantation. *Blood* 1986; **67**: 1302–1308.

Deeg HJ, Storb R, Weiden PL *et al*. Cyclosporin-A: effect on marrow engraftment and graft-versus-host disease in dogs.*Transplant Proc* 1981; **13**: 402-404.

Deeg HJ, Storb R, Thomas ED *et al*. Cyclosporin as prophylaxis for graft-versus-host disease: a randomized study in patients undergoing marrow transplantation for acute nonlymphoblastic leukemia. *Blood* 1985; **65**: 1325–1334.

Dickinson AM, Sviland L, Dunn J *et al*. Demonstration of direct involvement of cytokines in graft-versus-host reactions using an *in vitro* human explant model. *Bone Marrow Transplant* 1991; **7**: 209–216.

Doney KC, Weiden PL, Storb R, Thomas ED. Failure of early administration of antithymocyte globulin to lessen graft-versus-host disease in human allogeneic marrow transplant recipients. *Transplantation* 1981; **31**: 141–143.

Dulley FL, Kanfer EJ. Appelbaum FR *et al*. Veno-occlusive disease (VOD) of the liver after chemoradiotherapy and autologous bone marrow transplantation. *Transplantation* 1987; **43**: 870–873.

Essel JH, Thompson JM, Harman GS *et al*. Marked increase in veno-occlusive disease of the liver associated with methotrexate use for graft-versus-host disease prophylaxis in patients receiving busulfan/cyclophosphamide. *Blood* 1992 **79**: 2784–2788.

Ferrara JL, Guillen FJ, van Dijken PJ *et al*. Evidence that large granular lymphocytes of donor origin mediate acute graft-versus-host disease. *Transplantation* 1989; **47**: 50–54.

Filipovich AH, Vellera DA, Youle RJ *et al*. *Ex vivo* treatment of donor bone marrow with anti-T-cell immunotoxins for prevention of graft versus host disease. *Lancet* 1984; **1**: 469–472.

Gale RP, Bortin MM, van Bekkum DW *et al*. Risk factors for acute graft-versus-host disease. *Br J Haematol* 1987; **67**: 397–406.

Geller RB, Saral R, Piantadosi S *et al*. Allogeneic bone marrow transplantation after high-dose busulfan and cyclophosphamide in patients with acute nonlymphocytic leukemia. *Blood* 1989; **73**: 2209–2218.

Gluckman E, Horowitz MM, Champlin RE *et al*. Bone marrow transplantation for severe aplastic anemia: influence of conditioning and graft-versus-host disease prophylaxis regimens on outcome. *Blood* 1992; **79**: 269–275.

Goldman JM, Gale RP, Horowitz MM *et al*. Bone marrow transplantation for chronic myelogenous leukemia in chronic phase. *Ann Intern Med* 1988; **108**: 806–814.

Heit W, Bunjes D, Weisneth M *et al*. Ex vivo T-cell depletion with the monoclonal antibody Campath-1 plus human complement effectively prevents acute graft-versus-host disease in allogeneic bone marrow transplantation. *Brit J Haematol* 1986; **64**: 479–486.

Herve P. Depletion of T-lymphocytes in donor marrow with pan-T monoclonal antibodies and complement for prevention of acute graft-versus-host disease: a pilot study on 29 patients. *J Natl Cancer Inst* 1986; **76**: 1311–1316.

Herve P, Wijdenes J, Bergerat JP *et al*. Treatment of corticosteroid resistant acute graft-versus-host disease by *in vivo* administration of anti-interleukin-2 receptor monoclonal antibody (B-B10). *Blood* 1990; **75**: 1017–1023.

Herve P, Flesch M, Tiberghien P *et al*. Phase I–II trial of a monoclonal anti-tumor necrosis factor alpha antibody for the treatment of refractory severe acute graft-versus-host disease. *Blood* 1992; **79**: 3362–3368.

Hiraoka A, Masaoka T, Asano S *et al*. Phase II study of FK506 for allogeneic bone marrow transplantation. *Exp Hematol* 1992; **20**: 707.

Hood AF, Vogelsang GB, Black LP *et al*. Acute graft-versus-host disease: development following autologous and syngeneic bone marrow transplantation. *Arch Dermatol* 1987; **123**: 745–750.

Horowitz MM, Gale RP, Sondel PM *et al*. Graft-versus-leukemia reactions after bone marrow transplantation. *Blood* 1990; **75**: 555–562.

Hows JM, Palmer S, Gordon-Smith EC. Use of cyclosporin A in allogeneic bone marrow transplantation for severe aplastic anemia. *Transplantation* 1982; **33**: 382–386.

Hows JM, Chipping PM, Fairhead S *et al*. Nephrotoxicity in bone marrow transplant recipients treated with cyclosporin A. *Br J Haematol* 1983; **54**: 69–78.

Hows JM, Marsh J, Liu Yin J *et al*. Bone marrow transplantation for severe aplastic anaemia using cyclosporin: long-term follow-up. *Bone Marrow Transplant* 1989; **4**: 11–16.

Hunter AE, Bessell EM, Russell NH. Effective prevention of acute GvHD following allogeneic BMT with low leukaemic relapse using methotrexate and therapeutically monitored levels of cyclosporin A. *Bone Marrow Transplant* 1992; **10**: 431–434.

Irle C, van Rood JJ. Mismatched bone marrow transplantation in Europe: preliminary results. *Bone Marrow Transplant* 1987; **2** (Suppl 1): 285.

Jadus MR, Wepsic HT. The role of cytokines in graft-versus-host reactions and disease. *Bone Marrow Transplant* 1992; **10**: 1–14.

Jiang YZ, Kanfer EJ, Macdonald D *et al*. Graft-versus-leukaemia following allogeneic marrow transplantation: emergence of cytotoxic T-lymphocytes reacting to host leukaemia cells. *Bone Marrow Transplant* 1991; **8**: 253–258.

Jones RJ, Vogelsang GB, Hess AD et al. Induction of graft-versus-host disease after autologous bone marrow transplantation. *Lancet* 1989; **1**: 754–756.

Kalhs P, Lechner K, Stockschlader M et al. Pentoxifylline did not prevent transplant-related toxicity in 31 consecutive allogeneic bone marrow recipients. *Blood* 1992; **80**: 2683–2684.

Kaminski E, Sharrowck C, Hows J et al. Frequency analysis of cytotoxic T lymphocyte precursors—possible relevance to HLA-matched unrelated donor bone marrow transplantation. *Bone Marrow Transplant* 1988; **3**: 149–165.

Kirkman RL, Barrett LV, Gaulton GN et al. The effect of anti-interleukin-2 receptor monoclonal antibody on allograft rejection. *Transplantation* 1985; **40**: 719–722.

Korngold R, Sprent J. T cell subsets and graft-versus-host disease. *Transplantation* 1987; **44**: 335–339.

Kromke M, Leonard WJ, Depper JM et al. Cyclosporin A inhibits T-cell growth factor gene expression at the level of mRNA transcription. *Proc Natl Acad Sci USA* 1984; **81**: 5214–5218.

Maraninchi D, Gluckman E, Blaise D et al. Impact of T-cell depletion on outcome of allogeneic bone marrow transplantation for standard-risk leukaemias. *Lancet* 1987; **2**: 175–178.

Martin PJ, Hansen JA, Buckner CD et al. Effects of *in vitro* depletion of T cells in HLA-identical allogeneic marrow grafts. *Blood* 1985; **66**: 664–672.

Martin PJ. Increased disparity for minor histocompatibility antigens as a potential cause of increased GvHD risk in marrow transplantation from unrelated donors compared with related donors. *Bone Marrow Transplant* 1991; **8**: 217–223.

Mitsuyasu RT, Champlin R, Gale RP et al. Treatment of donor bone marrow with monoclonal anti-T-cell antibody and complement for the prevention of graft-versus-host disease. *Ann Intern Med* 1986; **105**: 20–26.

Morgan G, Linch DC, Knott LT et al. Successful haploidentical mismatched bone marrow transplantation in severe combined immunodeficiency: T cell removal using Campath-1 monoclonal antibody and E-rosetting. *Br J Haematol* 1986; **62**: 421–430.

Nevill TJ, Tirgan MH, Deeg HJ et al. Influence of post-methotrexate folinic acid rescue on regimen-related toxicity and graft-versus-host disease after allogeneic bone marrow transplantation. *Bone Marrow Transplant* 1992; **9**: 349–354.

O'Reilly RJ, Collins NH, Kernan N et al. Transplantation of marrow-depleted T cells by soybean lectin agglutination and E-rosette depletion: major histocompatibility complex-related graft resistance in leukemic transplant recipients. *Transplant Proc* 1985a; **17**: 455–459.

O'Reilly RJ, Shank B, Collins N et al. Increased total body irradiation (TBI) abrogates resistance to HLA-matched marrow grafts depleted of T-cells by lectin agglutination and E-rosette depletion (SBA-E-BMT). *Exp Hematol* 1985b; **13**: 406 #203.

Patterson J, Prentice HG, Brenner MK et al. Graft rejection following HLA matched T-lymphocyte depleted bone marrow transplantation. *Br J Haematol* 1986; **63**: 221–230.

Peralvo J, Bacigalupo A, Pittaluga PA et al. Poor graft function associated with graft-versus-host disease after allogeneic transplantation. *Bone Marrow Transplant* 1987; **2**: 279–285.

Potter MN, Pamphilon DH, Cornish JM, Oakhill A. Graft-versus-host disease in children receiving HLA-identical allogeneic bone marrow transplants with a low adjusted T lymphocyte dose. *Bone Marrow Transplant* 1991; **8**: 357–361.

Powles RL, Clink HM, Spence D et al. Cyclosporin A to prevent graft-versus-host disease in man after allogeneic bone marrow transplantation. *Lancet* 1980; **1**: 327–329.

Poynton CH. T cell depletion in bone marrow transplantation. *Bone Marrow Transplant* 1988; **3**: 265–279.

Prentice HG, Blacklock HA, Janossy G et al. Depletion of T lymphocytes in donor marrow prevents significant graft-versus-host disease in matched allogeneic leukaemic marrow transplant recipients. *Lancet* 1984; **1**: 472–476.

Reisner Y, Kapoor N, Kirkpatrick D et al. Transplantation for acute leukaemia with HLA-A and B non-identical parental marrow cells fractionated with soybean agglutinin and sheep red blood cells. *Lancet* 1981; **2**: 327–331.

Ringden O, Klaesson S, Sundberg B et al. Decreased incidence of graft-versus-host disease and improved survival with methotrexate combined with cyclosporin compared with monotherapy in recipients of bone marrow from donors other than HLA identical siblings. *Bone Marrow Transplant* 1992; **9**: 19–25.

Santos GW, Tutschka PJ, Brookmeyer R et al. Marrow transplantation for acute nonlymphocytic leukemia after treatment with busulfan and cyclophosphamide. *N Engl J Med* 1983; **309**: 1347–1353.

Santos GW, Tutschka PJ, Brookmeyer R et al. Cyclosporin plus methylprednisolone versus cyclophosphamide plus methylprednisolone as prophylaxis for graft-versus-host disease: a randomized double blind study in patients undergoing allogeneic marrow transplantation. *Clin Transplant* 1987; **1**: 21–29.

Schwarer AP, Jiang YZ, Brookes PA et al. The frequency of anti-recipient alloreactive helper T-cell precursors (HTLp) in donor blood predicts significant graft-versus-host disease after HLA-identical sibling bone marrow transplantation. *Lancet* 1993; **341**: 203–205.

Slavin S, Or R, Weshler Z et al. The use of total lymphoid irradiation for abrogation of host resistance to T-cell depleted marrow allografts. *Bone Marrow Transplant* 1986; **1**: (suppl 1) 98.

Slavin S, Ackerstein A, Naperstek E et al. The graft-versus-leukemia (GvL) phenomenon: is GvL separable from GvHD? *Bone Marrow Transplant* 1990; **6**: 155–161.

Storb R, Epstein RB, Graham TC, Thomas ED. Methotrexate regimens for control of graft-versus-host disease in dogs with allogeneic marrow grafts. *Transplantation* 1970; **9**: 240–246.

Storb R, Deeg HJ, Thomas ED *et al*. Marrow transplantation for chronic myelocytic leukemia: a controlled trial of cyclosporin versus methotrexate for prophylaxis of graft-versus-host disease. *Blood* 1985; **66**: 698–702.

Storb R, Deeg HJ, Farewell V *et al*. Marrow transplantation for severe aplastic anemia: methotrexate alone compared with a combination of methotrexate and cyclosporin for prevention of acute graft-versus-host disease. *Blood* 1986a; **68**: 119–125.

Storb R, Deeg HJ, Whitehead J *et al*. Methotrexate and cyclosporin compared with cyclosporin alone for prophylaxis of acute graft versus host disease after marrow transplantation for leukemia. *N Engl J Med* 1986b; **314**: 729–735.

Storb R, Deeg HJ, Pepe M *et al*. Methotrexate and cyclosporin versus cyclosporin alone for prophylaxis of graft-versus-host disease in patients given HLA-identical marrow grafts for leukemia: long-term follow-up of a controlled trial. *Blood* 1989; **73**: 1729–1734.

Sullivan KM, Deeg HJ, Sanders J *et al*. Hyperacute graft-versus-host disease in patients not given immunosuppression after allogeneic marrow transplantation. *Blood* 1986; **67**: 1172–1175.

Sullivan KM, Agura E, Anasetti C *et al*. Chronic graft-versus-host disease and other late complications of bone marrow transplantation. *Sem Hematol* 1991; **28**: 250–259

Talbot DC, Powles RL, Sloane JP *et al*. Cyclosporin-induced graft-versus-host disease following autologous bone marrow transplantation in acute myeloid leukaemia. *Bone Marrow Transplant* 1990; **6**: 17–20.

Thomas ED, Storb R, Clift RA *et al*. Bone marrow transplantation. *N Engl J Med* 1975; **292**: 895–902.

Thomas ED, Buckner CD, Banaji M *et al*. One hundred patients with acute leukemia treated by chemotherapy, total body irradiation, and allogeneic marrow transplantation. *Blood* 1977; **49**: 511–533.

Trigg ME, Gingrich R, Goeken N *et al*. Low rejection rate when using unrelated or haploidentical donors for children with leukemia undergoing marrow transplantation. *Bone Marrow Transplant* 1989; **4**: 431–437.

Vogelsang GB, Hess AD, Berkman AW *et al*. An *in vitro* predictive test for graft versus host disease in patients with genotypic HLA-identical bone marrow transplants. *N Engl J Med* 1985; **313**: 645–650.

Weiden PL, Doney K, Storb R, Thomas ED. Antihuman thymocyte globulin for prophylaxis of graft-versus-host disease: a randomized trial in patients with leukemia treated with HLA-identical sibling marrow grafts. *Transplantation* 1979; **27**: 227–230.

Weiner RS, Horowitz MM, Gale RP *et al*. Risk factors for interstitial pneumonia following bone marrow transplantation for severe aplastic anaemia. *Br J Haematol* 1989; **71**: 535–543.

Yau JC, LeMaistre CF, Zagars GK *et al*. Methylprednisolone, cyclosporin and methotrexate for prophylaxis of acute graft-versus-host disease. *Bone Marrow Transplant* 1990; **5**: 269–272.

Yeager AM, Vogelsang GB, Jones RJ *et al*. Induction of cutaneous graft-versus-host disease by administration of cyclosporin to patients undergoing autologous bone marrow transplantation for acute myeloid leukemia. *Blood* 1992; **79**: 3031–3035.

VIII Patient Conditioning

1. Total Body Irradiation

Peter Barrett-Lee

Total body irradiation (TBI) has been used for the treatment of malignant disease since the 1950s, but is now most commonly given prior to bone marrow transplantation in combination with chemotherapy. The benefits of TBI are threefold (**Table 35**). Firstly, conventional TBI doses of approximately 10 Gy produce around a 5-log cell kill. This complements the cell kill achieved by chemotherapy and may be more effective with cells in G_0 and those occupying 'sanctuary sites' such as the central nervous system and testes. Secondly, it has been calculated that relatively low doses of 2–3 Gy are capable of creating the necessary space within the bone marrow cavity to permit grafting of stem cells.

Finally, TBI at low doses of 3–6 Gy has been shown to be the single most effective immunosuppressive agent for bone marrow transplantation, and is superior to alkylating agents in this resect.

The intended target cells for TBI (leukaemic stem cells, lymphocytes and bone marrow stem cells) are widely dispersed, and thus the target volume is the entire body of the patient, including the skin. Since conventional radiotherapy units operating at 1 metre from the patient are capable of a maximum field size of only 40 × 40 cm, such units require modification to achieve the required limits, and this can be achieved in different ways (**198–203**).

Table 35. Benefits of TBI.

Benefit	Single dose TBI required
Tumour cell kill	10 Gy (5 log cell kill)
Creation of space	2–3 Gy
Immunosuppression	3–6 Gy

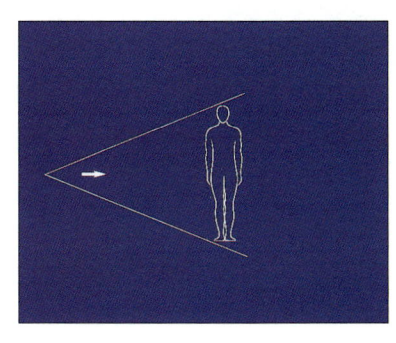

198 Single lateral source used at long treatment distance.

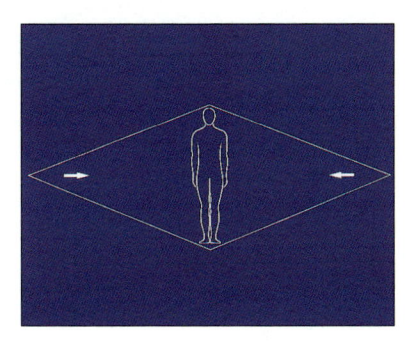

199 Dual source with opposed lateral beams.

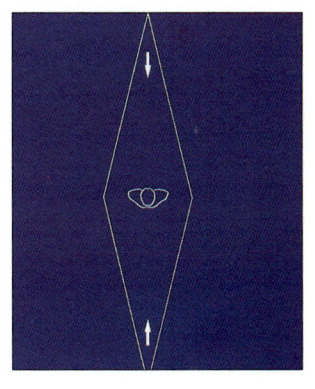

200 Dual source with opposed antero-posterior beams.

Bone Marrow Transplantation

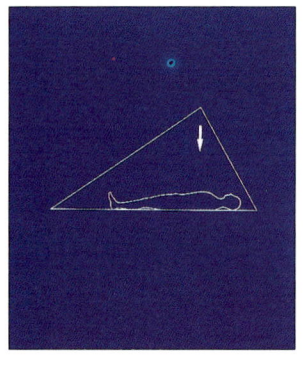

201 Single source modified for use at short treatment distance.

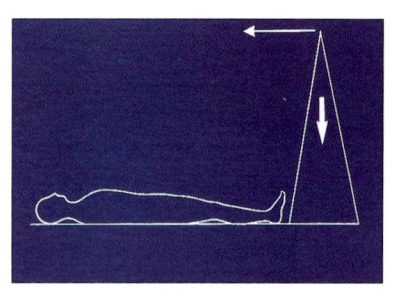

202 Single source, modified to scan the length of the patient.

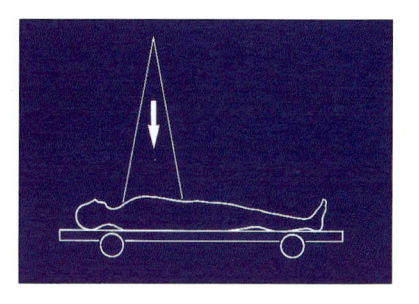

203 Single source with mobile couch.

Some centres have dedicated treatment facilities such as the dual ^{60}Co TBI unit at the Royal Marsden Hospital, Sutton, Surrey, UK. This consists of two track mounted opposing ^{60}Co units in a special room, capable of treating field sizes up to 200 × 65 cm, with a variable dose rate attainable by the use of custom-made attenuators (**204**). For treatment, the patient lies within the confines of a perspex cot and is aligned using lasers (**205**). Before TBI is commenced, a test dose of radiation is given over 1 min, and measured by placing semiconductors dosimeters at several site on the skin of the patient. This is repeated for the two treatment positions (**206, 207**) and the readings obtained are expressed as a dose distribution (**Table 36**). For maximum dose uniformity, especially across critical structures such as the lungs, a combination of positions is best. During the main treatment the patient is covered with a thin sheet for comfort (**208**) and is in communication with staff in the control room via a two-way microphone and closed-circuit television (**209**).

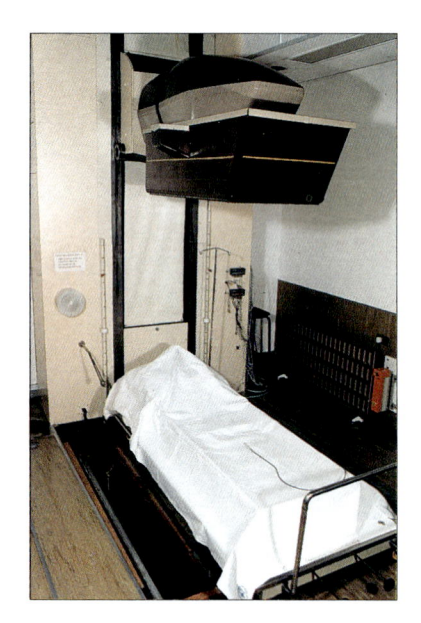

204 Dual ^{60}Co TBI unit, capable of treating field sizes up to 200 × 65 cms with variable dose rate.

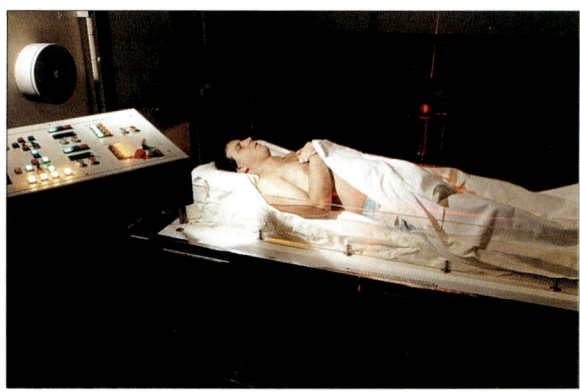

205 Perspex cot used for treatment. The patient is aligned using lasers.

Total Body Irradiation

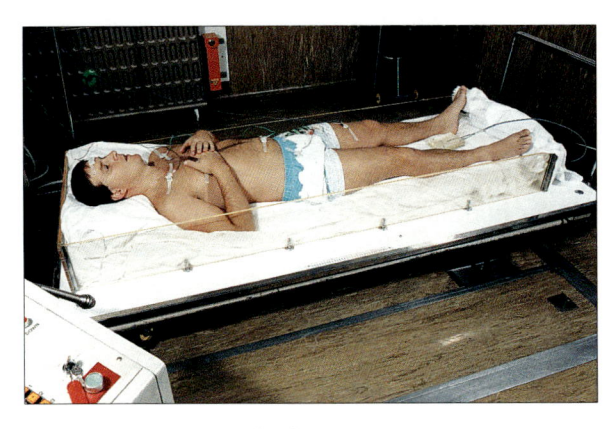

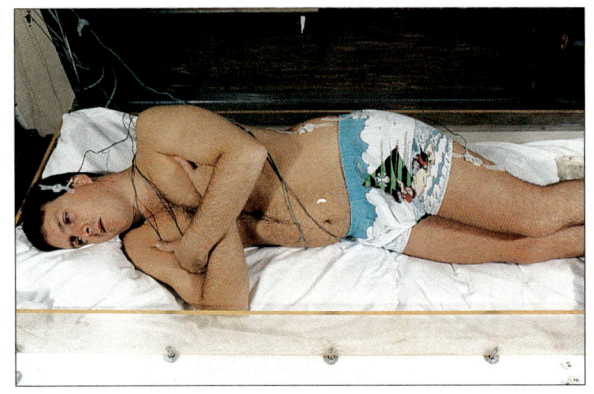

206, 207 A test dose of radiation is given over 1 minute and dosimeters placed at several skin sites measure this for the 2 treatment positions.

Table 36. Typical dose distribution during TBI as measured by semiconductor diodes. The figures are percentages normalised to 100 at the upper lungs.

Site	On site	Supine	Two-thirds on side, one-third supine
Head	92	107	97
Neck	104	112	107
Mediastinum	98	93	96
Upper lungs	100	100	100
Lower lungs	95	99	96
Abdomen	103	102	103
Pelvis	107	102	105
Ankle	105	116	109
Overall variation	92–107	93–116	96–109
Variation from ideal (%)	15	23	13
Variation across whole lungs (%)	5	7	4

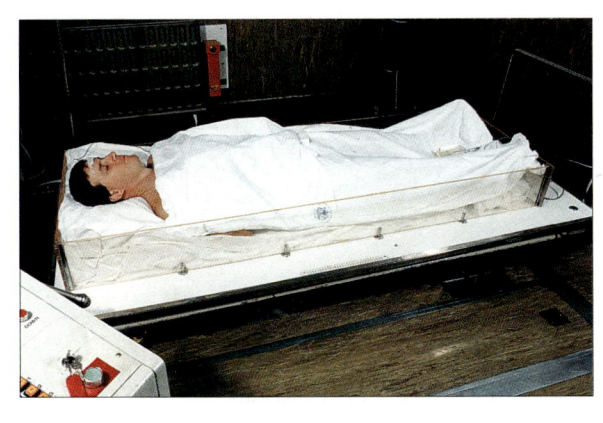

208 Patient receiving main treatment.

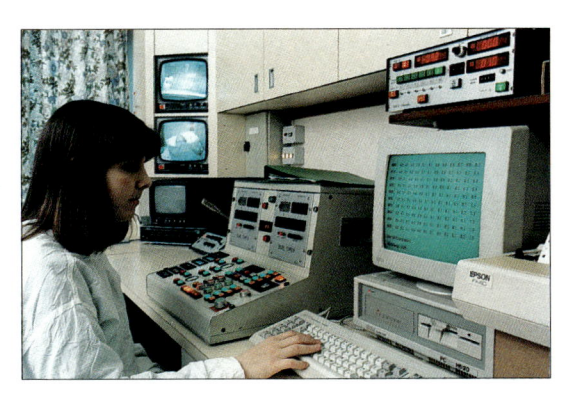

209 Control room staff can hear and see the patient by way of microphones and closed-circuit television.

TBI may be given in a single fraction over several hours (single fraction TBI), or in multiple smaller fractions over several days (fractionated TBI). Careful preparation of the patient is necessary, especially before single fraction TBI, where the overall treatment time may be 5–6 hours. The procedure and the likely side-effects are explained to the patient (Table 37). Adequate premedication before TBI dramatically reduces the attendant nausea and vomiting, and should be administered in all cases, and especially during single fraction TBI (Tiley *et al.* 1992) (Table 38).

The total dose and dose rate vary from centre to centre. In general, the total dose and dose rate are higher in fractionated TBI compared with single

Table 37. Side effects of TBI.

Side effect	Onset (hours)	Duration (days)
Acute		
Nausea and vomiting	During TBI	
Diarrhoea	48	10
Jaw pain (parotitis)	24	2
Skin erythema	24	10
Mucositis	24	10
Total alopecia	Complete after 10–14 days	
Somnolence syndrome	May occur after 6–8 weeks	
Veno-occlusive disease		
Late		
Sterility		
Hypothyroidism		
Cataracts		
Second malignancy		
Interstitial pneumonitis		

Table 38. Regime for preventing emesis during single fraction TBI in adults.

Patient fasting from previous midnight
Intravenous hydration
Phenobarbitone (80 mg/m^2) i.v. every 2 h
Hydrocortisone (80 mg/m^2) i.v. every 4 h
Diazepam (10 mg) i.v. for restlessness

Table 39. Examples of TBI fractionation regimes used in Europe and the USA.

Centre	Machine	Dose rate (cGy/min)	Dose (Gy)	Fractions
Royal Marsden Hospital, Surrey, UK	Dual 60 Co	4	10.5	single
Hammersmith Hospital London, UK	Linear accelerator	15	12	6 (2 × daily)
Middlesex Hospital London, UK	Linear accelerator	22	14.4	8 (2 × daily)
Istituto Nazionale per la Ricerca sul Cancro, Genova, Italy	Linear accelerator	6	9.9	3 (1 × daily)
Institut J Paoli 1 Calmettes, Marseille, France	Linear accelerator	4	11	5 (1 × daily)
University of Minnesota Minneapolis, USA	Linear accelerator	10	13.2	8 (2 × daily)
Fred Hutchinson Cancer Research Center, Seattle, USA	Dual 60 Co	4	12	6 (1 × daily)
Memorial Sloan-Kettering Cancer Centre, New York, USA	Linear accelerator	12	13.2	11 (3 × daily)

fraction TBI (**Table 39**). In a recent survey, over half of European centres used single fractions of 8–10 Gy, while the rest employed fractionated (Altschuler *et al.*, 1989; Kim *et al.*, 1990) or hyperfractionated (more than one fraction per day) radiotherapy (Cosset *et al.*, 1989).

The dose specification point is also important. The dose is most often prescribed to the mid-point of the abdomen, but some centres prefer to specify their dose to the maximum lung isodose, as the lungs are the critical dose-limiting structure in TBI (Deeg *et al.*, 1986; Weiner 1987). It should be noted that when TBI is given for non-malignant disorders the total dose is usually lower (5–6 Gy), reflecting the fact that tumour cell kill is unnecessary.

Many centres use lung shielding to limit the total dose to the lungs, while giving a higher dose to other parts of the body. However, this requires accurate positioning of the patient, which may be difficult to maintain during long treatment times. There is also the potential risk of shielding leukaemic cells.

It may also be necessary to administer additional booster radiotherapy to sanctuary sites such as the brain and testes. Testicular irradiation can be given simply by direct orthovoltage (250 kV) machines. Cranial irradiation is carried out with the patient positioned in a supine head shell using parallel opposed fields with lead shielding to the orbits and nasopharynx (**210, 211**). The whole cranium is treated on a linear accelerator using megavoltage photons to a dose of 18–24 Gy in 1.8–2.0 Gy fractions.

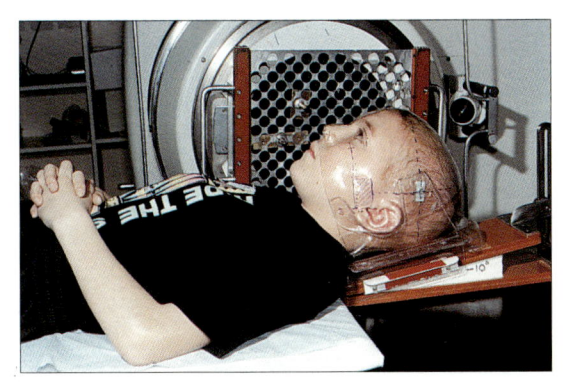

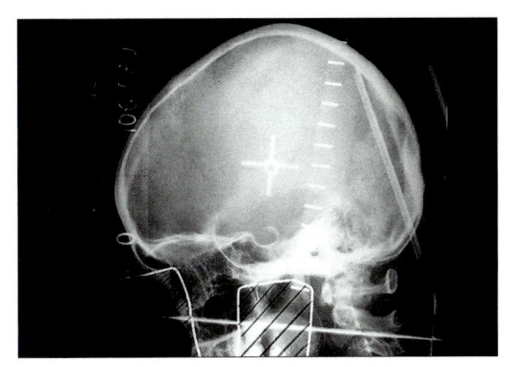

210, 211 Cranial booster radiotherapy may be used to treat sanctuary sites. A supine head shell is used with lead shielding to orbits and nasopharynx.

References

Altschuler C, Resbeut M, Maraninchi D *et al.* Fractionated total body irradiation and allogeneic bone marrow transplantation for standard risk leukaemia. *Radiat Oncol* 1989; **16**: 289–295.

Cosset JM, Baume D, Pico JL *et al.* Single dose versus hyperfractionated total body irradiation before allogeneic bone marrow transplantation: a non-randomized comparative study of 54 patients at the Institut Gustave-Roussy. *Radiat Oncol* 1989; **15**: 151–160.

Deeg HJ, Sullivan KM, Buckner CD *et al.* Marrow transplantation for acute nonlymphoblastic leukaemia in first remission: toxicity and long term follow-up of patients conditioned with single dose or fractionated total body irradiation. *Bone Marrow Transplant* 1986; **1**: 151-157.

Kim TH, McGlave PB, Ramsay NR.*et al.* Comparison of two total body irradiation regimes in allogeneic bone marrow transplantation for acute non-lymphoblastic leukaemia in first remission. *Int J Radiat Oncol Biol Phys* 1990; **19**: 889–897

Tiley C, Powles RL, Catalano J *et al.*Results of a double blind placebo controlled study of Ondasetron as an antiemetic during total body irradiation in patients undergoing bone marrow transplantation. *Leukaemia Lymphoma* 1992; **7**: 317-321.

Weiner RS. Interstitial pneumonitis following bone marrow transplantation. In: *Recent Advances in Bone Marrow Transplantation*, 1987. Eds: Gale RP, Champlin RE. Alan R Liss, New York, pp. 507–523.

2. Chemotherapy Conditioning Agents

Edward Kanfer

There are three principal objectives for bone marrow transplant (BMT) conditioning therapy: 'space-making', immunosuppression and disease eradication. The first of these involves competition between stem cells originating from the host and those of donor origin, although the precise biology of this competition has not been fully elucidated. It may, however, revolve around the presumed requirement for immature progenitor cells to occupy defined niches within the marrow stroma in order to obtain necessary nutrient and cytokine support for proliferation and differentiation, and the consequent necessity for existing stem cells to be eradicated in order for donor engraftment to take place. Pre-graft ablation is therefore an important prerequisite for patients with hyperplastic marrows as is the case in thalassaemia major, and it is of less importance in patients with a severely hypocellular marrow, as in aplastic anaemia. The principal agents used for this purpose are those with a major effect on stem cells, such as total body irradiation (TBI), busulphan, the nitrosoureas and melphalan. Conversely, cyclophosphamide, which is very commonly used in the BMT conditioning setting (see below), is not usually sufficient on its own to ablate the host marrow except in hypoplastic states.

Immunosuppression, as in solid organ transplantation, is required to prevent rejection of the donor allogeneic marrow and is clearly not necessary in the context of autologous BMT. The probability of marrow rejection is related to several factors:
- Closeness of match between the HLA types of donor and recipient (non-HLA identity increases rejection risk).
- Whether donor and recipient are related or unrelated (unrelated pairing increases risk).
- Whether the recipient has received multiple transfusions of blood products (most relevant in patients with aplastic anaemia).
- Whether the marrow has been T-lymphocyte depleted prior to transfusion into the recipient (which increases the risk of subsequent graft rejection).

The immunosuppressive conditioning agents most commonly used are high-dose cyclophosphamide and TBI, although by themselves these may not be sufficient to permit permanent donor marrow engraftment in some instances. Additional post-graft immunosuppression such as cyclosporin is usually given to prevent graft-versus-host disease (GvHD), and this has the added benefit of inhibiting the recipient from mounting an anti-donor rejection response.

In patients with malignancy, BMT is employed with curative intent, and the role of the cytotoxic conditioning therapy, in addition to that described above, is to eradicate neoplastic cells. Until the last few years it was assumed that the mechanism of cure resided entirely with this therapy, and that the transplant itself was a purely supportive measure designed to allow the patient to receive very high-dose supralethal anti-neoplastic treatment without suffering the permanent marrow aplasia that would otherwise result. However, analysis of the results of large numbers of transplants in patients with leukaemia strongly suggests that other mechanisms of cure are operative (Horowitz et al., 1990). Recipients of identical twin (syngeneic) grafts relapse more frequently than do allogeneic recipients, patients who develop GvHD after allogeneic BMT relapse less often than those who do not, and recipients of T-lymphocyte depleted marrow, an extremely effective method of preventing GvHD, have a significantly increased risk for disease relapse compared with patients receiving T-replete grafts. These findings point towards an allogeneic graft-versus-leukaemia (GvL) effect independent of the high-dose conditioning therapy employed, and the mechanisms of this remain uncertain. However, despite experimental and clinical evidence supporting an important role for GvL after allogeneic BMT, it appears that a percentage of both autologous and syngeneic BMT recipients are cured by the procedure and that the pre-graft cytotoxic therapy must be a major factor in these circumstances.

Complications of conditioning therapy

Early studies in patients with advanced haematological malignancy demonstrated a small but significant cure rate for allogeneic BMT of about 10–15%, an encouraging result in a heavily pre-treated end-stage population (Thomas et al., 1977). The major causes of treatment failure were GvHD, cytomegalovirus pneumonia and leukaemic relapse. However, it was also clear that a proportion of patients were experiencing considerable morbidity from the conditioning therapy, and that in some cases this toxicity was either fatal in itself or at least contributed very significantly towards an early post-BMT demise. This therapy-related mortality was primarily due to the development of idiopathic (toxic) interstitial pneumonitis and hepatic veno-occlusive disease. Additionally, toxic effects on the gastrointestinal, cardiovascular and neurological systems caused notable morbidity in a proportion of patients.

These problems have assumed increasing importance in current clinical BMT practice. Firstly, during the 1980s there was a trend towards intensifying conditioning therapies beyond the original Seattle 'gold standard' of cyclophosphamide (120 mg/kg) with TBI (10 Gy). Although some such studies suggested reduced leukaemic relapse rates, this was not a universal finding and early toxic mortality was often increased with, in some cases, an overall reduction in disease-free survival. Secondly, there has been an increasing tendency to utilise unrelated donors for allogeneic BMT in patients without a suitable related marrow source for the past few years, and also the median age of BMT recipients has been rising. Both of these factors increase the likelihood for early transplant-related morbidity and mortality. Thirdly, as mentioned above, it has become clear that donor immunocompetent cells may play a significant curative role after allogeneic BMT for leukaemia (GvL). For these reasons the intensification of conditioning therapies may be inadvisable in the allogeneic BMT setting and several centres have utilised non-TBI-containing preparative therapy, at least partly to reduce early toxicity. Advances in our understanding of GvL, and the ability to manipulate this clinically may allow an overall reduction in intensity of conditioning therapy in the future.

Individual agents

The great majority of transplants for non-malignant conditions, such as severe aplastic anaemia, haemoglobinopathies and inborn errors of metabolism, utilise either cyclophosphamide alone or cyclophosphamide with a space-making agent such as busulphan for conditioning therapy. For this reason the other agents discussed below are used almost exclusively in patients with haematological or other malignancies.

The early toxic complications which impact most significantly on survival and which include idiopathic interstitial pneumonitis and hepatic veno-occlusive disease are mentioned below and discussed in more detail elsewhere. However two almost universal immediate problems associated with the preparative therapy which should be noted here are emesis and mucositis, if only because they may be the cause of much misery for the patients affected.

Although the emetic potential of the cytotoxic drugs used varies, it is safest to assume that all conditioning therapies will induce vomiting in the majority of patients. For this reason anti-emetic therapy should be given prophylactically. The most effective of such agents currently available are the 5-HT3 (5-hyrdroxytryptamine) antagonists, and the combination of these with other anti-emetic drugs can prevent vomiting in nearly all patients.

Mucositis is a predictable result of the conditioning therapy and is particularly associated with TBI, busulphan, melphalan, cytosine arabinoside and the anthracycline antibiotics. Factors which may increase the severity of mucositis are the use of combinations of the above agents and the employment of methotrexate for GvHD prophylaxis. Liberal use of opiate analgesia may be necessary, and parenteral nutrition is often required if significant mucositis is prolonged. Additionally it is important to exclude superimposed infection, with, for example, herpes simplex virus or *Candida*, since the clinical features of these may be difficult to distinguish from the underlying chemotherapy-related toxicity.

Cyclophosphamide

Cyclophosphamide (CY) has been the most widely used drug in BMT conditioning therapy, principally because it has very useful immunosuppressive properties in addition to cytotoxic efficacy against a wide range of malignancies. The metabolism of CY by the liver produces several compounds with alkylating properties including phosphoramide mustard and aldophosphamide. Another metabolite, acrolein, is believed to be the major cause of haemorrhagic cystitis (see below).

CY alone and with TBI were the early standard conditioning therapies used in BMT for aplastic anaemia and leukaemia respectively (Thomas *et al.*, 1977; Storb *et al.*, 1980). While these remain the agents of choice for most patients with aplastic anaemia, various preparative protocols for leukaemia BMT studied subsequently have added other agents to these two, such as etoposide, cytosine arabinoside and busulphan.

The dose of CY used in the BMT context is usually in the range of 120–200 mg/kg. At this level of therapy the major toxicities encountered are myocardial damage and haemorrhagic cystitis. Cardiac toxicity associated with CY is well recognised (Gottdeiner *et al.*, 1981) and clearly dose-related (Goldberg *et al.*, 1986). Approximately one-third of patients receiving 120 mg/kg CY develop acute electrocardiographic changes (Kupari *et al.*, 1990b) although less than half of these demonstrate clinical evidence of impairment of cardiac function.

Long-term cardiac dysfunction appears to be uncommon (Kupari et al 1990a). Haemorrhagic cystitis following CY therapy is thought to be due to the ulcerative and vasculitic effects of acrolein on the urothelium (Cox, 1979). However, other agents such as radiation, additional cytotoxic drugs and viral infections have been implicated in the aetiology of haemorrhagic cystitis, and the specific protective agent (2-mercaptoethane sulphonate sodium, MESNA) is not universally effective in haemorrhagic cystitis prevention (Arcese, 1990).

Another complication of high-dose CY to be noted is inappropriate anti-diuretic hormone secretion (SIADH) which usually occurs during or shortly after conditioning therapy. This is commonly of short duration and frequently responds to simple measures such as fluid restriction.

Busulphan

The alkylating agent busulphan (Bu), and the closely related dimethylbusulphan, have been used as preparative agents in BMT for both malignant and non-malignant conditions (Santos *et al.*, 1983; Shaw *et al.*, 1986; Lucarelli *et al.*, 1987). The dose of Bu commonly used for this purpose is in the range of 14–16 mg/kg, usually given over 4 days. In the context of BMT for haematological malignancy Bu is often used as a substitute for TBI (Santos *et al.*, 1983), although it has been incorporated into regimens which include radiation (Petersen *et al.*, 1989). However, this latter strategy may result in unacceptable levels of toxicity (Kanfer *et al.*, 1987).

Important complications of high-dose Bu therapy are mucositis, interstitial pneumonitis, hepatic veno-occlusive disease and seizures. The mucositis experienced may be severe and prolonged. Idiopathic interstitial pneumonitis occurs in about 10% of patients following BMT conditioning therapy, and seems particularly related to the use of TBI or busulphan. Similarly, the incidence of veno-occlusive disease reflects the intensity of the conditioning regimen and is a complication associated with both TBI and Bu, although it is seen less frequently with other agents. Bu is well recognised as causing seizures (Marcus and Goldman, 1984) at this dosage and prophylaxis is commonly employed. Bu is also thought to contribute towards the development of haemorrhagic cystitis (Millard, 1981).

Melphalan

Melphalan is an alkylating agent belonging to the nitrogen mustard group of drugs. Its major use in the field of BMT conditioning has been as sole agent in autologous transplantation both for solid tumours (McElwain *et al.*, 1981; Lazarus *et al.*, 1983) and haematological malignancies, especially myeloma (Maraninchi *et al.*, 1986; Barlogie *et al*, 1986). However, it is also used in combination with TBI for allogeneic BMT (Helenglass *et al.*, 1988).

The dose of melphalan given is usually in the range of 100–180 mg/m^2. The important toxicities of melphalan when utilised at this dose are mucositis, which may be particularly severe, and renal impairment. In the context of BMT for myeloma this latter potential complication may prejudice its use.

Cytosine arabinoside

Cytosine arabinoside (Ara-C) is an antimetabolite which inhibits DNA synthesis and increases its susceptibility to degradation. It has been widely used both for primary therapy and in conditioning protocols for BMT in patients with haematological malignancy. In the latter situation it has been combined with TBI (Champlin et al 1985; Weyman et al., 1993), with CY and TBI (Trigg et al., 1989), and it has been used in several regimens excluding radiation such as BACT (Philip et al., 1985), BAVC (Mandelli et al., 1986) and LACE (Kanfer et al., 1992).

The dose of Ara-C used in BMT preparative therapy has varied widely from 4 to 36 g/m^2. Serious complications, which are generally dose related, include neurological, gastrointestinal, retinal and pulmonary toxicity. In addition, as with busulphan, there is some evidence to suggest that Ara-C may cause haemorrhagic cystitis (Renert et al., 1973).

Etoposide (VP-16-213)

Etoposide has become an increasingly utilised component of BMT cytotoxic preparative therapies. Like teniposide, it is a derivative of podophyllotoxin and is believed to act through the inhibition of cellular topoisomerase-II (Chow et al., 1988). It has been used in a variety of conditioning protocols for BMT in patients with acute lymphoblastic and myeloblastic leukaemias, lymphoma and myeloma in combination with TBI (Blume et al., 1987), BCNU, amsacrine and cytosine arabinoside (Mandelli et al., 1986), busulphan and CY (Spitzer et al., 1989), and BCNU with CY (Zander et al., 1987; Ventura et al., 1990).

The dose of etoposide used in these regimens has ranged from 450 mg/m^2 to 60 mg/kg. Serious toxicity with this agent is usually liver related, and haemorrhagic cystitis has been described (Blume et al., 1987).

BCNU/CCNU

The nitrosoureas are a group of alkylating agents which include BCNU (carmustine) and CCNU (lomustine). These drugs have principally found popularity in protocols for autologous BMT for patients with solid tumours as well as haematological malignancies. Examples of regimens used are BAVC (Mandelli et al., 1986), BACT (Philip et al., 1985), CBV (Zander et al., 1987), CCB (Peters et al., 1986) and LACE (Kanfer et al., 1992).

The doses of BCNU and CCNU used have ranged from 250 to 800 mg/m^2 and 200 to 500 mg/m^2, respectively. The nitrosoureas are amongst the most toxic of the commonly utilised conditioning agents, and serious hepatic, renal, neurologic and pulmonary complications may arise.

Thiotepa

Thiotepa is an alkylating agent of the aziridine group. Its main use in the context of conditioning therapy has been for patients with brain tumours receiving autologous BMT (Kalifa et al., 1992), although there has been recent experience of adding this agent to the cytoreductive preparation of patients with chronic myelogenous leukaemia. Neurotoxicity and skin eruptions are recognised complications of therapy.

Platinum compounds

The platinum-derived agents, cisplatin and carboplatin, have alkylating-like properties and have found a particular place in BMT for solid tumours, for example in combination with CY and BCNU (Peters et al., 1986), and with CY and etoposide (Guimaraes et al., 1992). The doses of cisplatin and carboplatin used have been in the region of 150 mg/m^2 and 1500 mg/m^2, respectively.

The principal toxicities of these agents are renal, auditory, neurological and symptomatic hypomagnesaemia. They are also notably emetogenic. However, carboplatin is substantially less likely to produce these complications than cisplatin.

Daunorubicin/doxorubicin

Daunorubicin and doxorubicin are anthracycline antibiotics, the mode of action of which appears to be topoisomerase-II inhibition. Although both of these agents are active against a wide variety of haematological and non-haematological tumours, they have not been used frequently in the BMT-conditioning context because of significant dose-limiting toxicities. The most important of these are cardiac and gastrointestinal.

Examples of regimens used are the combination of daunorubicin with TBI and CY (Goldman *et al.*, 1986), and the replacement of daunorubicin by idarubicin (Raemaekers *et al.*, 1989).

Combinations of cytotoxic agents

Although conditioning therapies with single agents have been used in the setting of autologous BMT, for example melphalan for myeloma and BCNU for malignant glioma, the majority of protocols employed have utilised several drugs in combination. This strategy has the advantages that resistance to all of the agents by the malignant cell population is less likely than it might be with monotherapy, and that toxicity profiles for the drugs used may reduce overall morbidity compared with the equivalent intensity provided by a single drug. In addition, the substitution of TBI by chemotherapeutic agents may lessen early significant toxicity without compromising the efficacy of the BMT procedure (Kanfer and McCarthy, 1989).

Examples of some of the more commonly used chemotherapy conditioning regimens have been mentioned above and are shown in **Table 40**.

Table 40. Examples of combination chemotherapy BMT conditioning regimens (see text for references).

BACT	BCNU 200 mg/m^2; cytosine arabinoside 800 mg/m^2; cyclophosphamide 200 mg/kg; 6 thioguanine 800 mg/m^2
BAVC	BCNU 800 mg/m^2; amsacrine 450 mg/m^2; etoposide 450 mg/m^2; cytosine arabinoside 900 mg/m^2.
BuCy	Busulphan 14–16 mg/kg; cyclophosphamide 120–200 mg/kg.
BuCyVP	Busulphan 16 mg/kg; cyclophosphamide 120 mg/kg; etoposide 30 mg/kg.
CBV	Cyclophosphamide 6 g/m^2; BCNU 300 mg/m^2; etoposide 600 mg/m^2.
CCB	Cyclophosphamide 5.625 g/m^2; cisplatin 165 mg/m^2; BCNU 600 mg/m^2.
CCE	Cyclophosphamide 80–120 mg/kg; carboplatin 1500 mg/m^2; etoposide 1200–1800 mg/m^2.
LACE	CCNU 200 mg/m^2; cytosine arabinoside 4 g/m^2; cyclophosphamide 5.4 g/m^2; etoposide 1 g/m^2.
Bu/Thio	Busulphan 600 mg/m^2; thiotepa 950 mg/m^2.

Conclusions

As the number of diseases for which BMT becomes a therapeutic option increases, it is likely that the variety of conditioning protocols in use will enlarge. Hopefully the incorporation of newer, more effective and less toxic agents will reduce procedure-related morbidity and mortality and ultimately improve the long-term results achievable with this increasingly utilised therapy.

References

Arcese W. Hemorrhagic cystitis in allogeneic bone marrow transplantation—Gruppo Italiano Trapianto Medollo Osseo. *Bone Marrow Transplant* 1990; **5** (suppl 2): 19.

Barlogie B, Hall R, Zander A et al. High-dose melphalan with autologous bone marrow tranplantation for multiple myeloma. *Blood* 1986; **67**: 1298–1301.

Blume KG, Forman SJ, O'Donnell MR et al. Total body irradiation and high-dose etoposide: a new preparatory regimen for bone marrow transplantation in patients with advanced hematologic malignancies. *Blood* 1987; **69**: 1015–1020.

Champlin R, Jacobs A, Gale RP et al. High-dose cytarabine in consolidation chemotherapy or with bone marrow transplantation for patients with acute leukemia: preliminary results. *Semin Oncol* 1985; **12**: (suppl 3): 190–195.

Chow K-C, Macdonald TL, Ross E. DNA binding by epipodophyllotoxins and *N*-acyl anthracyclines: implications for mechanism of topoisomerase-II inhibition. *Mol Pharmacol* 1988; **34**: 467–473.

Cox PJ. Cyclophosphamide cystitis: identification of acrolein as the causative agent. *Biochem Pharmacol* 1979; **28**: 2045–2049.

Goldberg MA, Antin JH, Guinan EC, Rappeport JM. Cyclophosphamide cardiotoxicity: an analysis of dosing as a risk factor. *Blood* 1986; **68**: 1114–1118.

Goldman JM, Apperley JF, Jones L et al. Bone marrow transplantation for patients with chronic myeloid leukemia. *N Eng J Med* 1986; **314**: 202–207.

Gottdeiner JS, Appelbaum FR, Ferrans VJ et al. Cardiotoxicity associated with high-dose cyclophosphamide therapy. *Arch Intern Med* 1981; **141**: 758–763.

Guimaraes A, Camba L, Hall G et al. High dose chemotherapy followed by autologous bone marrow transplant for refractory germ cell tumours. *Leukemia Lymphoma* 1992; **7**: (suppl): 65–68.

Helenglass G, Powles RL, McElwain TJ et al. Melphalan and total body irradiation (TBI) versus cyclophosphamide and TBI as conditioning for allogeneic matched sibling bone marrow transplants for acute myeloblastic leukaemia in first remission. *Bone Marrow Transplant* 1988; **3**: 21–31.

Horowitz MM, Gale RP, Sondel PM et al. Graft-versus-leukemia reactions after bone marrow transplantation. *Blood* 1990; **75**: 555–562.

Kalifa C, Hartmann O, Demeocq F et al. High-dose busulfan and thiotepa with autologous bone marrow transplantation in childhood malignant brain tumors: a Phase II study. *Bone Marrow Transplant* 1992; **9**: 227–233.

Kanfer EJ, McCarthy DM. Cytoreductive preparation for bone marrow transplantation in leukaemia: to irradiate or not? *Br J Haematol* 1989; **71**: 447–450.

Kanfer EJ, Buckner CD, Fefer A et al. Allogeneic and syngeneic marrow transplantation following high dose dimethylbusulfan, cyclophosphamide and total body irradiation. *Bone Marrow Transplant* 1987; **1**: 339–346.

Kanfer EJ, Macdonald I, Hall G et al. Poor prognosis acute myeloid leukaemia treated by matched unrelated donor marrow transplant without preceding total body irradiation. *Bone Marrow Transplant* 1992; **9**: 67–69.

Kupari M, Volin L, Suokas A, et al. Cardiac involvement in bone marrow transplantation: serial changes in left ventricular size, mass and performance. *J Intern Med* 1990a; **227**: 259–266.

Kupari M, Volin L, Suokas A et al. Cardiac involvement in bone marrow transplantation: electrocardiographic changes, arrhythmias, heart failure and autopsy findings. *Bone Marrow Transplant* 1990b; **5**: 91–98.

Lazarus HM, Herzig RH, Graham-Pole J, et al. Intensive melphalan chemotherapy and cryopreserved autologous bone marrow transplantation for the treatment of refractory cancer. *J Clin Oncol* 1983; **1**: 359–367.

Lucarelli G, Galimberti M, Polchi P et al. Marrow transplantation in patients with advanced thalassemia. *N Eng J Med* 1987; **316**: 1050–1055.

Mandelli F, Rizzoli V, Carella AM. Massive cytoreductive therapy and autologous BMT after intensive conventional chemotherapy. *Bone Marrow Transplant* 1986; **1** (suppl 1): 259–260.

Maraninchi D, Pico JL, Hartmann O et al. High-dose melphalan with or without marrow transplantation: a study of dose–effect in patients with refractory and/or relapsed leukaemia. *Cancer Treat Rep* 1986; **70**: 445–448.

Marcus RE, Goldman JM. Convulsions due to high-dose busulphan. *Lancet* 1984; **2**: 1463.

McElwain TJ, Hedley DW, Burton G et al. Marrow autotransplantation accelerates haematological recovery in patients with malignant melanoma treated with high-dose melphalan. *Br J Cancer* 1981; **40**: 72–80.

Millard RJ. Busulphan-induced hemorrhagic cystitis. *Urology* 1981; **18**: 143–144.

Peters WP, Eder JP, Henner WD et al. High-dose combination alkylating agents with autologous bone marrow support: a Phase I trial. *J Clin Oncol* 1986; **4**: 646–654.

Petersen FB, Buckner CD, Appelbaum FR et al. Busulfan, cyclophosphamide and fractionated total body irradiation as a conditioning regimen for marrow transplantation in patients with advanced hematological malignancies: a Phase I study. *Bone Marrow Transplant* 1989; **4**: 617–623.

Philip T, Biron P, Maraninchi D et al. Massive chemotherapy with autologous bone marrow transplantation in 50 cases of bad prognosis non-Hodgkin's lymphoma. *Br J Haematol* 1985; **60**: 599–609.

Raemaekers J, de Witte T, Schattenberg A et al. Prevention of leukemic relapse after transplantation with lymphocyte depleted marrow by intensification of the conditioning regimen with a 6-day infusion of anthracyclines. *Bone Marrow Transplant* 1989; **4**: 167–171.

Renert WA, Berdon WE, Baker DH. Haemorrhagic cystitis and vesicoureteric reflux secondary to cytotoxic therapy for childhood malignancies. *Am J Roentgenol* 1973; **117**: 664–669.

Santos GW, Tutschka PJ, Brookmeyer R et al. Marrow transplantation for acute nonlymphocytic leukemia after treatment with busulfan and cyclophosphamide. *N Engl J Med* 1983; **309**: 1347–1353.

Shaw PJ, Hugh-Jones K, Hobbs JR et al. Busulphan and cyclophosphamide cause little early toxicity during displacement bone marrow transplantation in fifty children. *Bone Marrow Transplant* 1986; **1**: 193–200.

Spitzer TR, Cottler-Fox M, Torrisi J, et al. Escalating doses of etoposide with cyclophosphamide and fractionated total body irradiation or busulfan as conditioning for bone marrow transplantation. *Bone Marrow Transplant* 1989; **4**: 559–565.

Storb R, Thomas ED, Buckner CD et al. Marrow transplantation in thirty untransfused patients with severe aplastic anemia. *Ann Intern Med* 1980; **92**: 30–36.

Thomas ED, Buckner CD, Banaji M et al. One hundred patients with acute leukemia treated by chemotherapy, total body irradiation, and allogeneic marrow transplantation. *Blood* 1977; **49**: 511–533.

Trigg ME, Gingrich R, Goeken N et al. Low rejection rate when using unrelated or haploidentical donors for children with leukemia undergoing marrow transplantation. *Bone Marrow Transplant* 1989; **4**: 431–437.

Ventura GJ, Barlogie B, Hester JP et al. High-dose cyclophosphamide, BCNU and VP-16 with autologous blood stem cell support for refractory multiple myeloma. *Bone Marrow Transplant* 1990; **5**: 265–268.

Weyman C, Graham-Pole J, Emerson S et al. Use of cytosine arabinoside and total body irradiation as conditioning for allogeneic marrow transplantation in patients with acute lymphoblastic leukemia: a multicenter survey. *Bone Marrow Transplant* 1993; **11**: 43–50.

Zander AR, Culbert S, Jagannath S et al. High-dose cyclophosphamide, BCNU, and VP-16 (CBV) as a conditioning regimen for allogeneic bone marrow transplantation for patients with acute leukemia. *Cancer* 1987; **59**: 1083–1086.

IX Problems Following Bone Marrow Transplantation

1. Pulmonary Complications

Susan Height and Michael Shields

Pulmonary complications following bone marrow transplantation (BMT) account for considerable procedure-related morbidity and mortality, affecting between 40 and 60% of patients. They can be divided broadly into acute and chronic according to the time they develop following the transplant.

Complications occurring in the immediate post-transplant phase and up to 100 days are termed 'acute'. They arise mainly secondary to conditioning regimen toxicity and the marrow aplasia which inevitably follows. During this period, the patient is particularly susceptible to bacterial and fungal infections, this risk being somewhat reduced once successful marrow engraftment has occurred.

The 'chronic' complications occur from 100 days post-transplant onwards. The majority of chronic complications arise in allograft recipients receiving long-term immunosuppression who may also develop chronic graft versus host disease (GvHD). Both of these factors contribute to pulmonary disease.

The commonest complications will be described, approximately in the order in which they are likely to occur.

Pneumothorax

Pneumothorax may be associated with invasive procedures, such as Hickman line insertion, and thus may occur pretransplant. However, spontaneous pneumothorax or pneumomediastinum (**212**) may also occur as a complication of BMT in both the acute and chronic phase. Predisposing factors include the use of high-dose steroids, total body irradiation (TBI) and poor nutrition with recent weight loss. It may also be associated with the development of pneumonitis (Hill *et al*, 1987) (**213**).

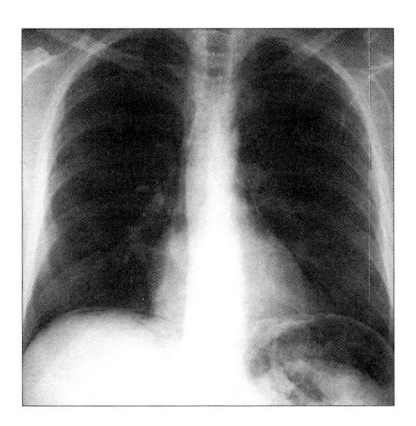

212 (left) Chest X-ray showing spontaneous pneumomediastinum and pneumoperitoneum.

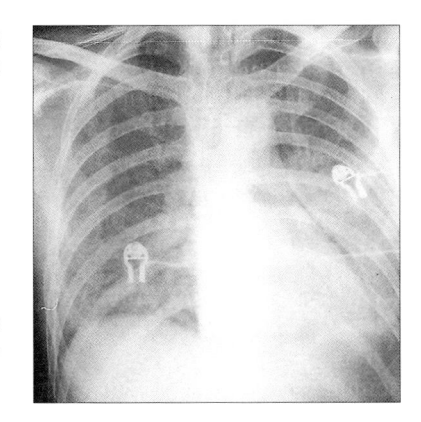

213 (right) Chest X-ray showing pneumomediastinum with pneumonitis.

Pulmonary oedema

Pulmonary oedema due to fluid overload is often seen in the first few days following BMT and may be exacerbated by previous exposure to anthracyclines and the use of cyclophosphamide and total body irradiation during conditioning (Hamilton and Pearson, 1986).

Pulmonary haemorrhage

Pulmonary haemorrhage is usually associated with infection and thrombocytopenia. It appears as alveolar shadowing on the chest X-ray (**214**). More rarely, it may be associated with the development of acute haemorrhagic pulmonary oedema, which occurs typically in patients receiving high doses of cyclosporine who are undergoing matched–unrelated transplants. The clinical features are those of fluid retention, acute renal failure, hypotension, hypoalbuminaemia and a low central venous pressure. This syndrome has a high mortality. Pathologically, there is alveolar and interstitial oedema with fibrin exudation and red cells in the alveolar spaces (Sloane *et al*, 1983) (**215**).

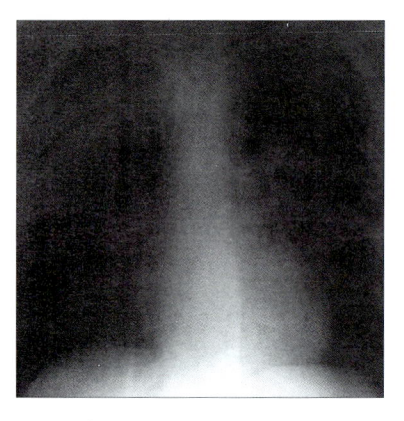

214 Chest X-Ray showing widespread alveolar haemorrhage.

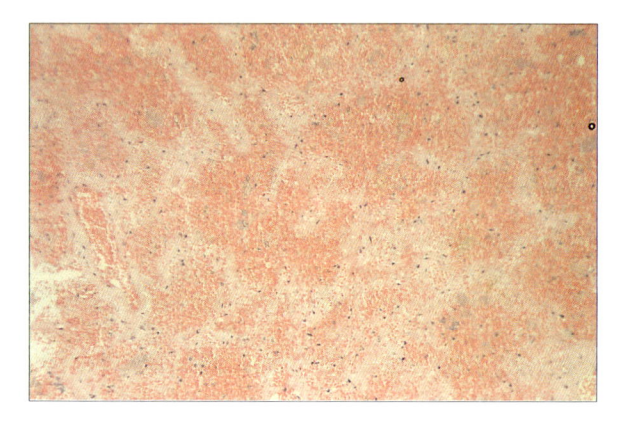

215 Lung biopsy showing intra-alveolar haemorrhage.

Pulmonary embolus

Transient hypoxia may occur at the time of marrow infusion due to the presence of small particles of bone and fat in the marrow. However, chronic endothelial changes and thickening of the intima in pulmonary vessels has been demonstrated, possibly related to radiation damage. This may predispose to thrombotic events at a later stage. Pulmonary thrombi have been found at post-mortem in up to 50% of BMT patients, although they may not have been of clinical significance during life (Krowka *et al*, 1985).

Infections

Bacterial infections

Acute Phase

During the acute phase following BMT, bacterial respiratory infections occur frequently (20–50%) (Cordonnier *et al*, 1986), particularly during neutropenia. There may be few clinical or radiological signs.

Oropharyngeal mucositis is a common complication, and colonization by Gram-positive or Gram-negative organisms, particularly *Pseudomonas* sp., *Klebsiella*, *Serratia* and *Enterobacter* sp. frequently occurs. Spread to the lungs may be direct by aspiration or indirect by bacteraemia, leading to lower respiratory tract infection.

Atypical organisms—including *Mycoplasma pneumoniae*, *Legionella* (**216**) and *Chlamydia*—have also been implicated in both the acute and chronic post-transplant phase.

Most antibiotic regimens are designed to provide good Gram-positive and Gram-negative cover and are usually commenced empirically when patients become febrile. Early intervention with antibiotic therapy results in the prompt resolution of some bacterial infections. However, if the patient does not respond clinically and develops signs of pulmonary infection it may be necessary to perform bronchoscopy with bronchoalveolar lavage in order to identify the causative organisms. Transbronchial biopsy or open lung biopsy are no longer performed routinely. While results are pending, further antibiotic treatment may be added in order to cover atypical organisms and fungi. Rarely, mycobacterial species may be isolated.

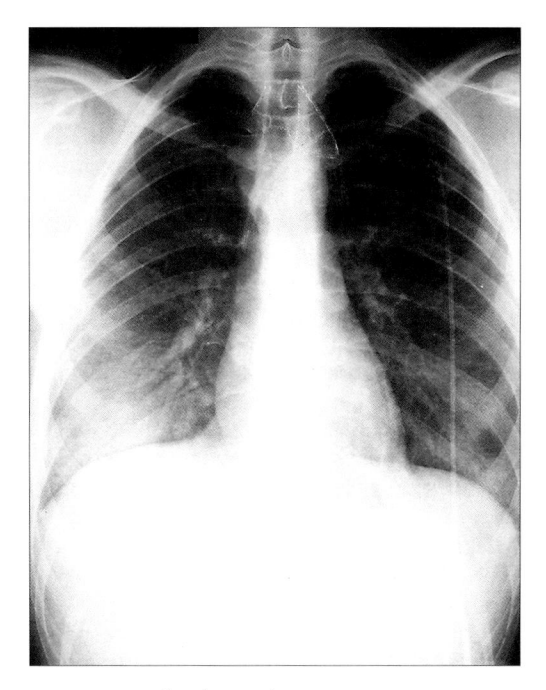

216 Legionella chest infection.

Chronic phase

Following TBI, effective splenic function is lost and patients are vulnerable to infection by capsulated organisms, especially *Streptococcus*. It is now common practice to give patients prophylactic penicillin V for one to two years following BMT until splenic function is regained. Many respiratory infections which occur during the chronic phase are due to *Streptocccus* sp., *Staphylococcus* sp., and *Haemophilus influenzae*. Chronic GvHD is a predisposing factor. The widespread use of co-trimoxazole prophylaxis for *Pneumocystis carinii* may help to reduce the overall incidence of Gram-negative pulmonary infections, although patients who have obstructive airways disease are more prone.

Viral infections

The herpes virus family accounts for the majority of viral respiratory infections post-BMT, cytomegalovirus (CMV) being found most commonly. However, the other herpes viruses are responsible for up to 7% of infectious pneumonitis (Chan *et al*, 1990); herpes simplex pneumonitis occurs mainly in the first few weeks post-BMT, whilst varicella zoster pneumonitis is usually a late complication.

Other respiratory viruses, particularly respiratory syncytial virus (RSV), the parainfluenzae viruses and adenovirus have been implicated in episodes of pneumonitis.

Cytomegalovirus

CMV infection is associated with a high morbidity and mortality in allogeneic BMT recipients. Interstitial pneumonitis is a serious complication occurring in 15–20% of patients with a mortality of 85%, and CMV is implicated in up to 70% of these cases. The peak time for the development of CMV pneumonitis is from 100 days post-transplant onwards.

Among adults, 80% are CMV positive, and in this group re-infection or re-activation of latent virus may occur during immunosuppression associated with transplant conditioning. In CMV-negative patients the virus may be acquired as a primary infection at the time of transplant if a CMV-positive donor is used, or as a result of CMV transmission via leukocytes in blood products. Primary infection is most likely to cause symptoms in the early post-transplant period, whereas re-activation may remain subclinical until later.

Risk factors for development of CMV pneumonitis include increasing age of the patient, the presence and severity of graft versus host disease (GvHD), and also CMV-negative recipients of CMV-positive marrow (Levin, 1990).

Clinically, CMV pneumonitis is not distinguishable from other causes (see below) and is associated with dyspnoea, a dry cough, and infiltrates on the chest X-ray (**217**). These may progress rapidly with the development of respiratory failure.

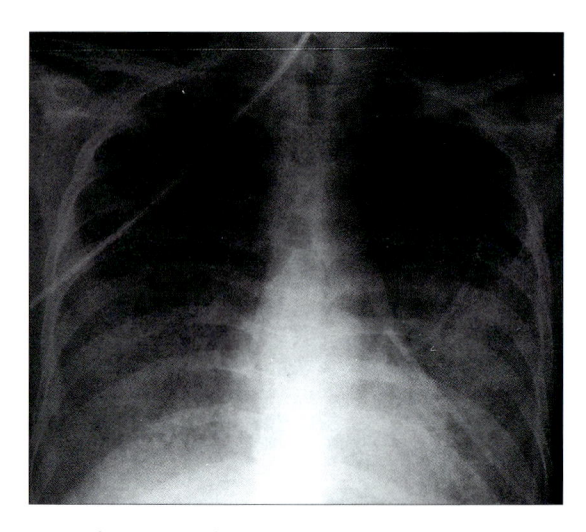

217 Chest X-ray showing CMV pneumonitis.

Diagnosis
Determining whether or not CMV is responsible for pneumonitis occurring in a patient known to be CMV-positive can be difficult. If the diagnosis is suspected, fibreoptic bronchoscopy and bronchoalveolar lavage are performed as soon as possible. The presence of CMV in the lavage fluid may be detected rapidly by the use of monoclonal antibodies, with CMV culture providing confirmation with a high degree of sensitivity and specificity (95–100% and 80–100% respectively) (Chan *et al*, 1988). However, the virus may be isolated from lavage fluid in CMV-positive patients who do not have pneumonitis (Ruutu *et al*, 1990). The results of lavage analysis must therefore be interpreted in the context of the clinical picture. CMV inclusion bodies may be seen on biopsy (**218**), but transbronchial biopsies are not usually performed in these patients due to thrombocytopenia and haemostatic problems. *In situ* hybridization may also detect virus in tissue (Spector, 1990). Isolation of CMV from buffy coats, urine and throat washings may provide further evidence of active infection.

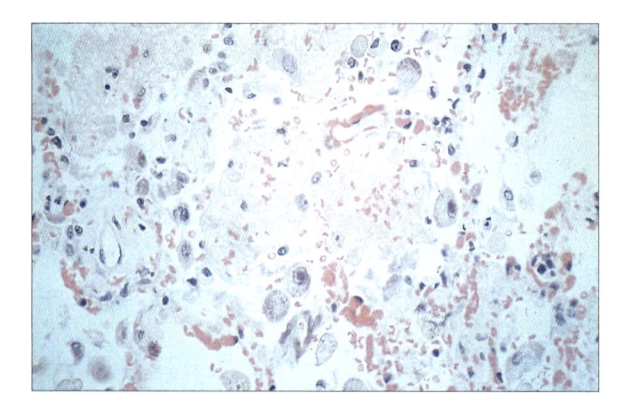

Serology is not a reliable guide to infection in post-transplant patients because of the global impairment of antibody responses during the first few months. An exception to this generalization is the demonstration of a fourfold rise in anti-CMV IgM titres, since this strongly suggests a primary CMV infection in a CMV-negative recipient.

Pathology
CMV pneumonitis is characterized by oedema and an inflammatory infiltrate with little evidence of viral replication in the affected tissue. It appears that the pulmonary damage is not a direct result of local tissue infection, but is due to a local immune response triggered by the virus (Grundy *et al*, 1987). CMV is known to alter cell-mediated immunity via its effects on T-cell populations. This may cause abnormal immune activation following CMV infection which may be exacerbated by the presence of other factors mentioned above, including GvHD. There is evidence that CMV antigens interact with HLA antigens and this may be important in fuelling the inflammatory process in individuals with GvHD who develop CMV pneumonitis (Grundy *et al*, 1988). Further evidence that GvHD is central to the development of CMV pneumonitis is the finding that in a series of 100 syngeneic transplants none developed CMV pneumonitis compared with 16% of allogenic transplants (Appelbaum *et al*, 1982)

Treatment and prophylaxis
Ganciclovir inhibits CMV DNA replication and has been useful in the treatment of AIDS-associated CMV pneumonitis and retinitis. However, as a single agent

218 Lung biopsy showing CMV pneumonitis with CMV inclusion bodies.

it has been less successful in the treatment of CMV pneumonitis in BMT patients. Treatment starts with an induction phase at high dose and is followed by a lower maintenance dose that is continued for 10 weeks to 6 months. High-dose intravenous immunoglobulin has been used in combination with ganciclovir, and this approach seems to be more successful and various regimens are being evaluated (Emanuel, 1990). Marrow toxicity is a major drawback, however, and 50% of BMT patients are unable to tolerate ganciclovir. More recently, there have been reports of ganciclovir-resistant CMV (Drobyski *et al*, 1991).

Foscarnet is an alternative to ganciclovir and has the advantage of not being marrow toxic. It can, however, cause reversible dose-dependent renal impairment and this may preclude its use in some BMT patients. As yet it is not licensed for use in CMV patients.

High-dose intravenous anti-CMV immunoglobulin has also been used as an adjunct to ganciclovir in patients with proven CMV pneumonitis (Reed *et al*, 1988), but it is still under evaluation.

Preventive measures are taken to reduce the risk of primary CMV infection occurring at the time of transplantation in the 20% of CMV-negative recipients. CMV-negative donors are used whenever possible and CMV-negative or leukocyte-depleted blood products are used for support. In spite of these measures, up to 3% of CMV-negative patients with CMV-negative donors become seropositive following BMT (Bowden *et al*, 1986). Possible methods of preventing re-activation or re-infection occurring in CMV-positive patients are currently under evaluation; passive immunization with anti-CMV immunoglobulin does not seem to be of benefit in BMT patients. Prophylactic high-dose acyclovir has been found to be beneficial (Winston and Gale, 1991). Ganciclovir and foscarnet are currently being investigated as prophylaxis in CMV-positive patients (Bowden and Meyers, 1990) and ganciclovir may also have a role in the treatment of patients who become buffy coat positive for CMV post-transplant (Schmidt, 1991).

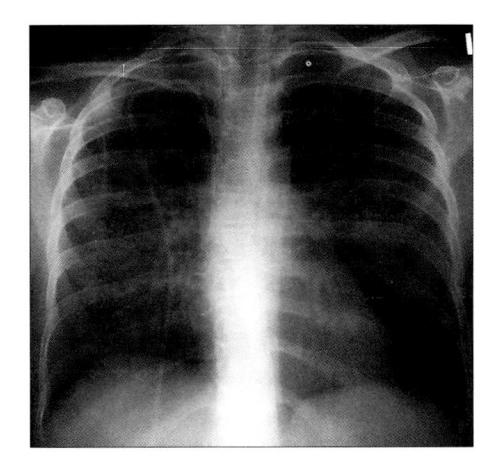

Herpes simplex

Herpes simplex Types I and II may give rise to a clinical picture similar to that of CMV pneumonitis (**219**), usually in the early post-transplant period. In one series all the patients who developed herpes simplex pneumonitis had pre-existing oral or genital herpes. Direct spread from the oropharynx or viraemia may occur to cause pulmonary infection. The use of prophylactic acyclovir may help to prevent this complication.

219 Chest X-ray of a patient with overwhelming herpes pneumonitis.

Respiratory syncitial virus (RSV)

RSV causes a diffuse, severe giant-cell pneumonitis in BMT patients. This is usually preceded by symptoms of an upper respiratory tract infection with otitis and sinusitis occurring in 40% (Foulliard *et al*, 1992). Typically, RSV pneumonitis presents with low-grade fever and dry unproductive cough, and may progress to respiratory failure. The chest X-ray may show diffuse infiltrates and, rarely, pleural effusions.

Diagnosis
Diagnosis is confirmed by bronchoscopy with bronchoalveolar lavage and detection of viral antigen in the lavage fluid. The virus may also be cultured, but this takes several days and therefore is not sufficiently rapid for diagnosis in BMT patients.

The infection is transmitted by direct contact or fomites. During the winter, 3–5% of adults in the general population may develop an RSV infection and transmission from staff may play a role in infections arising in the transplant unit.

Treatment
Treatment of RSV pneumonitis is with nebulized ribavirin, a synthetic nucleoside which inhibits DNA replication in DNA and RNA viruses. It is initially administered continuously for at least 18 hours per day for 4 days. Some patients find this intolerable,

and an alternative regimen involves use of high-dose ribavirin for shorter periods, several times per day (Engleund et al, 1990). RSV infections occurring in the early post-transplant period are associated with a worse outcome than those occurring after marrow engraftment.

Parainfluenza viruses

This group of viruses may cause both upper and lower respiratory tract infections. All four serotypes have been implicated in BMT patients, and the median time for occurrence of the infection is 3 weeks after transplant, although it may occur much later (Wendt et al, 1992). Like RSV, parainfluenza infection causes a giant-cell pneumonitis and can lead to respiratory failure. The virus may be isolated from nasopharyngeal aspirates, but bronchoalveolar lavage is usually required. This may reveal the presence of other infective organisms (Lehner et al, 1992). Ribavirin has been used to treat these patients, but its effectiveness has yet to be fully evaluated.

Adenovirus

Adenovirus causes multisystem infection including pneumonitis in the BMT patient. The only consistent risk factor, found in one series, was the occurrence of acute GvHD (Shields et al, 1985). Reverse-barrier nursing did not make any difference to the overall incidence of infection, and it has been suggested that latent virus undergoes re-activation following BMT. There is no specific agent available for treatment of adenovirus infections.

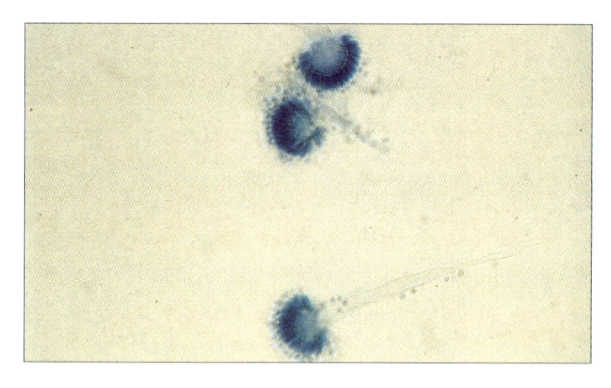

Fungal infections

Bone marrow transplant patients are susceptible to respiratory fungal infections which are mainly due to *Aspergillus* sp. (**220**), *Candida* sp. (**221**) and occasionally *Cryptococcus neoformans* (**222**).

In the acute phase, the risk of developing a fungal infection is directly related to the duration and severity of neutropoenia. During the first 3 weeks the risk of developing *Aspergillus* infection has been estimated at 1% per day, with the risk increasing to 4.3% per day after day 22 (Gerson et al, 1984). Bone marrow transplant patients remain at risk even after neutrophil recovery because of intensive transplant

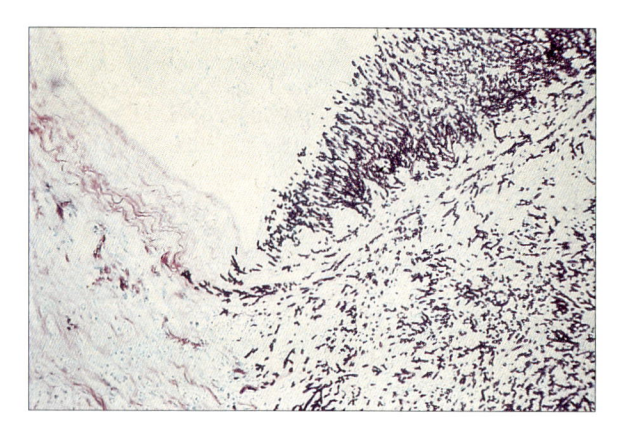

220 Microscopic appearance of *Aspergillus* sp. with hyphae formation.

221 *Candida* shown with Grocott stain.

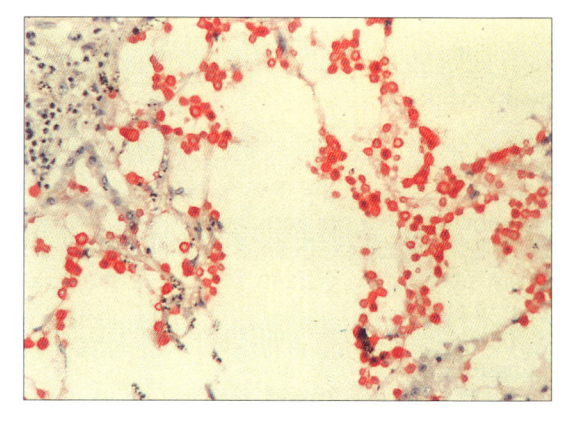

222 *Cryptococcus* identified in a lung biopsy specimen by mucicarmine stain.

conditioning and the prolonged administration of cyclosporine.

The onset of fungal infection may be insidious, often with fever unresponsive to antibacterials and no localizing symptoms or signs, although pleuritic chest pain may be a feature. The chest X-ray findings are usually non-specific and up to 25% of patients with fungal infection have normal chest X-rays at the onset. In these patients a chest computed tomography may detect early lesions (Kuhlman, 1991). However, the chest X-ray is abnormal in most cases and may demonstrate a lobar pneumonia, disseminated nodules or patchy infiltrates which change slowly and do not respond to antibacterial agents.

Aspergillus

The development of invasive pulmonary aspergillosis is associated with invasion of pulmonary vessels (**223**), usually small arterioles, and this causes haemorrhagic infarction of lung tissue. Intra-alveolar haemorrhage may occur, which appears as diffuse alveolar shadowing (**224**). Larger vessels may also be invaded leading to rapid exsanguination.

The outcome of invasive pulmonary aspergillosis depends on the timing of marrow engraftment and the re-appearance of granulocytes. With prolonged marrow aplasia, the pulmonary infiltrates progress with development of overwhelming systemic infection. However, an aspergilloma (**225**) may form. The infarcted pulmonary tissue forms a sequestrum which cavitates in the presence of granulocytes to produce a characteristic X-ray appearance, the 'air crescent' sign (Curtis *et al*, 1979). Haemorrhage may occur at this time with massive haemoptysis and disappearance of the air crescent as the air space fills with blood. In the BMT population, it is sometimes necessary to resect these lesions because of the risk of uncontrollable bleeding and further infection.

Diagnosis
Diagnosis of pulmonary aspergillosis in the early stages is difficult; sputum is positive for *Aspergillus* in less than 10% of patients and is not a diagnostic finding. Bronchoalveolar lavage may detect it in only 50% of patients with active infection (Gefter *et al*, 1985). As yet there is no generally available, reliable method of antigen detection, and in many cases treatment is commenced empirically. As mentioned above, computed tomographic scanning may be a useful adjunct in diagnosis.

Treatment and prophylaxis
Amphotericin B is started at a low dose which is then rapidly escalated. The major problems associated with its use are renal toxicity and hypokalaemia. It causes reversible abnormalities of liver function and can cause fever and rigors in some patients. Recently a liposomal form of amphotericin B has been developed which is currently under evaluation. Even with prompt treatment, the mortality of invasive fungal infections is very high.

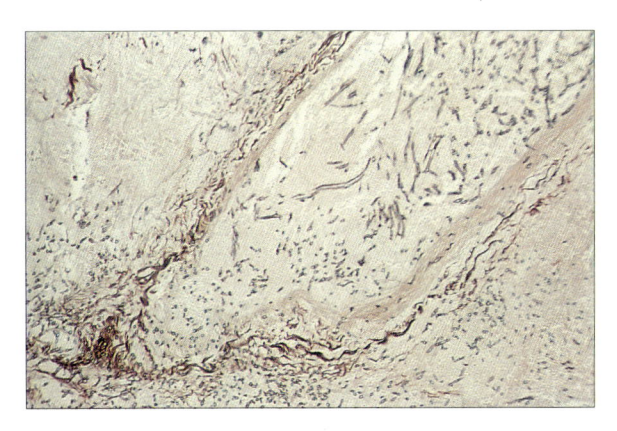

223 Invasive *Aspergillus* on lung biopsy.

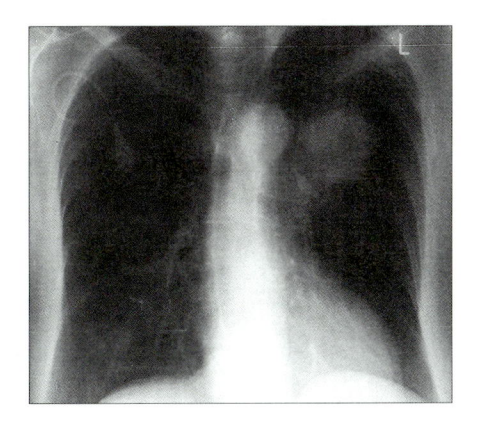

224 Chest X-ray showing an aspergilloma in a neutropenic patient.

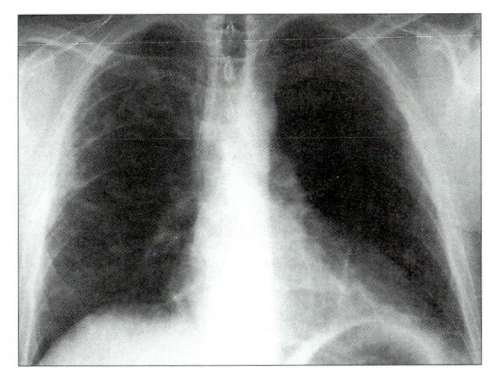

225 Chest X-ray showing intra-alveolar haemorrhage with invasive aspergillosis.

Aspergillus is a spore-forming organism which is air-borne. An important part of the prophylaxis of fungal infection in the BMT patient entails isolation and use of high-efficiency particulate air filters and laminar airflow facilities. In some units, low-dose prophylactic amphotericin from the time of conditioning has been used (Rousey *et al*, 1991).

Other significant infections

Pneumocystis carinii pneumonia

Pneumocystis carinii is an opportunistic organism which causes a desquamative alveolitis in immunocompromised patients with defective T-cell function. The peak time for development of *Pneumocystis carinii* pneumonia (PCP) post-transplant is between 30 and 100 days, and the organism is implicated in up to 4% of cases of infectious pneumonitis (Hamilton and Pearson, 1986).

The symptoms of dyspnoea and an unproductive cough with or without fever are characteristic, but not specific, for PCP. The physical signs may be few, although the patient is usually hypoxic. The classical chest X-ray appearance is of bilateral, diffuse perihilar shadowing with an alveolar pattern also described as 'ground glass' (**226**), but this may not be apparent for several days after the development of symptoms and hypoxia.

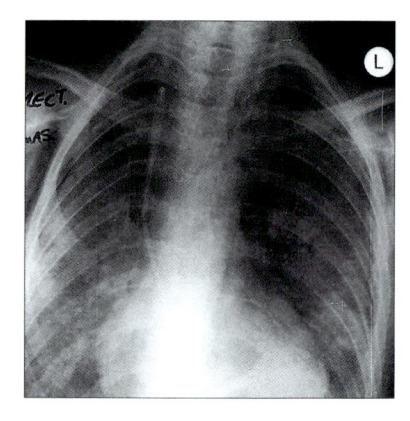

226 Chest X-ray of a patient with *Pneumocystis carinii* pneumonia.

Diagnosis
The diagnosis of PCP is confirmed by identification of the organism in washings obtained by fibreoptic bronchoscopy and bronchoalveolar lavage using either a silver stain (**227**) or indirect immunofluorescence. Transbronchial biopsy is not usually performed in this group of patients due to thrombocytopenia. Induced sputum obtained using nebulized hypertonic saline may yield a positive result (Leigh *et al*, 1989), but a negative result using this technique does not exclude the diagnosis.

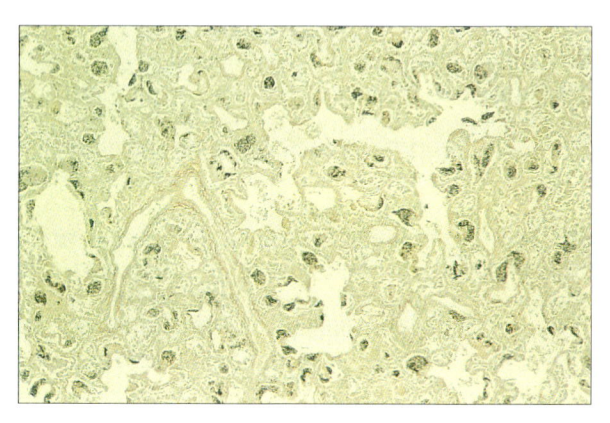

227 Lung biopsy with silver stain showing multiple pneumocysts.

Treatment and prophylaxis
Treatment of PCP involves high-dose intravenous co-trimoxazole and respiratory support to maintain the PaO_2 above 8 kPa. The mortality of PCP in BMT is high, and patients surviving one episode are at increased risk of a recurrence.

The incidence of PCP in transplant patients was approximately 10% before the routine use of prophylaxis. It is policy in some units to use nebulized pentamidine (Mahon *et al*, 1990) every 2–4 weeks after transplant until the neutrophil count exceeds $0.5 \times 10^9/l$. Patients then commence co-trimoxazole 960 mg orally b.d. 3 days per week and continue for

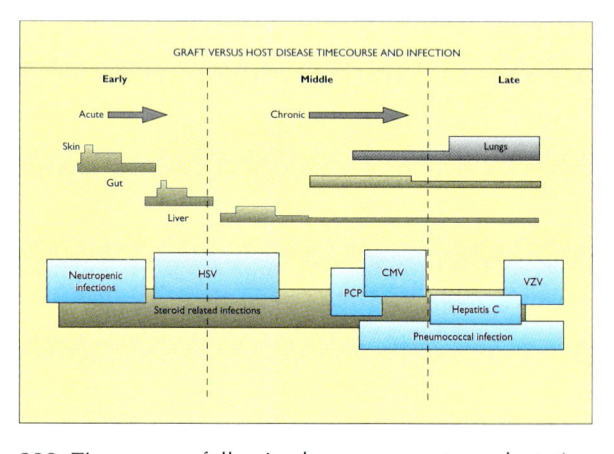

228 Time course following bone marrow transplantation when individual infections are most likely.

at least one year. Allogeneic BMT recipients with chronic GvHD at this stage are still at increased risk and need further prophylaxis.

Patients who require an alternative to co-trimoxazole, either because of allergy or intolerance due to cytopenia, may continue to receive regular nebulized pentamidine. This may be inconvenient and does not provide protection from systemic infection. Additional alternatives include dapsone (100 mg twice per week), with or without trimethoprim, or fansidar (Smith and Gazzard, 1991).

The approximate time course following bone marrow transplantation when particular infections are most likely to occur is shown in **228**.

Idiopathic pneumonitis

Interstitial pneumonitis occurs most frequently between 30 and 100 days following BMT. Clinically, it presents with breathlessness, a non-productive cough and fever, and the chest X-ray usually shows patchy infiltration (**229**). The incidence varies in different series but figures quoted range from 20 to 65%. Approximately half the cases are associated with CMV infection, and of the remainder only a few cases can be shown to be due to other infective agents. The group in whom no cause can be identified are termed 'idiopathic'.

Pathologically, pneumonitis is a tissue reaction. It is characterized by alveolar infiltration and thickening and the formation of a hyaline membrane (**230**) which later progresses to fibrosis (**231**). At bronchoalveolar lavage, excessive numbers of activated cytotoxic lymphocytes can be detected (Milburn *et al*, 1990).

Risk factors for idiopathic pneumonitis include:
- The type of chemotherapy used in the conditioning regime.
- Pre-existing pulmonary abnormality.

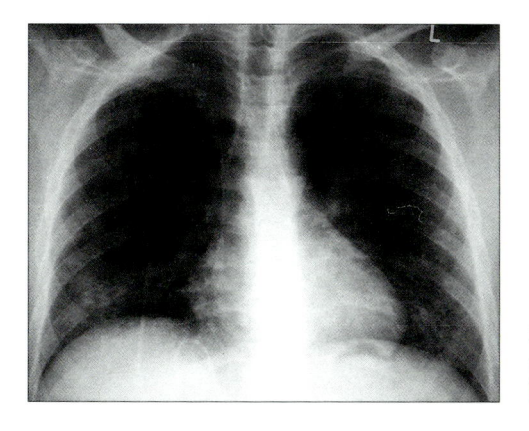

229 Chest X-ray of a patient with idiopathic pneumonitis—no organism was identified at bronchoscopy.

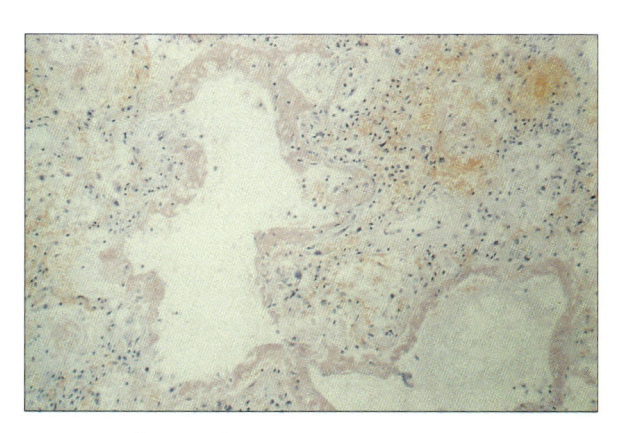

230 Lung biopsy showing early changes of idiopathic pneumonitis with hyaline membrane formation.

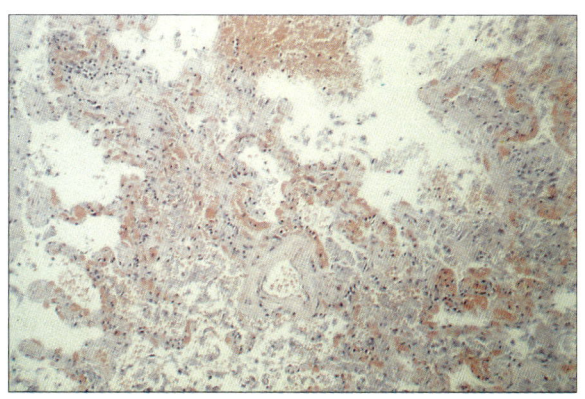

231 Lung biopsy showing idiopathic pneumonitis at a later stage with fibrosis.

- Increasing patient age.
- The use of TBI as part of the conditioning regime.
- The use of methotrexate as anti-GvHD prophylaxis.
- Severe GvHD (Weiner *et al*, 1986).

The pulmonary toxicity of TBI may be reduced by delivering fractionated doses at low dose rates.

Lung function tests reveal a reduction in lung volume and compliance. Arterial blood gases demonstrate Type I respiratory failure with hypoxia and a $Paco_2$ which may be normal or reduced. Occasional patients may respond to treatment with steroids, although most do not. The mortality of BMT patients with pneumonitis who require intubation and mechanical ventilation is greater than 90%.

Bronchoalveolar lavage has become the 'gold standard' for diagnosis of pneumonitis after BMT, and open lung biopsy is now very rarely used. The high mortality of pneumonitis remains a challenge, and efforts are being directed towards early diagnosis and identification of any infective agents to attenuate disease progression. To this end, a policy of surveillance fibreoptic bronchoscopy and bronchoalveolar lavage has been adopted in some units (Vaughan *et al*, 1991).

Long-term pulmonary complications

Both restrictive and obstructive defects have been identified in long-term survivors of BMT. A restrictive defect of mild-to-moderate severity has been found in 20% of patients at one year following transplant (Fyles *et al*, 1988). The aetiology of this is likely to be related to previous chemotherapy exposure, the use of TBI, and infection. Some patients improved over a two-to-three year period.

Follow-up of asymptomatic BMT patients over a two-year period shows that there is a reduction in diffusing capacity of 11.9% per year from the predicted value. This does not appear to be related to the age of the patient, their smoking habits, acute GvHD or the type of GvHD prophylaxis used. Patients transplanted for CML were a distinct group who had a more marked fall in diffusing capacity (Prince *et al*, 1989).

Patients with chronic GvHD have been found to be predisposed to develop a progressive obstructive defect. In a minority, the progression is relentless and irreversible, terminating in respiratory failure and death. Pathologically, this process resembles obliterative bronchiolitis (Ostrow and Buskard, 1985).

The chest X-ray may be normal, or show hyperinflation, and spontaneous pneumothoraces may occur (**232**). Treatment is with steroids and azathioprine, but the mortality is high.

Patients with either obstructive or restrictive lung disease following BMT are at risk of recurrent infective episodes which may compromise their pulmonary function further. The long-term management of these complications remains a challenge.

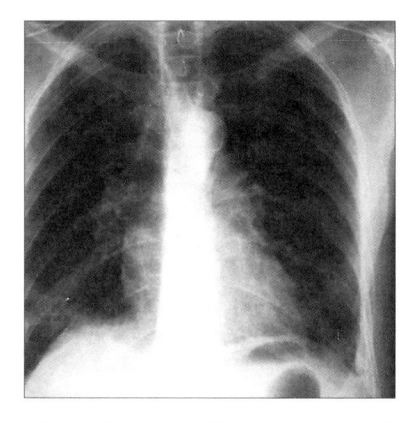

232 Pulmonary fibrosis post-BMT with a spontaneous pneumothorax.

References

Appelbaum FR, Meyers JD, Fefer A et al. Nonbacterial nonfungal pneumonia following marrow transplantation in 100 identical twins. *Transplantation* 1982; **33**: 265–268.

Bowden RA, Meyers JD. Prophylaxis of cytomegalovirus infection. *Semin Hematol* 1990; **27** (suppl 1): 7–21.

Bowden RA, Sayers M, Flourney N et al. Cytomegalovirus immune globulin and seronegative blood products to prevent primary cytomegalovirus infection after bone marrow transplants. *N Engl J Med* 1986; **314**: 1006–1010.

Chan CK, Kasupski GJ, Steale J. Rapid immunodiagnosis of cytomegalovirus pulmonary complications by bronchoalveolar lavage after allogeneic bone marrow transplantation. *Chest* 1988; **94**: 578–582.

Chan CK, Hyland RH, Hutcheon MA Pulmonary complications following bone marrow transplantation. *Clin Chest Med* 1990; **11**: 323–332.

Cordonnier C, Bernaudin J-F, Bierling P et al. Pulmonary complications occurring after allogeneic bone marrow transplantation: A study of 130 consecutive transplanted patients. *Cancer* 1986; **58**: 1047–1054.

Curtis AM, Smith GJW, Ravin CE. Air crescent sign of invasive aspergillosis. *Radiology* 1979; **133**: 17–21.

Drobyski WR, Knox KK, Carrigan DR, Ash CR. Foscarnet therapy of ganciclovir-resistant cytomegalovirus in marrow transplantation. *Transplantation* 1991; **52**: 155–157.

Emanuel D. Treatment of cytomegalovirus disease. *Semin Hematol* 1990; **27** (suppl 1): 22–27.

Engleund JA, Piedra PA, Jefferson LS et al. High-dose, short duration ribavarin aerosol therapy in children with suspected respiratory syncytial virus infection. *J Pediatr* 1990; **117**: 313–320.

Foulliard L, Mouthon L, Laporte JP et al. Severe respiratory syncytial virus pneumonia after autologous bone marrow transplantation—a report of three cases and review of the literature. *Bone Marrow Transplant* 1992; **9**: 97–100.

Fyles G, Chan CK, Hyland RH. Restrictive ventilatory defect after allogeneic bone marrow transplantation. *Am Rev Respir Dis* 1988; **137** (suppl): 313.

Gefter WB, Albeda SM, Talbot GH et al. Invasive pulmonary aspergillosis and acute leukaemia. Limitations in the diagnostic utility of the air crescent sign. *Radiology* 1985; **157**: 605–610.

Gerson SL, Talbot GH, Hurwitz S. Prolonged granulocytopenia; the major risk factor for invasive pulmonary aspergillosis in patients with acute leukaemia. *Ann Intern Med* 1984; **100**: 345–351.

Grundy JE, Shanley JD, Griffiths PD. Is cytomegalovirus interstitial pneumonitis in transplant patients an immunopathological condition? *Lancet* 1987; **2**: 996–999.

Grundy JE, Ayles HM, McKeating JA et al. Enhancement of Class 1 HLA antigen expression by cytomegalovirus: role in amplification of virus infection. *J Med Virol* 1988; **25**: 483–495.

Hamilton PJ, Pearson ADJ. Bone marrow transplantation and the lung. Editorial. *Thorax* 1986; **41**: 497–502.

Hill G, Helenglass G, Powles R et al. Mediastinal emphysema in marrow transplant recipients. *Bone Marrow Transplant* 1987; **2**: 315–320.

Krowka ML, Rosenow EC III, Hoagland HC. Pulmonary complications of bone marrow transplantation. *Chest* 1985; **87**: 237–246.

Kuhlman J. The role of chest CT in the evaluation of the febrile bone marrow transplant recipient. *Chest* 1991; **99**: 794–795.

Leigh TR, Hume C, Gazzard B. Sputum induction for diagnosis of *Pneumocystis carinii* pneumonia. *Lancet* 1989; **2**: 205–206.

Lehner PJ, Rawal B, Hoyle C, Cohen J. Dual infection with *Pneumocystis carinii* and respiratory viruses complicating bone marrow transplantation. *Bone Marrow Transplant* 1992; **9**: 213–215.

Levin M. Current approaches to the prevention and treatment of CMV disease after bone marrow transplantation: An overview. *Semin Hematol* 1990; **27** (suppl 1): 1–4.

Mahon FX, Sadoun A, Benz-Lemoine E et al. Possible prevention of *Pneumocystis carinii* pneumonia by pentamidine aerosol after bone marrow transplantation (Letter). *Bone Marrow Transplant* 1991; **8**: 64–65.

Milburn HJ, Du Bois RM, Prentice HG, Poulter LW. Pneumonitis in bone marrow transplant recipients results from a local immune response. *Clin Exp Immunol* 1990; **81**: 232–237.

Ostrow D, Buskard N. Bronchiolitis obliterans complicating bone marrow transplantation. *Chest* 1985; **87**: 828–830.

Prince DS, Wingard JR, Saral R. Longitudinal changes in pulmonary function following bone marrow transplantation. *Chest* 1989; **96**: 301–306.

Reed EC, Bowden RA, Dandliker PS, Lilleby K, Meyers JD. Treatment of cytomegalovirus pneumonia with ganciclovir and intravenous cytomegalovirus immunoglobulin in patients with bone marrow transplants. *Ann Intern Med* 1988; **109**: 783–788.

Rousey SR, Russler S, Gottlieb M, Ash RC. Low-dose amphotericin B prophylaxis against invasive *Aspergillus* infections in allogeneic marrow transplantation. *Am J Med* 1991; **91**: 484–492.

Ruutu P, Ruutu T, Volin L et al. Cytomegalovirus is frequently isolated in bronchoalveolar lavage fluid of bone marrow transplant recipients without pneumonia. *Ann Intern Med* 1990; **112**: 913–916.

Schmidt GM, Horak DA, Niland JC. A randomised controlled trial of prophylactic ganciclovir for cytomegalovirus infections in recipients of allogeneic bone marrow transplants. *N Engl J Med* 1991; **324**: 1005-1011.

Shields AF, Hackman RC, Fife KH et al. Adenovirus infections in patients undergoing bone marrow transplantation. *N Engl J Med* 1985; **312**: 529–533.

Sloane JP, Depledge MH, Powles RL. Histopathology of the lung after bone marrow transplantation. *J Clin Pathol* 1983; **36**: 546–554.

Smith D, Gazzard B. Treatment and prophylaxis of *Pneumocystis carinii* pneumonia in AIDS patients. *Drugs* 1991; **42**: 628–639.

Spector SA. Diagnosis of cytomegalovirus infection. *Semin Hematol* 1990; **27** (suppl 1): 1–6.

Vaughan W, Linder J, Robbis R. Pulmonary surveillance using bronchoscopy and bronchoalveolar lavage during high-dose antineoplastic therapy. *Chest* 1991; **99**: 105–111.

Weiner RS, Bortin MM, Gale RP *et al*. Interstitial pneumonitis after bone marrow transplantation. *Ann Intern Med* 1986; **104**: 168–175.

Wendt CH, Weisdorf DJ, Jordan MC. Parainfluenza virus respiratory infection post bone marrow transplant. *N Engl J Med* 1992; **326**: 921–925.

Winston DJ, Gale RP. Review: Prevention and treatment of cytomegalovirus infection and disease after bone marrow transplantation in the 1990s. *Bone Marrow Transplant* 1991; **8**: 7–11.

2. Cerebral Infections

Rosemary Barnes

Central nervous system (CNS) infections occurring in bone marrow transplant (BMT) patients are listed in **Table 41**. The type of infection seen will be determined by the immune function of the patient. During the early neutropenic phase, Gram-negative meningitis secondary to septicaemia may occur. If the neutropenia is prolonged, fungal infections with *Candida*, *Aspergillus* and *Mucoraceae* species (**233**, **234**) may supervene. In the intermediate transplant period, when cell-mediated immunity is most

Table 41. Central nervous system infections in BMT patients.

Bacteria	Fungi	Viruses	Protozoa/Parasites
Meningitis			
Streptococcus pneumoniae	*Cryptococcus neoformans*	HSV	*Toxoplasma gondii*
Haemophilus influenzae	*Candida* spp.	VZV	
Listeria monocytogenes			*Strongyloides stercoralis*
Meningoencephalitis			
Listeria monocytogenes	*Cryptococcus neoformans*	VZV	*Toxoplasma gondii*
		HSV	
		Papovavirus	
Abscess			
Listeria monocytogenes	*Aspergillus* spp.		*Toxoplasma gondii*
Nocardia spp.	*Mucoraceae*		

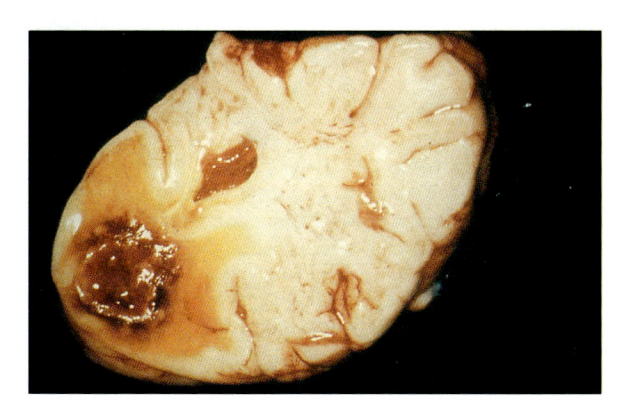

233 Large abscess with extensive infarction and necrosis of the cerebral cortex following disseminated *Aspergillus* infection in a BMT patient. The brain is frequently involved following dissemination from the lung. Neurological symptoms may be the presenting feature. Invasion of blood vessels with resulting thrombosis, haemorrhage and infarction is characteristic of this infection and also of CNS mucormycosis (see **234**)

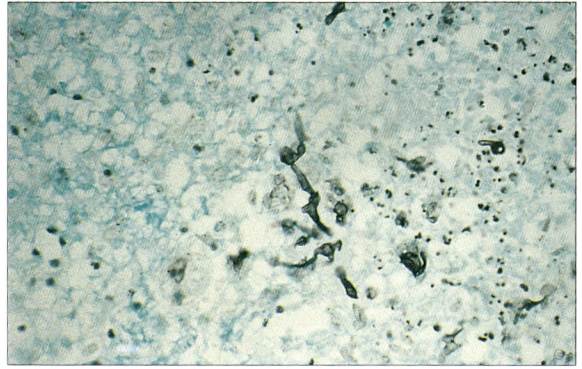

234 Section of brain tissue (methenamine–silver nitrate stain) showing broad (20 µm diameter), irregularly shaped hyphae with right-angle branching characteristic of *Mucor* species. Infection is usually initiated following deposition of inhaled spores in the nasal turbinates and direct extension of the infection into the brain. Facial pain and headache are frequent presenting features, and the orbit may be involved.

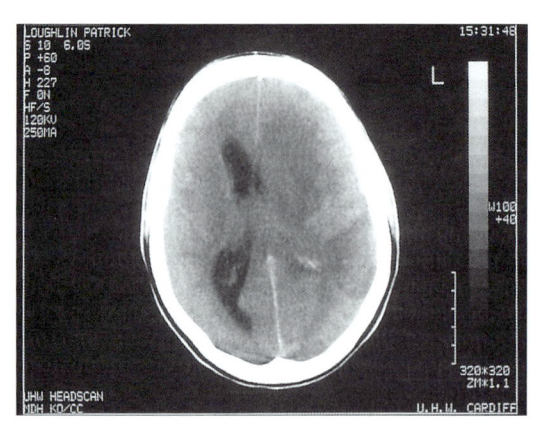

235 Herpes simplex encephalitis demonstrated by computer tomographic (CT) scanning. Haemorrhagic necrosis and oedema are characteristic; localization over the temporal lobes is best demonstrated by electroencephalography.

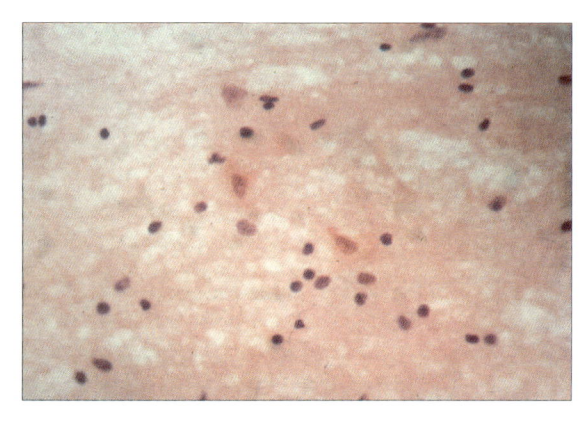

236 Brain biopsy from a case of herpes simplex encephalitis with typical intranuclear inclusions. (H & E stain.)

affected, re-activation of herpes viruses may occasionally cause meningitis or encephalitis (**235, 236**). Diagnosis may be difficult but culture of cerebrospinal fluid (CSF) may yield the virus which can be identified by specific immunofluorescence of the cell culture (**237**). *Listeria monocytogenes* causes meningitis and also encephalitis with multiple abscess formation (**238**). *Toxoplasma* infections occur during this period due either to re-activation or to donor-transmitted infection (**239, 240**). In the late transplant period, infections due to capsulate bacteria such as *Streptococcus pneumoniae* (**241**) or *Haemophilus influenzae* occur due to deficiencies in IgG subclasses and poor opsonic activity of the patient's serum. Whilst bacterial meningitis may be the classic presentation, atypical infections can occur, which are often fulminant. If the patient remains immunocompromised due to the presence of chronic graft-versus host disease and concomitant steroid and/or cyclosporin treatment, any of the infections listed may occur and the risk of otherwise rare infections caused by *Nocardia* (**242**) and *Cryptococcus neoformans* (**243, 244**) increases.

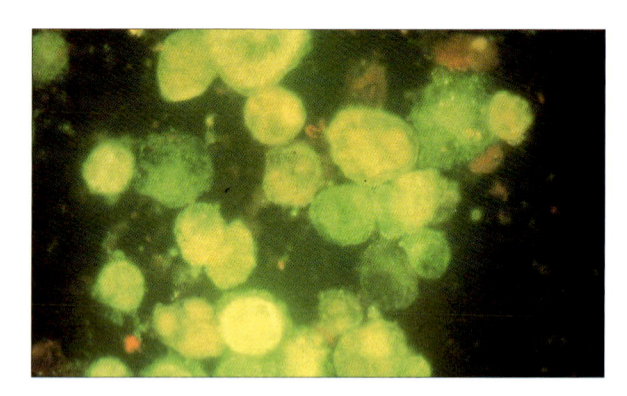

237 Herpes simplex virus from the CSF identified by specific immunofluorescence in tissue culture. Note the characteristic nuclear fluorescence pattern.

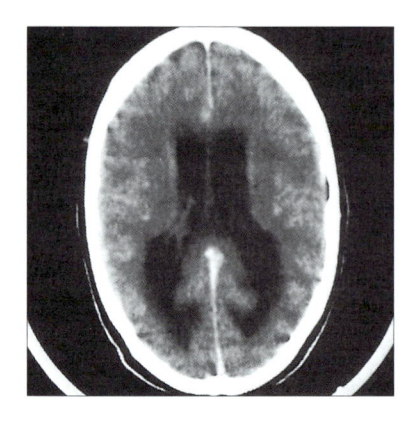

238 CT scan from a patient with meningoencephalitis due to *Listeria monocytogenes* showing enlargement of the ventricles and multiple low-density areas in the cerebral cortices. These were initially thought to be lymphomatous deposits but were subsequently shown to be due to early abscess formation.

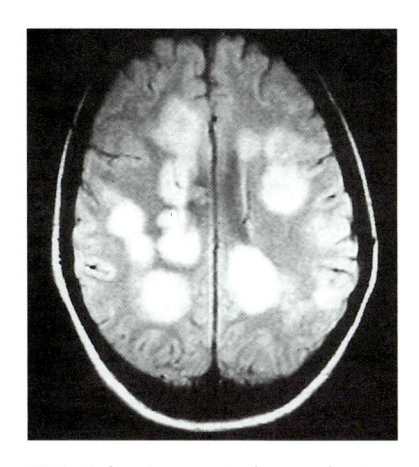

Cerebral Infections

239 Enlarging central mass lesions demonstrated by magnetic resonance imaging (MRI) in a patient with CNS toxoplasmosis. The patient presented with a diffuse encephalopathy and impaired consciousness. Cerebrospinal fluid examination was unhelpful.

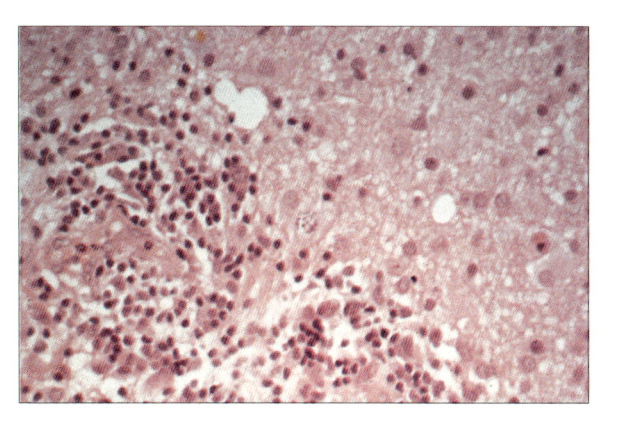

240 Brain biopsy from **239** revealed a non-specific inflammatory infiltrate surrounding a cyst of *Toxoplasma gondii*. The patient responded to pyrimethamine and sulphadiazine treatment. (H & E stain.)

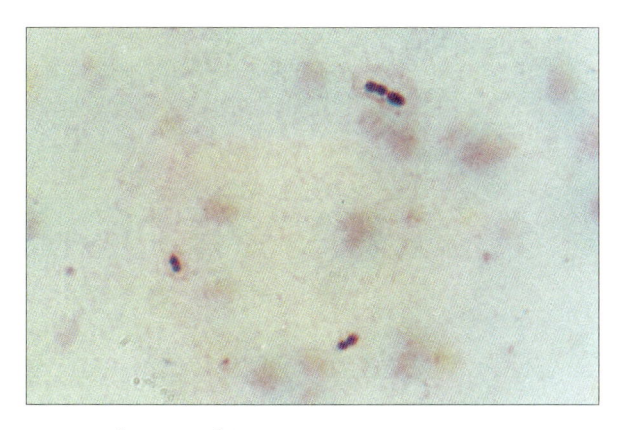

241 Diplococci of *Streptococcus pneumoniae* in a wet preparation of CSF. The polysaccharide capsule can be clearly seen. The classic features of bacterial meningitis with pleocytosis of the CSF and reduced glucose concentration may be absent in BMT patients, whose cellular responses are often impaired.

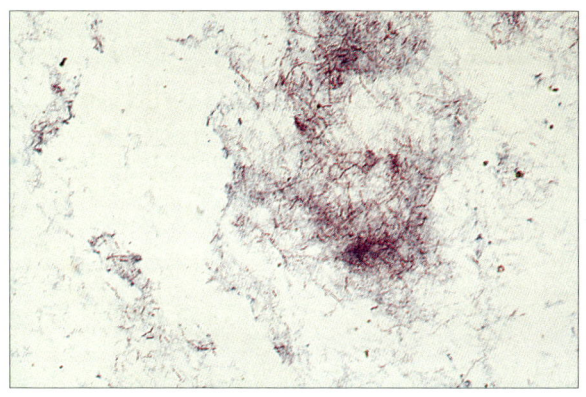

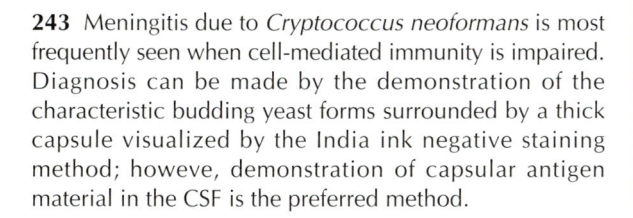

242 *Nocardia asteroides* (ZN stain) is a weakly acid-fast branching bacterium related to the *Mycobacterium* and *Actinomyces* genera. It may cause cerebral abscesses in patients with impaired T-cell function following dissemination from the lungs. Infections are usually sporadic but, like air-borne fungal infections, outbreaks have been reported associated with building construction.

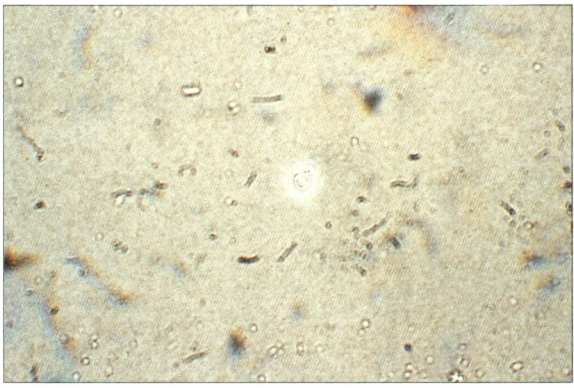

243 Meningitis due to *Cryptococcus neoformans* is most frequently seen when cell-mediated immunity is impaired. Diagnosis can be made by the demonstration of the characteristic budding yeast forms surrounded by a thick capsule visualized by the India ink negative staining method; howeve, demonstration of capsular antigen material in the CSF is the preferred method.

Other rare infections have been reported in BMT patients: progressive multifocal leukoencephalopathy has been attributed to papovavirus-Jakob Creutzfeldt infection and is manifested as a slowly progressive generalized disease with marked cortical atrophy. Diagnosis is made by brain biopsy but there is no effective treatment.

Overwhelming hyperinfection with *Strongyloides stercoralis* can also occur in endemically infected individuals following immunosuppression. Massive invasion of the gut leads to disseminated infection which may involve the CNS causing aseptic meningitis (**245**).

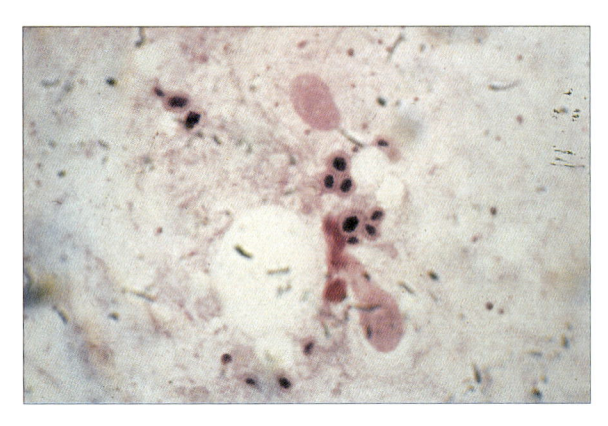

244 The aseptic meningitis caused by *Cryptococcus neoformans* may have a chronic course over a number of weeks and there is frequently evidence of underlying cerebritis with Gram-positive yeasts present in the brain tissue. Calcification within the cortex may occur.

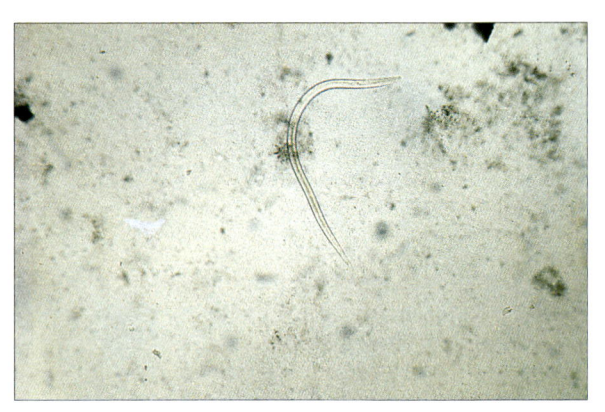

245 In the rare cases of hyperinvasive *Strongyloides stercoralis* infection, rhabdoid larval forms may be demonstrable in the CSF.

3. Graft-Versus-Host Disease

Jane Norton

Graft-versus-host disease (GvHD) affects up to 50% of allogeneic bone marrow transplant (BMT) recipients and contributes significantly to the morbidity of the BMT procedure (Gale, 1985). GvHD is divided into acute and chronic forms. Acute GvHD occurs approximately 10–40 days after BMT, manifesting as a clinical triad of dermatitis, diarrhoea and cholestatic jaundice (Glucksberg et al., 1974). Chronic GvHD is defined as occurring more than 100 days after BMT and has a spectrum of clinical manifestations similar to those seen in systemic collagen–vascular disorders such as scleroderma, Sjögren's syndrome and primary biliary cirrhosis (Shulman et al., 1978) **(Table 42)**. Chronic GvHD may follow persistent or exacerbated acute GvHD or arise *de novo* with no preceding acute phase. Both acute and chronic forms are associated with immune impairment and increased susceptibility to infection (Glucksberg et al., 1974; Noel et al., 1978). See also Section VII.

Table 42. Manifestations of acute and chronic graft-versus-host disease.

Acute	*Chronic*
Lichenoid skin rash	Skin rash, lichenoid or sclerodermatous
Diarrhoea	Weight loss, diarrhoea Malabsorption, wasting Oral mucositis Oesophagitis
Chronic liver disease	Sicca syndrome Arthralgia Joint contractures Restrictive and obstructive lung disease Pleural and peri-cardial effusions

Clinical features

The clinical features of GvHD vary greatly and a grading system based on the severity of disease and the number of organs affected is used (Thomas et al., 1975) **(Tables 43, 44)**.

Table 43. Clinical staging of graft-versus-host disease according to organ system.

Stage	Skin	Liver (serum bilirubin, mmol/l)	*Intestinal tract* (diarrhoea volume/day)
+	Maculopapular rash, <25% body surface	34–50	>500 ml
++	Maculopapular rash, 25–50% body surface	51–102	>1000 ml
+++	Generalized erythroderma	103–255	>1500 ml
++++	Generalized erythroderma with bullous formation and desquamation	>255	>2000 ml with ileus and abdominal pain

Table 44. Overall clinical grading of severity of graft-versus-host disease.

Grade	Degree of organ involvement
I	+ to ++ skin rash; no gut involvement; no liver involvement; no decrease in clinical performance
II	+ to +++ skin rash; + gut involvement or + liver involvement (or both); mild decrease in clinical performance
III	++ to +++ skin rash; ++ to +++ gut involvement or ++ to ++++ liver involvement (or both); marked decrease in clinical performance
IV	Similar to Grade III with ++ to ++++ organ involvement and extreme decrease in clinical performance

Skin

Cutaneous manifestations of acute GvHD usually precede intestinal and hepatic involvement and are easy both to observe and to biopsy. Skin rashes develop after BMT for many reasons, including the effects of cytotoxic drugs, irradiation, antibiotics and infections. Confirmation of the diagnosis of GvHD by biopsy is thus essential and sufficient tissue can be obtained by punch biopsy with minimal discomfort. Biopsies should be taken from an affected site, preferably before any immunosuppressive therapy is commenced. Repeat samples may be required in equivocal cases if the diagnostic histological features are not identified (see later).

Acute GvHD classically affects the hands, feet, face and trunk. Itching, tenderness and redness of the palms and soles may precede the morbilliform or erythematous maculopapular rash which becomes more diffusely distributed on the trunk, limbs, face and neck (**246–248**). Early disease involving only hair follicles may appear punctate. In

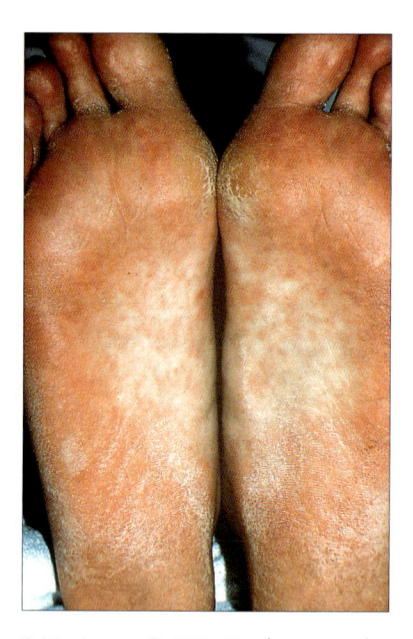

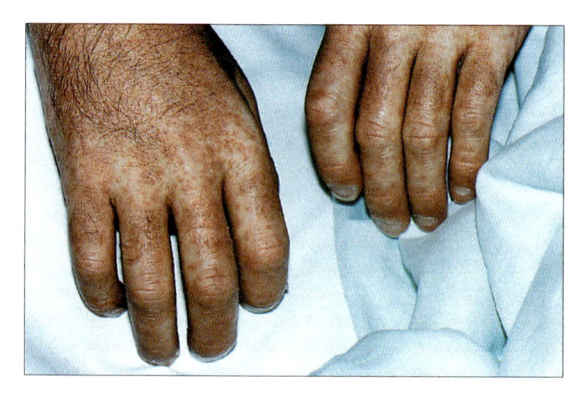

246 Acute GvHD. Erythema and a papular rash on the soles of the feet.

247 Acute GvHD. Typical lichenoid papular eruption on the back of the hands.

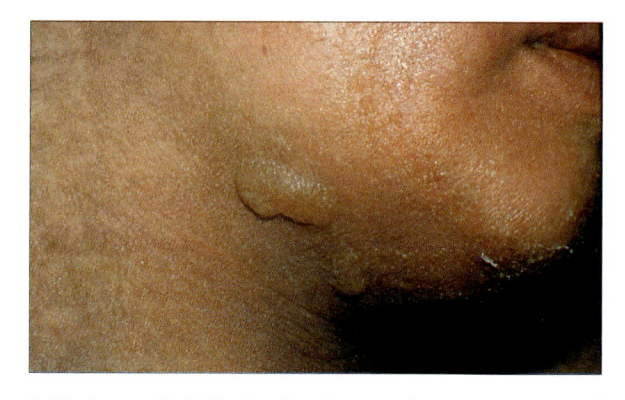

248 Acute GvHD. Erythroderma, desquamation and blistering on the neck.

Graft-Versus-Host Disease

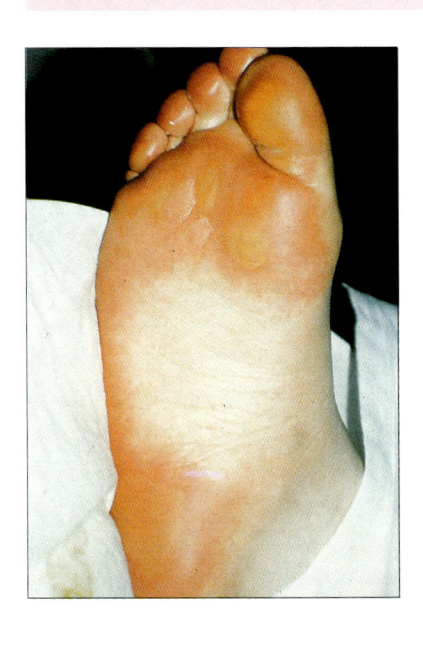

249 Acute GvHD. Blistering of the soles of the feet.

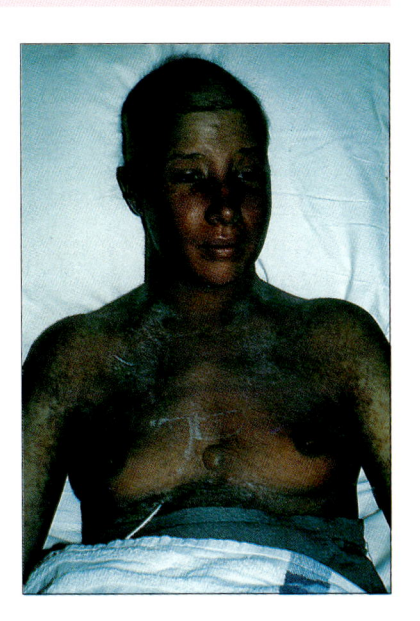

250 Acute GvHD. Widespread maculopapular rash, erythroderma of the face and trunk and blister formation on the anterior chest wall.

severe cases acute GvHD progresses to generalized erythroderma with blistering and epidermal sloughing; manifestations resembling toxic epidermal necrolysis (**249, 250**). The maculopapular rash and erythroderma may wax and wane and the skin may become dry and scaling. Residual areas of altered pigmentation may remain for several days after dissolution of the rash.

Chronic cutaneous GvHD may be localized or diffuse and show a spectrum of changes from a lichenoid dermatitis to scleroderma (Shulman and Sale, 1984). An erythematous maculopapular rash is often accompanied by scaling and altered pigmentation (hypo- and hyperpigmentation) (**251**). The skin may become progressively dry and atrophic with hair loss. In later phases poikiloderma, telangectasia and scarring with loss of dermal elasticity are common resulting in contractures and tight hidebound skin.

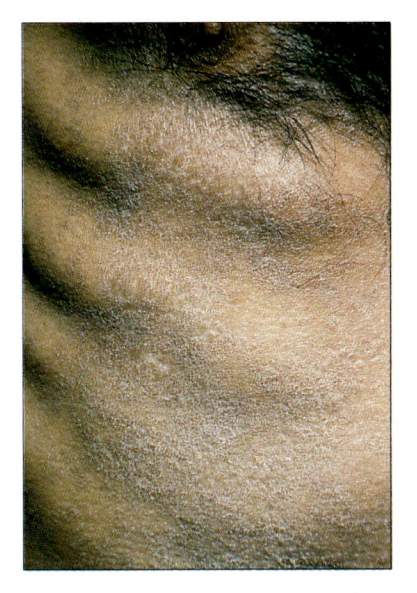

251 Chronic GvHD. Dry, scaling eruption with hypopigmentation.

Gastrointestinal tract

Intestinal GvHD typically presents with watery diarrhoea and cramping abdominal pain. It is most often, but not exclusively, seen in patients with some evidence of skin involvement. Upper gastrointestinal symptoms of anorexia, nausea and vomiting, or intestinal ileus may occur. The diarrhoea is watery and greenish, containing mucus and cellular debris, and several litres per day may be passed. Occult blood is usually present but rarely there may be significant intestinal haemorrhage requiring transfusion (Beschorner 1984).

Radiology of the bowel in acute GvHD, including barium studies, demonstrates mucosal and submucosal oedema with ulceration. Later the bowel may appear ribbon-like due to total effacement of mucosal folds.

Acute GvHD can affect the entire gastrointestinal tract but autopsy studies have shown that involvement of the ileum, colon and rectum exceeds that of other sites. The macroscopic appearances of the bowel reflect the severity and duration of the GvHD. In the early stages mild mucosal oedema, erythema and focal ulceration are seen on sigmoidoscopy. Descriptions of the later stages include complete mucosal denudation, large ulcers, oedema of the bowel wall and haemorrhage (Sale *et al.*, 1979).

Chronic GvHD frequently affects the upper gastrointestinal tract with oral mucositis (**252**), dysphagia, malabsorption and weight loss. In the mouth, lesions similar to those seen in lichen planus are commonly present, together with loss of papillae of the tongue and oral ulceration. Oesophageal involvement includes generalized epithelial desquamation and stricture formation. Patchy submucosal fibrosis and stenosis may be seen anywhere throughout the bowel.

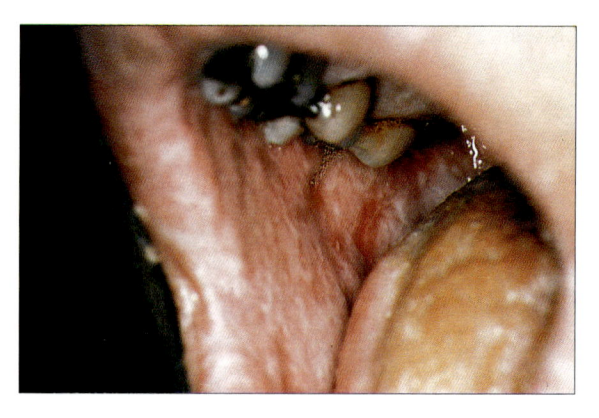

252 Chronic GvHD. Lichenoid eruption on the oral mucosa.

Liver

Abnormalities of liver function are common following allogeneic BMT with many possible causes including chemotherapy, radiation, hepatitis, opportunistic infections and veno-occlusive disease. Hepatic GvHD usually occurs secondary to skin or gut disease, at approximately 25–100 days after BMT, but may occur in isolation. Clinical signs are predominantly those of cholestatic jaundice. Hepatomegaly, if present, is only moderate and painless. There is a progressive rise in serum bilirubin, with a variable rise in alkaline phosphatase and transaminase (Farthing *et al.*, 1982).

Liver disease of varying severity is seen in approximately 90% of patients with chronic GvHD. Patients may have fluctuating icterus, anorexia and weight loss (McDonald *et al.*, 1986). Despite prolonged disturbance of liver function, hepatic failure, portal hypertension and cirrhosis are unusual. Liver biopsy may be required to exclude other causes of liver disease, mainly viral infections and hepatotoxic reactions to drugs in the late stages after BMT.

Histological features

The clinical features described above are reflected histologically by epithelial cell damage and lymphocytic infiltration in affected tissues. The histological picture seen in acute and chronic GvHD may overlap although the latter tends to have a more pronounced lymphocytic infiltrate and evidence of fibrosis. The histological changes in skin, gut and liver are graded according to their

Table 45. Histopathological grade of graft-versus-host disease according to organ system.

Grade	Skin	Liver	Intestinal tract
I	Epidermal basal cell vacuolation	<25% abnormal small bile ducts	Apoptotic cells at base of crypts
II	I and eosinophilic necrosis of epidermal cells	25–50%	I and loss of entire crypts
III	II and confluent necrosis with bullae	50–75%	II and mucosal ulceration
IV	Epidermal sloughing	>75%	Mucosal denudation

severity (**Table 45**). Careful clinicopathological correlation is needed in interpretation of biopsies taken from BMT recipients. The features of GvHD may be mimicked to varying degrees by the effects of cytotoxic drugs and irradiation of the conditioning regimen and also by viral infections, particularly CMV, resulting in false positive changes in biopsies. Alternatively, false negative results may be obtained from biopsies taken from early GvHD, disease of patchy distribution, or after the administration of immunosuppressive drugs.

Skin

The classical histological picture seen in acute cutaneous GvHD is that of an interface dermatitis with epidermal basal cell vacuolation and necrosis, and a lichenoid lymphocytic infiltrate at the dermal–epidermal junction (Lerner *et al.*, 1974) (**253**). Similar changes may be seen affecting hair follicles. The dead epidermal cells have pyknotic nuclei, or are anucleate, with deeply eosinophilic cytoplasm, so-called eosinophilic bodies. With increasing severity there is bullous formation (**254**) and, in the most severe cases, total necrosis of the epidermis. This is the basis for the histological grading of GvHD (**Table 45**). Epidermal basal cell damage may be seen as a consequence of the conditioning regimen, particularly in the first 10 days after transplantation, and should be interpreted with caution. Lymphocytic infiltration, while diagnostic, may be very scanty, especially in biopsies taken soon after the onset of a rash. Diagnosis of early disease can therefore be difficult but the expression of HLA-DR antigens on epidermal keratinocytes, detected by immunohistochemical staining, has proven useful as a disease marker (Lampert *et al.*, 1981; Sloane *et al.*, 1988). The mononuclear cells infiltrating the skin in acute GvHD comprise a mixed population of CD4 and CD8 positive lymphocytes, macrophages and natural killer cells (Elliott *et al.*, 1988). After administration of immunosupressive therapy the biopsy may show basal cell changes with vacuolation and eosinophilic bodies, but no evidence of lymphocytic infiltration. After clinical resolution of the rash residual histological changes include hyperkeratosis, melanin incontinence and epidermal atrophy.

Chronic cutaneous GvHD may have lichenoid histological features similar to those seen in the acute phase, although the epidermis is often hyperplastic, and the lymphocytic infiltrate more pronounced with frequent involvement of hair follicles. Sclerodermatous changes are best demonstrated on deep incisional biopsies (**255**). The normal dermal collagen, elastic and adipose tissue is replaced by dense fibrosis, and adnexal stuctures, especially hair follicles and sweat glands, are lost. The epidermis becomes atrophic and there may be evidence of continuing lymphocytic infiltration with ongoing basal cell damage.

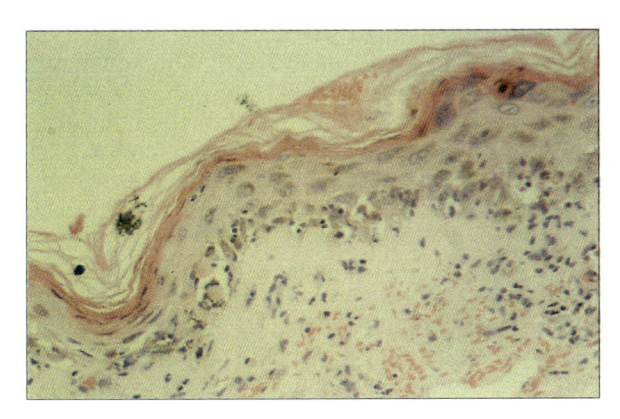

253 Acute GvHD. Skin biopsy showing degeneration of the basal layer of the epidermis with eosinophilic bodies and a lymphocytic infiltrate at the dermal–epidermal junction (histological Grade II).

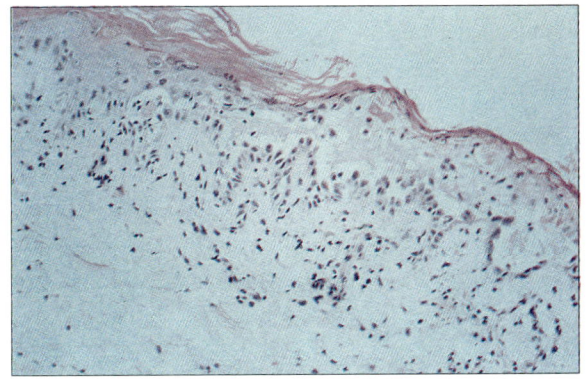

254 Acute GvHD. Skin biopsy with confluent epidermal necrosis and formation of a bullous (histological Grade III).

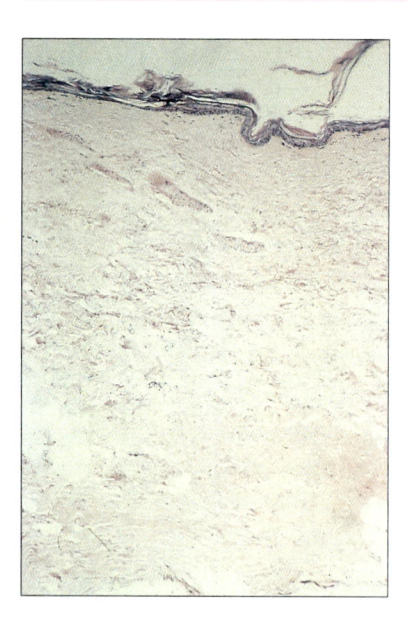

255 Chronic GvHD. Skin biopsy. The epidermis is atrophic with loss of rete ridges. Hair follicles are destroyed and there is dense dermal fibrosis.

Gastrointestinal Tract

A rectal biopsy is most often used to confirm the diagnosis of intestinal GvHD. The characteristic feature seen is the so-called exploding crypt. Apoptosis of individual epithelial cells at the base of crypts leaves fragments of nuclear and cytoplasmic debris (**256**). Progressively severe changes lead to loss of glands, although enterochromaffin cells alone survive (Lampert *et al.*, 1985) (**257**). Surface ulceration may be followed by total denudation of the epithelium and bacterial colonization.

The histological changes seen in GvHD are closely mimicked by the effects of the conditioning regimen, although not to the same degree. Features indistinguishable from Grades I or II acute GvHD are seen in rectal biopsies from all patients 7–10 days after transplantation, but in the absence of a skin rash or diarrhoea the changes resolve by day 20 (Epstein, 1980). CMV colitis can also induce identical histological features, and should be carefully excluded (Snover, 1985).

The leukocytes in the epithelium and lamina propria in GvHD comprise predominantly CD8+ lymphocytes (Dilly and Sloane, 1987). HLA-DR antigens are expressed on affected epithelium, and may be of diagnostic use in early GvHD (Sviland *et al.*, 1988).

In gastric and small bowel biopsies similar histological features are seen, with single-cell necrosis, crypt dilatation and crypt abscess formation. Intestinal metaplasia may be seen in the stomach and villous atrophy in the small bowel. The squamous epithelium of the mouth and oesophagus shows similar histological changes to those seen in the skin.

Chronic GvHD affecting the gastrointestinal tract has rather non-specific histological features. Increased numbers of lymphocytes and plasma cells are seen in the lamina propria. Fibrosis and stenosis of the submucosal and serosal layers may be seen throughout the bowel.

Incisional lip biopsies can be used to show the changes in the oral mucosa and salivary glands in chronic GvHD. Lymphocytic infiltration and necrosis of squamous cells in the mucosa are seen together with Sjögren-like damage to salivary gland ductular epithelium and eventual atrophy of acini and fibrosis.

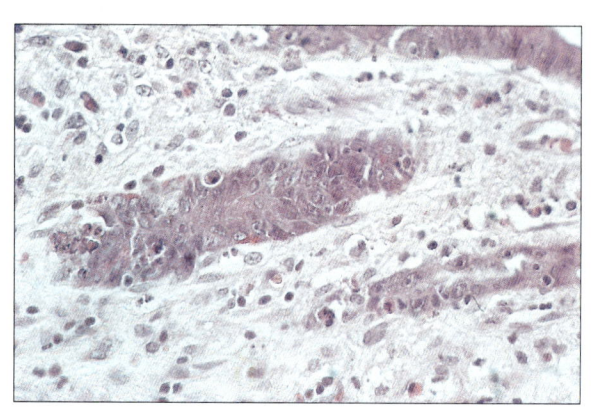

256 Acute GvHD. Rectal biopsy. Several basal crypt cells show apoptosis with fragments of cellular debris (histological Grade I).

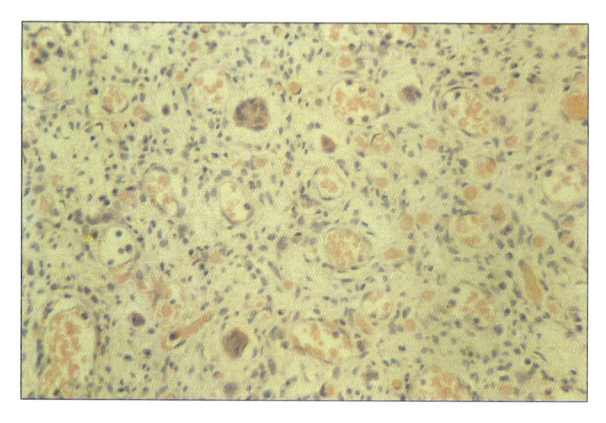

257 Acute GvHD. Rectal biopsy. Grade IV changes with loss of entire glands. Only enterochromaffin cells survive.

Liver

The most consistent histological feature of hepatic GvHD is small bile duct damage which is almost always seen in association with cholestasis (Sloane *et al.*, 1986). Epithelial cell necrosis and nuclear atypia or anucleate cells are seen lining small bile ducts, which may contain necrotic debris in their lumens (**258**). The small bile duct atypia correlates well with clinical evidence of GvHD, and unlike the epithelial damage in the skin and gut, does not appear to be induced by chemoradiation. Other less specific histological features include mononuclear cell infiltration of portal tracts and parenchyma and individual hepatocyte necrosis. The latter has been shown not to correlate closely with clinical GvHD (Shulman and McDonald, 1984, Shulman *et al.*, 1988). Needle biopsies of the liver are useful in differentiating between GvHD and other causes of jaundice, particularly infections and veno-occlusive disease. The biopsy may, however, give false-negative results either because the bile duct lesions are patchily distributed and missed with sampling error, or because the characteristic histological changes appear relatively late after disease onset. Histological grading of hepatic GvHD is based on the percentage of affected bile ducts (**Table 45**), but this cannot be reliably assessed on a small biopsy specimen.

Chronic hepatic GvHD shows essentially similar changes to the acute form. Lymphocytic infiltration is more prominent with portal tract fibrosis and, very rarely, cirrhosis (Yau *et al.*, 1986; Knapp *et al.*, 1987). With progressive disease, small bile ducts may be lost completely, the so-called vanishing bile duct syndrome, leading to fatal liver failure.

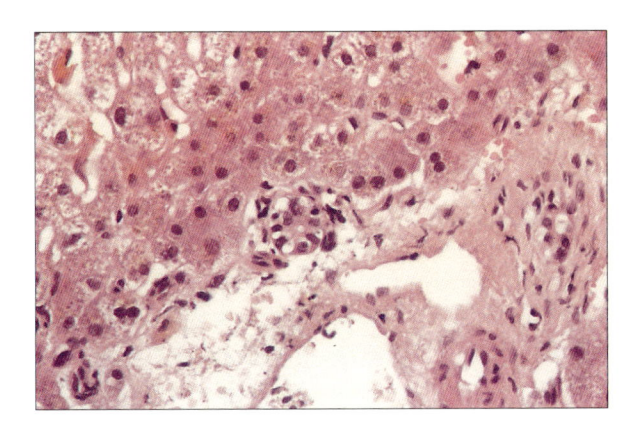

258 Acute GvHD. Liver biopsy. Small bile ducts show nuclear pyknosis and cytoplasmic vacuolation of lining epithelial cells. A scanty lymphocytic infiltrate is present in the portal tract.

References

Beschorner WE. Destruction of the intestinal mucosa after bone marrow transplantation and graft-versus-host disease. *Surv Synth Path Res* 1984; **3**: 264–274.

Dilly SA, Sloane JP. Changes in rectal leucocytes after allogeneic bone marrow transplantation. *Clin Exp Immunol* 1987; **67**: 151-158.

Elliott CJ, Sloane JP, Pallett CD, Sanderson, KV. Cutaneous leucocyte composition after human allogeneic bone marrow transplantation: relationship to marrow purging, histology and clinical rash. *Histopathology* 1988; **12**: 1–16.

Epstein RJ, McDonald GB, Sale GE *et al*. The diagnostic accuracy of the rectal biopsy in acute graft-versus-host disease: a prospective study of thirteen patients. *Gastroenterology* 1980; **78**: 764–771.

Farthing MJG, Clark ML, Sloane JP *et al*. Liver disease after bone marrow transplantation. *Gut* 1982; **23**: 465–474.

Gale RP. Graft-versus-host disease. *Immunol Rev* 1985; **88**: 193–224.

Glucksberg H, Storb R, Fefer A *et al*. Clinical manifestations of graft-versus-host disease in human recipients of marrow from HLA-matched sibling donors. *Transplantation* 1974; **18**:295–304.

Knapp AB, Crawford JM, Rappeport JM, Gollan JL. Cirrhosis as a consequence of graft-versus-host disease. *Gastroenterology* 1987; **92**: 513–519.

Lampert IA, Suitters AJ, Chisholm PM. Expression of Ia antigen on epidermal keratinocytes in graft-versus-host disease. *Nature* 1981; **293**: 149–150

Lampert IA, Thorpe P, van Noorden S *et al*. Selective sparing of enterochromaffin cells in graft-versus-host disease affecting the colonic mucosa. *Histopathology* 1985; **9**: 875–886.

Lerner KG, Kao GF, Storb R *et al*. Histopathology of graft-vs-host reaction (GvHR) in human recipients of marrow from HLA-matched sibling donors. *Transplant Proc* 1974; **6**: 367–371.

McDonald GB, Shulman HM, Sullivan KM, Spencer GD. Intestinal and hepatic complications of human bone marrow transplantation. *Gastroenterology* 1986; **90**: 460–77.

Noel DR, Witherspoon RP, Storb R *et al*. Does graft-versus-host disease influence the tempo of immunologic recovery after allogeneic human marrow transplantation? An observation on 56 long-term survivors. *Blood* 1978; **51**: 1087–1105.

Sale GE, Shulman HM, McDonald GB, Thomas ED. Gastro-intestinal graft-versus-host disease in man. A clinicopathological study of the rectal biopsy. *Am J Surg Pathol* 1979; **3**: 291–299.

Shulman HM, Sale GE, Lerner KG, *et al*. Chronic cutaneous graft-versus-host disease in man. *Am J Pathol* 1978; **91**: 545–570.

Shulman HM, Sale GE. Pathology of acute and chronic cutaneous GvHD. In: *The Pathology of Bone Marrow Transplantation*, 1984 Eds: Sale GE, Shulman HM. Masson, New York, pp..

Shulman HM, McDonald GB. Liver disease after marrow transplantation. In: *The Pathology of Bone Marrow Transplantation*, 1984. Eds: Sale GE, Shulman HM. Masson, New York, pp. 104–135.

Shulman HM, Sharma P, Amos D *et al*. A coded histological study of hepatic graft-versus-host disease after human bone marrow transplantation. *Hepatology* 1988; **3**: 463–470.

Sloane JP, Farthing MJG, Powles RL. Histopathological changes in the liver after allogeneic bone marrow transplantation. *J Clin Pathol* 1986; **33**: 344–350.

Sloane JP, Elliott CJ, Powles R. HLA-DR expression in epidermal keratinocytes after allogeneic bone marrow transplantation. *Transplantation* 1988; **46**: 840–844.

Snover DC. Mucosal damage simulating acute graft-versus-host reaction in cytomegalovirus colitis. *Transplantation* 1985; **39**: 669–670.

Sviland L, Pearson ADJ, Eastham EJ *et al*. Class II antigen expression by keratinocytes and enterocytes—an early feature of graft-versus-host disease. *Transplantation* 1989; **48**: 402–406.

Thomas ED, Storb R, Clift RA *et al*. Bone marrow transplantation. *N Engl J Med* 1975; **292**: 832–902.

Yau JC, Zander AR, Srigley JR *et al*. Chronic graft-versus-host disease complicated by micronodular cirrhosis and oesophageal varices. *Transplantation* 1986; **41**: 129–130.

X Late Effects of Bone Marrow Transplantation

Jennifer Treleaven

Since an increasing number of patients who undergo bone marrow transplantation (BMT) may be expected to live for many years, it is clearly essential that the potential side effects of the procedure are explained, recognised, and remedied where possible. This is particularly important where children are concerned, since as transplantation occurs while they are still growing and probably prior to puberty, it is important to ascertain that growth continues at an acceptable rate, and that patients enter puberty at an appropriate age.

Table 46 shows the commonest late effects seen following principally allogeneic BMT; with autologous transplantation, side effects attributable to chronic graft-versus-host disease are obviously lacking.

The late effects of bone marrow transplantation are largely attributable to the high-dose chemoradiotherapy used for conditioning and the effects of chronic graft-versus-host disease (GvHD).

It is essential that careful monitoring of all patients who have undergone BMT is carried out (**Table 47**).

Table 46. Late effects of bone marrow transplantation.

General	*Liver function*	*Neurological and psychological*
Secondary malignancies	Chronic active hepatitis	Multifocal leukoencephalopathy
Infective (due to hyposplenia and chronic lung damage)	Biliary cirrhosis	Impairment of psychological development in children
Autoimmune phenomena	*Gut*	Re-adaptation difficulties
	Malabsorption with weight loss and diarrhoea	Polyneuropathy
Skin		Myasthenia gravis
Depigmentation, sclerosis, thinning		Sexual dysfunction
Lichenoid changes in mucosal surfaces	*Endocrine*	
	Growth failure	*Ophthalmic*
Sicca syndrome—dry eyes and mouth	Premature menopause	Cataracts
	Testicular failure	Sicca syndrome
Poor hair and nail growth	Infertility	
Premature dental deterioration	Thyroid hypofunction	*Bone problems*
		Osteoporosis
Pulmonary	*Renal*	Aseptic necrosis
Interstitial pneumonitis	Late-onset anaemia, hypertension and fluid retention	
Obliterative bronchiolitis		*Musculoskeletal*
Recurrent bronchitis and bronchopneumonia	Impaired glomerular filtration	Myositis
	Haemorrhagic cystitis	Arthritis

Bone Marrow Transplantation

Table 47. Investigations during follow-up of patients previously having undergone BMT.

Full blood count (Hb; WBC and differential; platelets)
Liver and renal fuction (U & E; LFTs)
Thyroid function (TSH and T_3)
FSH, LH, oestrogen, growth hormone, testosterone
T-cell subsets; immunoglobulins
Blood grouping and antibody titres where ABO-incompatibile BMT has taken place
Chest X-ray
Pulmonary function assessment
Check bone marrow at 6 months and 1 year
Inspect skin, teeth, buccal mucosa, eyes and joints for chronic GvHD
Gynaenocology clinic for hormone replacement and smear test
Psychological assessment for general re-adaptation, sexual problems
Growth clinic for children. Height and weight plotted on Tanner growth chart
Weigh adults regularly
Ophthalmology clinic to assess cataract formation

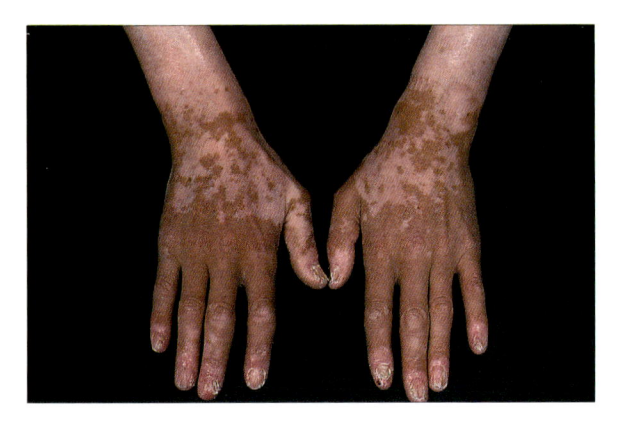

Chronic graft-versus-host disease

Chronic GvHD is seen in 30–50% of patients after HLA sibling-matched transplants (Atkinson, 1990). The commonest manifestations are skin changes, including depigmentation, thinning and sclerosis (**259–261**), and lichenoid mucosal lesions (**262**). Disturbances of liver function may be present, representing a degree of sclerosis within the liver parenchyma and biliary system, and there may be an increased susceptibilty to infection secondary to impairment of immune function. However, most patients with chronic GvHD are relatively disability-

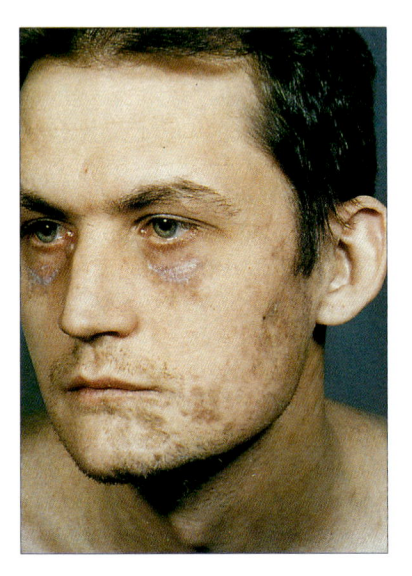

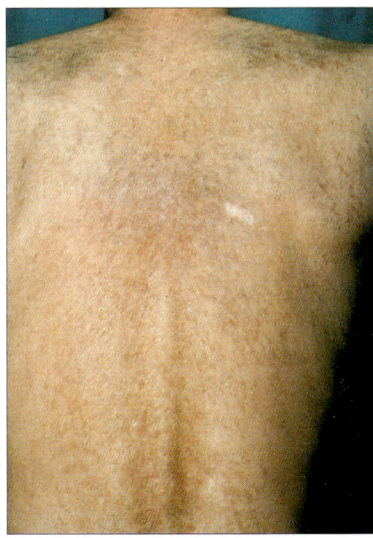

259 Chronic graft-versus-host disease of the skin, showing patchy depigmentation and poor nail growth.

260, 261 Chronic graft-versus-host disease of the skin showing dryness and thinning. There are depigmented patches with hyperpigmentation in previously scarred areas.

262 Chronic graft-versus-host disease of the buccal mucosa, showing thickened, lichenoid plaques which may be confused with candidiasis.

free if immunosuppressive agents are started sufficiently early, but a proportion of patients progress in the face of immunosuppressive therapy to develop severe joint contractures and sclerosis affecting most tissues (**263**).

Growth and development

Radiation is associated with growth retardation after BMT, the spine being particularly affected (Shalet et al., 1987). Development of dentition and the facial skeleton are also commonly impaired in children under 6 years of age who receive radiation (Sanders et al 1986). The younger the patient when irradiated, the greater skeletal disproportion that may result, and it is possible but not conclusive that growth retardation may be minimized by using fractionated rather than single dose total body irradiation (TBI) (Kolb et al., 1989). The impaired growth seen in children with chronic GvHD may be partially attributable to prolonged use of corticosteroids or to the catabolic effect of chronic GvHD, since growth problems also occur in children conditioned with chemotherapy alone, although less so (Urban et al., 1988).

Supplementation with growth hormone may improve growth velocity, and growth hormone secretion may be stimulated by administration of growth hormone releasing hormone, implying that the hypothalamus may suffer more from damage by

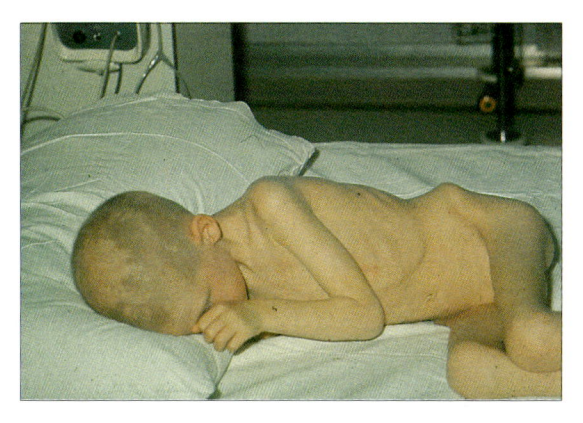

263 Severe chronic graft versus host disease showing marked wasting and joint contractures.

radiation than the pituitary gland itself (Blacklay et al., 1986). The growth chart of a child conditioned for BMT with single-fraction TBI, and his progress after institution of growth hormone supplements, is shown in **264**.

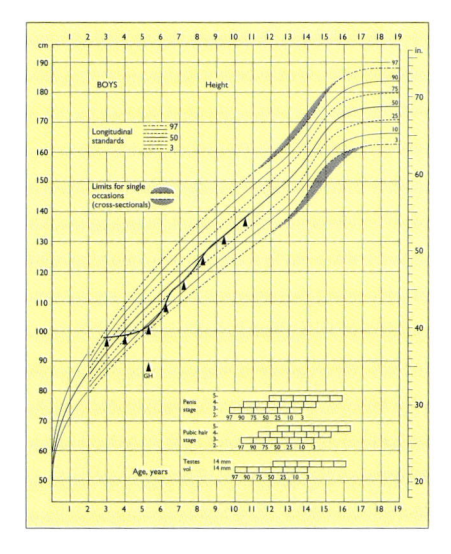

264 The growth chart of a boy conditioned for bone marrow transplantation with total body irradiation (TBI). Prior to therapy he was 39 inches tall and in the 90th centile for his age of just over 3 years; had he continued to grow at this rate his adult height would have been 72 inches. Following TBI his growth fell off until growth hormone therapy (GH) was started. Growth then resumed until he caught up to the 50th centile.

His father is 68 inches tall, which puts him on the 50th centile. The boy is therefore now growing at an acceptable rate and his final height should approximate that of his father, although had he not undergone bone marrow transplantation and the attendant growth retardation he would have been tall in relation to his father's height.

Fertility

Spontaneous puberty is invariably delayed or absent in irradiated females, with only a minority of girls achieving menarche. Most patients have raised gonadotropin levels and require sex hormone replacement. However, boys commonly recover Leydig cell function and produce testosterone, unless their testicles have received additional irradiation. They usually do not require hormone replacement (Barrett *et al.*, 1987).

In adults, infertility is almost universal. The incidence of pregnancy after TBI in women is so small that women need not use contraception. Following TBI, Sanders *et al.* (1988) reported a very low rate of return of ovarian function, with only 9 of 144 women transplanted for leukaemia having return of menses 3–7 years after treatment. All irradiated women develop primary ovarian failure as evidenced by raised luteinizing hormone (LH) and follicle stimulating hormone (FSH) levels, and low oestradiol levels. The rate of ovarian failure following TBI increases with patient age (Cumber and Whittaker, 1989), and hormone replacement therapy should be instituted (Cust *et al.*, 1989).

Occasional pregnancies have been reported (Buskard *et al.*, 1988; Russell *et al.*, 1989) in women who received doses of less than 8 Gy, and two of these spontaneously aborted, suggesting an increased incidence of congenital abnormalities after TBI. A number of pregnancies have been reported after cyclophosphamide-only conditioning for allogeneic transplantation and three have been described after high-dose melphalan conditioning (Milliken *et al.*, 1990). However, none has been reported after combination chemotherapy regimens.

More than 90% of men have permanent azoospermia after receiving TBI. However, rarely return of spermatogenesis is seen as late as 6 years after TBI (Sullivan *et al.*, 1984). Return of fertility after cyclophosphamide-only conditioning is variable, with low to normal sperm counts reported in 20 of 31 men (Sullivan *et al.*, 1984). Testosterone levels are normal even after irradiation, and LH levels may well recover. FSH levels remain elevated in about 75% of men. Animal experiments indicate that single-dose irradiation is less deleterious to testicular function than is fractionated TBI, and normal children have been fathered by both irradiated and busulphan-treated males.

Continuing GvHD, age, postural drop in diastolic blood pressure and low prolactin levels have been shown to be associated with sexual dysfunction in males undergoing BMT, although dysfunction may also occur in the absence of chronic illness (Baruch *et al.*, 1991).

Ophthalmic complications

The incidence of cataracts following TBI has been reported to be as high as 75% at 6 years after single fraction TBI, but is less after fractionated TBI (Tichelli *et al.*, 1987), or single fraction TBI using low dose rates (Barrett *et al.*, 1987). Most patients eventually require surgery, and use of corticosteroids to treat acute GvHD may compound the problem. Dry eyes may result either from reduced tear formation following radiation, or as part of the 'sicca syndrome' that occurs with chronic GvHD.

Respiratory function

Interstitial pneumonitis develops in approximately 30% of patients after allogeneic BMT and accounts for more than 20% of deaths. The majority of such problems occur in the immediate post-BMT period, but they may also occur later on, even after cessation of immunosuppressive therapy. They are more likely to occur in patients with evidence of chronic GvHD. The majority are caused by cytomegalovirus (CMV). A smaller incidence of pneumonitis is seen after autograft, sometimes attributable to CMV infection (Winston *et al.*, 1990). The mortality rate from CMV pneumonitis has dropped since the introduction of ganciclovir, which, when used with CMV hyperimmune globulin, may reduce the incidence to around 60%.

Mild restrictive lung abnormalities occur in all patients after TBI (Depledge *et al.*, 1983), although this defect is subclinical in most patients. Lung abnormalities may include late-onset interstitial pneumonitis and obliterative bronchiolitis.

Infection

Bacterial sepsis is most frequent in the early weeks due to neutropenia, but can occur late due to post-irradiation hyposplenia (Kahls et al., 1988) and chronic GvHD (Atkinson, 1990). Long-term penicillin or co-trimoxazole should be given to patients with chronic GvHD, and probably to all patients following TBI, since they have a predisposition to overwhelming sepsis from encapsulated organisms (Atkinson, 1990).

Viral and fungal infections are a long-term risk, exacerbated by the delay in immune reconstitution, pre-existing lung damage, and hyposplenia induced by conditioning therapy. A profound combined immunodeficiency is present after conditioning (265), and recovery of adequate B- and T-cell function may take more than 12 months (Atkinson, 1990). Oral fungal overgrowth, herpes simplex re-activation, cytomegaloviral and *Pneumocystis* pneumonitis are commonly encountered. Herpes zoster re-activation occurs in 50% of allogeneic transplants and after many autografts. Re-activation can be prevented with the use of oral acyclovir, but infections are still seen after cessation at 6 months (Selby et al., 1989). The approximate time course for the occurrence of different infections following BMT is shown in **266**.

Patients should be aware of the late susceptibility to infections, the importance of taking prophylactic medication and of seeking medical attention early if infection is suspected. Restricting contact with persons with known viral illnesses and avoiding crowds is advisable for some months after BMT since patients can be re-infected with diseases such as measles, mumps and chicken pox. Influenza can be a life-threatening illness.

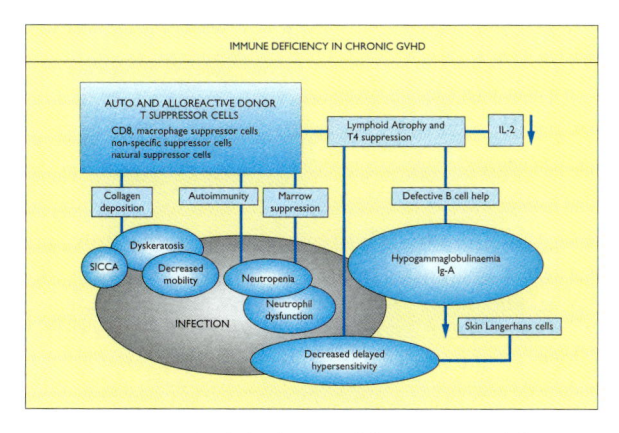

265 Diagrammatical depiction of the immune deficiency which occurs after bone marrow transplantation, particularly in the context of chronic graft-versus-host disease.

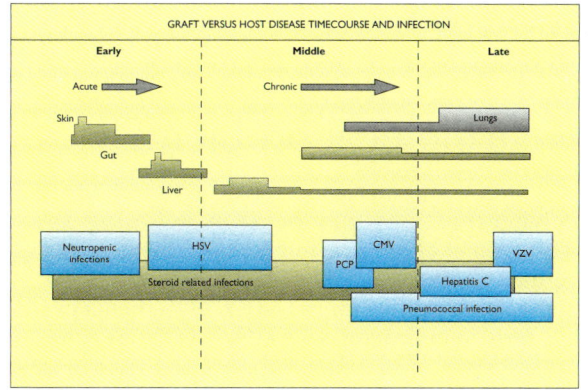

266 The time course for the occurence of various infections after bone marrow transplantation. Presence of graft-versus-host disease exacerbates the liklihood of these occuring.

Second malignancies

The incidence of second malignancies after BMT is low, and is related to the use of chemotherapy, particularly alkylating agents, radiotherapy and prolonged immunosuppression. The risk seems to be higher in patients older than 40 years, in those receiving intensive chemotherapy, and in those receiving a high dose rate of unfractionated irradiation. Lymphomas, solid tumours and recurrence of leukaemia in donor cells have been reported (Witherspoon et al., 1989). It has been suggested that there is a six- to sevenfold tumour incidence in BMT recipients compared with normal individuals (Deeg et al., 1984). However, the carcinogenic potential of various conditioning regimens is, to date, unknown.

Autoimmune disorders and thyroid dysfunction

There have been several reported cases of transmission of allergic or autoimmune disease to recipients of allogeneic BMT. It is also possible that such illnesses may incidentally be cured by BMT. Transfer of autoimmune thyroiditis (Wyatt et al., 1990; Aldouri et al., 1990), asthma and IgE hypersensitivity (Agosti et al., 1988) have been described from donor to recipient. Since donors may be able to transmit some disorders, a completely fit sibling should be used if possible.

Clinical hypothyroidism occurs in 8% of long-term survivors after TBI, although this is less frequent after fractionated TBI (Lio et al., 1988) and does not appear to occur after drug-only conditioning regimens (Sklar et al., 1982). Thyroid abnormalities are reported in up to 40% of BMT recipients, and mainly take the form of elevated thyroid stimulating hormone (TSH) levels. However, hyperthroidism with decreased response to thyroid-releasing hormone (TRH) stimulation has also been observed.

Bone problems and musculoskeletal dysfunction

Osteoporosis occurs commonly following BMT, related to prolonged use of steroids, premature menopause or chronic GvHD. It may result in pathological fractures. Aseptic osteonecrosis occurs in up to 10% of transplant recipients and commonly affects several joints (Russell et al., 1989). It is associated with chronic GvHD, and is to some extent treatable with steroids.

Neurological problems

Polyneuropathies may be seen following BMT (Granena et al., 1983), but isolated dysfunction of peripeheral nerves is most commonly due either to herpes zoster or to severe GvHD. Myasthenia gravis is a rare complication of chronic GvHD (Witznitzer et al., 1984), although thymic examination shows no evidence of neoplasia or hyperplasia (Bolger et al., 1986), and acute idiopathic demyelating polyneuritis (Guillain–Barré syndrome) has also been reported (Perry et al., 1994; Openshaw et al., 1991).

Renal function

Impaired glomerular filtration may persist in some patients after cessation of nephrotoxic agents such as cyclosporin, antifungals and nephrotoxic antibiotics, and late-onset renal dysfunction with anaema, oedema and hypertension has been described in transplant recipients (Bergstein et al., 1986; Tarbell et al., 1988). In such patients, the combination of radiotherapy and chemotherapy with agents such as melphalan or cyclophosphamide may have a contributory role. Haemorrhagic cystitis, commonly seen in the vicinity of administration of high-dose cyclophosphamide as conditioning therapy, may recur late after transplantation. Such viruses as the BK virus may be concurrently found in the urine (Arthur et al., 1986). Although bladder cancer has been recognised as occurring subsequent to high-dose cyclophosphamide administration (Stillwell and Benson, 1988), it has not so far been reported following BMT with high-dose cyclophosphamide conditioning therapy.

Hepatic function

The most frequent causes of chronic liver disease following BMT are chronic GvHD (Shulman et al., 1980) and chronic active hepatitis (Vernant, 1986). Occasionally, biliary cirrhosis may be seen secondary to progression of chronic GvHD (Knapp et al., 1987).

References

Agosti JM, Sprenger JD, Lum LG et al. Transfer of allergen-specific IgE-mediated hypersensitivity with allogeneic bone marrow transplantation. *N Eng J Med* 1988; **319**: 1623–162.

Aldouri MA, Ruggier R, Epstein O, Prentice HG. Adoptive transfer of hyperthyroidism and autoimmune thyroiditis following allogeneic bone marrow transplantation for chronic myeloid leukaemia. *Br J Haematol* 1990; **74**: 118–120.

Arthur RR, Shah KV, Baust SJ et al. Association of BK viruria with haemorrhagic cystitis in recipients of bone marrow transplant. *N Engl J Med* 1986; **315** 230–234.

Atkinson K. Chronic graft-versus-host disease. *Bone Marrow Transplant* 1990; **5**: 69-82.

Barrett A, Nicholls J, Gibson B. Late effects of total body irradiation. *Radiother Oncol* 1987; **9**: 131–135.

Baruch J, Benjamin S, Treleaven J, Wilcox H, Barron J, Powles RL. Male sexual function following bone marrow transplantation *Bone Marrow Transplant* 1991; **7** (suppl): 52.

Bergstein J, Andreoli SP, Provisor AJ, Yum M. Radiation nephritis following total body irradiation and cyclophosphamide in preparation for bone marrow transplantation. *Transplantation* 1986; **41**: 63–66.

Blacklay A, Grossmann A, Ross RJ et al. Cranial irradiation for cerebral and nasopharyngeal tumours in children: evidence for the production of a hypothalamic defect in growth hormone release. *J Endocrinol* 1986; **108**: 25–29.

Bolger GB, Sullivan KM, Spence AM et al. 1986 Myasthenia gravis after allogeneic bone marrow transplantation: relationship to chronic graft-versus-host disease. *Neurology* 1986; **36**: 1087–1091.

Buskard N, Ballem P, Hill R, Fryer C. Normal fertility after total body irradiation and chemotherapy in conjunction with a bone marrow transplant for acute leukaemia. *Clin Invest* 1988; **2**: (suppl): C57.

Cumber PM, Whittaker JA. Ovarian failure after total body irradiation. *Br Med J* 1989; **300**: 464.

Cust MP, Whitehead MI, Powles R et al. Consequences and treatment of ovarian failure after total body irradiation for leukaemia. *Br Med J* 1989; **299**: 1494-1497.

Deeg HJ, Sanders J, Martin P et al. Secondary malignancies after bone marrow transplantation. *Exp Hematol* 1984; **12**: 660-666.

Depledge M, Barrett A, Powles RL. Lung function after bone marrow grafting. *Int J Radiat Oncol Biol Phys* 1983; **9**: 145-151.

Granena A, Grau JM, Carreras E et al. Subacute sensori-motor polyneuropathy in a recipient of an allogeneic marrow graft. *Exp Hematol* 1983; **13** (suppl): 10–12.

Kahls P, Panzer S, Kletter K et al. Functional asplenia after bone marrow transplantation. *Ann Intern Med* 1988; **109**: 461–464.

Knapp AB, Crawford JM, Rappeport JM, Gollan JL. Cirrhosis as a consequence of graft-versus-host disease. *Gastroenterology* 1987; **392**: 513–519

Kolb HJ, Bender-Gotze CH, Haas RJ. Late effects in marrow transplanted patients—results of the AG-KMT, Munich *Bone Marrow Transplant* 1989; **4** (suppl 2): 269.

Lio S, Arcese W, Papa G, D'Armiento M. Thyroid and pituitary function following allogeneic bone marrow transplantation. *Arch Intern Med* 1988; **148**: 1066–1071.

Milliken S, Powles R, Parikh P et al. Successful pregnancy following bone marrow transplantation for leukaemia. *Bone Marrow Transplant* 1990; **1**: 135–137.

Openshaw H, Hinton DR, Slatkin NE et al. Exacerbation of inflammatory demyelinating polyneuropathy after bone marrow transplantation. *Bone Marrow Transplant* 1991; **7**: 411–414

Perry A, Mehta J, Iverson T et al. Guillain–Barré syndrome after bone marrow transplantation. *Bone Marrow Transplant* 1994 (In press).

Russell JA, Hanley DA. Full-term pregnancy after allogeneic transplantation for leukemia in a patient with oligomenorrhea. *Bone Marrow Transplant* 1989; **4**: 579–580.

Russell JA, Blakey WB, Stuart TA et al. Avascular necrosis of bone in bone marrow transplant recipients. *Med Paediatr Oncol* 1989; **17**: 140-143.

Sanders JE, Pritchard S, Mahoney P et al. Growth and development following marrow transplantation for leukemia. *Blood* 1986; **68**: 1129–1135.

Sanders JE, Buckner CD, Amos D et al. Ovarian function following marrow transplantation for aplastic anemia or leukemia. *J Clin Oncol* 1988; **6**: 813–818.

Selby PJ, Powles RL, Easton D et al. The prophylactic role of intravenous and long-term oral acyclovir after allogeneic bone marrow transplantation. *Br J Cancer* 1989; **59**: 434–438.

Shalet SM, Gibson B, Swindell R, Pearson D. Effect of spinal irradiation on growth. *Arch Dis Child* 1987; **62**: 461–464.

Shulman H, Sullivan KM, Weiden PL. Chronic graft-versus-host syndrome in man. A long-term clinicopathological study of 20 Seattle patients. *Am J Med* 1980; **69**: 204–217.

Sklar CA, Kim TH, Ramsay NK. Thyroid dysfunction among long-term survivors of bone marrow transplantation. *Am J Med* 1982; **73**: 5. 688–694.

Stillwell TJ, Benson RC. Cyclophosphamide-induced haemorrhagic cystitis. A review of 100 patients. *Cancer* 1988; **61**: 451–457.

Sullivan KM, Deeg HJ, Sanders JE et al. Late complications after marrow transplantation. *Semin Hematol* 1984; **21**: 53–63.

Tarbell NJ, Guinan EC, Niemeyer C et al. Late onset of renal dysfunction in survivors of bone marrow transplantation. *Int J Radiat Biol Phys* 1988; **15**: 99–104.

Tichelli A, Gratwohl A, Wursch A et al. Cataract formation after bone marrow transplantation (BMT) with and without irradiation: therapeutic implications. *Bone Marrow Transplant* 1987; **2** (suppl 1): 250.

Urban C, Schwingshandle J, Slavc I et al. Endocrine function after bone marrow transplantation without the use of preparative total body irradiation. *Bone Marrow Transplant* 1988; **3**: 291–296.

Vernant JP For the Leukaemia Working Party of the EBMT. Hepatitis B and non-A, non-B hepatitis after allogeneic bone marrow transplantation in leukaemia. *Bone Marrow Transplant* 1986; **1** (suppl 1): 183–184.

Winston DJ, Ho WG, Champlin RE (1990) Cytomegalovirus infections after allogeneic bone marrow transplantation. *Rev Infect Dis* 1990; 12 (suppl): 776–792.

Witherspoon RP, Fisher LD, Schock G et al. 1989 Secondary cancers after bone marrow transplantation for leukemia or aplastic anemia. *N Engl J Med* 1989; **321**: 784–789.

Witznitzer M, Packer RJ, August CS, Burkey ED. Neurological complications of bone marrow transplantation in childhood. *Ann Neurol* 1984; **16**: 569–576.

Wyatt DT, Lum LG, Casper J et al. Autoimmune thyroiditis after bone marrow transplantation. *Bone Marrow*

Index

NB Page numbers in *italics* refer to figures and tables.
Bone marrow transplantation is abbreviated to BMT.

A

Ableson proto-oncogene (ABL) 67
ABO compatible allografts 109
acetabulum 25
acute idiopathic demyelating polyneuritis 198
acute lymphoblastic leukaemia (ALL) 65–7
  BMT 65, 66, 67
  chemotherapy 65
  common 15
  maintenance therapy 66
  stem cell origin 66
  survival 65, 66, 67
acute myeloid leukaemia (AML) 63–5
  bone marrow purging 122
  chemotherapy 63, 64
  FAB type 63–4
  survival 64, *65*
acute promyelocytic leukaemia *63*
acyclovir 173, 197
adenosine deaminase (ADA) deficiency 57, 59, 60
adenovirus 174
adrenaline 121
Adriamycin 81
  see also doxorubicin
adult respiratory distress syndrome *106*, 107
agranulocytosis, infantile genetic 59
airways obstruction 30
alkaline phosphatase 188
alkyl lysophospholipids 121
allogeneic BMT 9
  acute GvHD 143
  acute myeloid leukaemia (AML) 64, *65*
  aplastic anaemia 49-51
  chronic granulocytic leukaemia (CGL) 68
  conditioning 10
  cyclosporin use 146
  Fanconi anaemia 32–3
  graft-versus-leukaemia effect 161
  GvHD disease problems 143
  haematological malignancies 19
  Hodgkin's lymphoma 70
  incidence of GvHD 185
  morbidity 185
  multiple myeloma 72
  myelodysplastic syndromes 64
  pre-graft cytotoxic conditioning 161
  recent history 10–11
  relapse rate with GvHD 161
  T-cell subset elimination 124
  unrelated donors 162
allogeneic haemopoietic stem cell infusions 10
allografts 13, 16
  ABO compatible 109
  acute lymphoblastic leukaemia (ALL) 66
  age 17
  donors 13
amphoterocin B 175, 176
Anthony Nolan Research Centre 14
anti-A removal 110
anti-B removal 110
anti-CD3 antibody 149
anti-CD34 MAb 126, *127*
anti-CMV immunoglobulin 173
anti-cytokine agents 149–50
anti-emetic therapy 162
anti-interleukin-2 receptor antibody (aIL-2-ra) 149
anti-lymphocyte globulin (ALG) 40
anti-T-cell MAbs 149
anti-TNF agents 150
antibiotic therapy 135
antilymphocyte globulin (ALG) 49, 149
antithymocyte globulin (ATG) 40, 49
aplastic anaemia 15, 19
  correction 10
  pre-graft ablation 161
  very severe 49
aplastic anaemia, severe 49–52, *53*
  allogeneic BMT 49-51
  cause of death 51
  fungal infections 52, *53*
  prognosis 49
  syngenetic BMT *53*
  treatment 49
arrhythmia
  catheter tip position 138
  central venous catheter insertion 135
aspergilloma 175
aspergillosis, pulmonary 175
Aspergillus 52, 175, 176
  cerebral infection 181
asplenia, functional 44
asthma transfer 198
astrocytoma 93, 95
atom bomb survivors 9
Auer rods *63*
autograft transplantation 14
  acute lymphoblastic leukaemia (ALL) 66
  age 17
  multiple myeloma 72
  no allogeneic donor 15
autoimmune disorders 58, 198
autologous blood donation 101–02
autologous BMT
  brain tumours 93, *94*, 95
  breast carcinoma 82, *83–4*, 85
  chronic granulocytic leukaemia (CGL) 68
  drug escalation 81
  germ cell tumour therapy 86, *87*, 88–99
  GvHD 144–5
  malignant cell detection 117–18
  marrow purging 116
  melanoma therapy 90, 91
  non-Hodgkin's lymphoma 71–2
  ovarian carcinoma 85–6
  plus combination chemotherapy 79–80
  plus high-dose chemotherapy 82, *83–4*, 85–6, *87*, 88-91, *92*, 93, *94*, 95–7
  solid tumours 77
  solid tumours of childhood 96–7
  tumour therapy 15
autologous bone marrow, cryopreservation 40
5-azacytidine 44
azathioprine 178

B

B-cell function, post-transplant 58
B-cell leukaemia/lymphoma immunotherapy 124
B-lymphocyte proliferative disease 59
bacterial sepsis 197

201

BCNU (carmustine) 164
BCR/ABL gene 67
bile duct damage 191
bilirubin 188
blast crisis 67, 68
bleomycin 81
blood cell development *13*
blood samples, BMT monitoring 129
BMT
  autologous 9
  children 16, 17
  complications 16
  conditioning therapy 16, 161
  course 16
  development effects 195
  fertility effects 196
  follow-up investigations *194*
  goals 15
  growth effects 195
  history 9–10
  HLA-identical 29
  indications for 15, *16*
  infection 197
  late effects 193-9
  mortality 17
  ophthalmic complications 196
  respiratory function effects 196
  results 17
  second malignancies 197
  survival 17
  thalassaemia 39–40
  types 13–14
bone marrow
  buffy coat separation 109
  clonogenic assay 112, *113*
  hypoplasia 30
  liquid nitrogen storage 112
  plasma depletion 110
  processing 109–12, *113*, 114–16
  red cell depletion 109–10
  stem cell recovery 109
bone marrow harvesting 101–7
  colony forming unit measurement 105
  complications *105*
  donor preparation 101–2
  nucleated cell count 105
  procedure 102, *103*, 104–5
bone marrow infusion
  conditioning chemotherapy 106
  morbidity 107
  pulmonary toxicity *106*, 107
  reinfusion 106-7
bone marrow purging 115–16
  chemical techniques 122
  immunological techniques 123–8
  physical techniques *120*, 121
brain tumours 93, *94*, 95
breakpoint cluster region (BCR) 67
breast cancer
  adenocarcinoma 80
  bone marrow purging 122
  chemotherapy plus autologous BMT 82, *83–4*, 85
  combination chemotherapy 80
  combination chemotherapy plus ABMT 80
  complete response (CR) rate 82
  dose intensification 80–81
  metastatic *83–4*
  operable 85
British Bone Marrow and Platelet Donor Panel 14
broncheolar lavage 177, 178

Broviac catheter 131
buffy coat
  cytomegalovirus isolation 172
  separation 109
busulphan 19, 40
  chemotherapy conditioning 162, 163
  conditioning for chronic granulocytic leukaemia BMT 68
  conditioning for primary immunodeficiency diseases BMT 57
  cyclophosphamide (BuCy) 72
  pre-graft ablation 161
  preconditioning for sickle cell anaemia BMT 44

C

calorie intake during BMT 129
Candida 52, 162, 181
carboplatin
  brain tumour therapy 95
  breast cancer therapy 80
  chemotherapy conditioning 164
  ovarian carcinoma therapy 86
  testicular carcinoma 86, *87*, 88, *89*
cardiac dysfunction 163
cardiomyopathy *27*
  Hurler's disease (MPS-IH) *23*
carmustine
  brain tumour therapy 93, 95
  breast cancer therapy 82, 85
  melanoma therapy 90, 91
  solid tumours of childhood 96
castor bean plant 123
cataract 196
catheter-related sepsis 130
CCNU (lomustine) 164
CD4+ cells 145
CD4 antigen 12
CD8+ cells 145
CD34+ cells *126*, 127, *128*
CD34
  harvested marrow 105
  positivity 64
central nervous system infections 181
central venous catheters 130–38
  bleeding with insertion 134–5
  catheter tip migration *137*, 138
  complications 133–8
  cuff extrusion 138
  duration of use 133
  embolization 137
  extravasation 138
  infection 135-6
  insertion 131-3
  local anaesthesia 132, 133
  non-tunnelled lines 130
  occlusion 136
  patient position 137
  patient preparation 131
  split sheath introducer *132*, 133
  traction accidents 138
  tunnel formation 133
  tunnel infection 135
  tunnelled lines 130–31
centrifugal elutriation 121
cerebral infections 181–2, *183*, 184
cerebral sulci 25
Ceredase 29
chelation, sickle cell anaemia 44
chemoradiotherapy late effects 193
chemotherapy
  acute lymphoblastic leukaemia 65

chemotherapy *cont*
  acute myeloid leukaemia (AML) 63, 64
  high-dose plus autologous BMT 82, *83–4*, 85-6, *87*, 88–91, *92*, 93, *94*, 95–7
  Hodgkin's lymphoma 70
  non-Hodgkin's lymphoma 71, 72
chemotherapy, combination
  dose-response effect 80–81
  plus autologous BMT 79, 79–80
chemotherapy conditioning 106, 164–5
  agents 161–3
  combination 165
  complications 162
  emetic potential 162
  intensification 162
  morbidity 162
chest syndrome, acute *44*
  sickle cell anaemia 46
childhood solid tumours, chemotherapy plus autologous BMT 96–7
children
  BMT 16, 17
  central venous catheters 132, 138
  growth effects 195
  pretransplant conditioning 19
Chlamydia 171
chlorambucil 85
cholestasis 191
chromosome 6, 11
chronic granulocytic leukaemia (CGL) 67–8
  blastic transformation 67, 68
  conditioning regimes 68
  GvHD attenuation 68
chronic myeloid leukaemia (CML) 15
  graft-versus leukaemia effect 143
  pulmonary complications 178
chymopapain *127*
cisplatin
  brain tumour therapy *94*
  breast cancer therapy 82, *83*, 85
  chemotherapy conditioning 164
  dose intensification 81
  germ cell tumour therapy 86, *87*, 90
  melanoma therapy 91, *92*
  ovarian carcinoma therapy 85
clavicle, osteomyelitis 135
clonogenic assay 112, *113*
⁶⁰Co unit 156
co-trimoxazole 171, 176–7, 197
common acute lymphoblastic leukaemia 15
common variable immunodeficiency 59
complement-mediated purging 123, 124
consanguinous marriage 39
corneal clouding 24
corticosteroids 49
cryopreservation
  rate of freezing 112
  stem cells 110, *111*, 112, *113*, 114, *115*
  temperature profile 112
  without programmable freezer 114
Cryptococcus neoformans cerebral infection 182, *183*, 184
Cryptosporidium 52
cyclophosphamide 19
  aplastic anaemia BMT 51, *53*
  breast cancer therapy 80, 81, 82, 85
  chemotherapy conditioning 162, 163
  conditioning chemotherapy for infusion 106
  conditioning for chronic granulocytic leukaemia BMT 68
  conditioning for primary immunodeficiency diseases BMT 57
  fertility effects 196
  germ cell tumour therapy 90
  graft failure 51
  GvHD prophylaxis 146
  immunosuppressive conditioning 161
  melanoma therapy 90
  multiple myeloma 73
  ovarian carcinoma therapy 85, 86
  preconditioning for sickle cell anaemia BMT 44
  pretransplant immunosuppression 40
  renal function 198
  solid tumours of childhood 96
cyclosporin 13
  aplastic anaemia treatment 49
  autologous GvHD 145
  GvHD in aplastic anaemia BMT 52
  GvHD prophylaxis 40, 44, 64, 146, *147*, 148, 161
  side effects 146, *147*, 148
cyclosporin A 33
cystitis, haemorrhagic 32, 33, 163, 198
cytokines 145
cytomegalovirus 196, 197
  AIDS-associated 172
  diagnosis 172
  hyperimmune globulin 196
  idiopathic pneumonitis 177
  inclusion bodies 172
  interstitial pneumonitis 52, 171, 172
  pathology 172
  prevention 173
  thalassaemia 39
  treatment 172–73
cytoreductive therapy, venous access 129
cytosine arabinoside, chemotherapy conditioning 164
cytotoxic drugs
  dose escalation *78*, 79–80
  dose-response effect 77
cytotoxic T lymphocytes 57

D
dacarbazine 90
dapsone 177
daunorubicin 165
dermatitis 185
desferrioxamine 38
development effects of BMT 195
diarrhoea 185, 187
dimethylsulphoxide (DMSO) 106, 107, 110, 112, 114
disodium EDTA 136
donor T lymphocytes 143
donors
  allografting 13
  blood transfusion 101–2
  characteristics and acute GvHD 143
  HLA-matched 144
  preparation 101–2
  sibling 13, 14
  sickle cell anaemia BMT 44
  T-cell depletion 68
  thalassaemia 39
doxorubicin 165
  see also Adriamycin
DR typing 12
Dynal Detachbead system *127*
dysosotosis multiplex *26*, *27*

E
embryonal cell carcinoma *87–8*
encephalitis 182
encephalopathy *183*

endocarditis 130, 136
Enterobacter 171
enterochromaffin cells 190
Epstein-Barr virus-associated polyclonal B-lymphocyte proliferation 59
Epstein-Barr-associated lymphoma 59
erythrocyte
  pheresis 42
  sickled *46*
ethnic minorities, donor matching 14
etoposide
  brain tumour therapy 95
  breast cancer therapy *84*
  chemotherapy conditioning 164
  dose intensification 81
  familial haemophagocytic lymphohistiocytosis 57
  germ cell tumour therapy 90
  ovarian carcinoma therapy 85
  testicular carcinoma 86, *87*, 88, 89
external jugular vein 132

F
falciparum malaria 43
familial haemophagocytic lymphohistiocytosis 57
Fanconi anaemia 30–33
  allogeneic BMT 32–3
  chromosomal abnormalities *32*
  cytogenetic abnormalities 32
  diagnosis criteria 32
  oesophageal stricture 33
  phenotypic expression 32
  survival rate 33
Fanconi facies 30
fansidar 177
femoral vein 132
fertility effects of BMT 196
fetal liver 58
fibrin
  intravascular formation 136
  sheath formation 138
fibrinolytic therapy 135, 136, 137
FK-506 147
5-fluoruracil 80, 81
folinic acid 145
foscarnet 172
freezer, programmed *111*, 112
fucosidosis dogs 20
fungal infection 174–6, 197
  aplastic anaemia 52, *53*
  central venous catheters 135, 136
  cerebral 181
Fusarium 53

G
G6PD (glucose 6-phosphate dehydrogenase) deficency 45
ganciclovir 172
gastrointestinal tract
  GvHD manifestations 187–8
  histological features of GvHD 190
Gaucher cells 28–9
Gaucher's disease 28–9
  Type I 19, 21
gene therapy for immune deficiency diseases 60
gene transfer, retroviral-mediated 60
germ cell tumours
  chemotherapy plus autologous BMT 86, *87*, 88–90
  dose intensification 81
Giardia 52
glioma *94*
globin chain synthesis 40, *41*, *42*

globin isoelectricfocusing 40, *42*
glomerular filtration 198
glucocerebroside 28
glycerol 110
glycogen storage disease Type II *28*
glycosaminoglycans
  storage 20
  urinary excretion 22
gonadotropin levels 196
graft rejection 9
  aplastic anaemia BMT 51
  immune deficiency disorders 57
  immunosuppression 161
  T-cell depletion 149
  thalassaemia 40
graft-versus leukaemia effect 10, 13, 14, 15, 77, 143
  allogeneic BMT 161
  chronic granulocytic leukaemia (CGL) 68
  marrow purging 115
graft-versus-host disease (GvHD) 10, 11, 143–50, 185–91
  acute 143, 185, 186–7
  aetiology 144–5
  allografting 13
  aplastic anaemia BMT 51, 52
  autoimmune manifestations 144, 145
  chronic 143–4, 185, 187, 188
  clinical features 185–8
  cytomegalovirus infection 172
  Fanconi anaemia 33
  gastrointestinal tract manifestations 187–8
  graft-versus-leukaemia coexistence 68
  histological features 188–91
  hyperacute 143
  idiopathic pneumonitis 178
  immune deficiency 57–8, *197*
  immunosuppression 144, 195
  infection prophylaxis 144
  intravenous support 129
  late effects of chronic 193, 194–5
  morbidity 185
  onset 143
  pathogenesis 12
  prevention *145*
  prophylaxis 40, 44
  pulmonary complications 178
  rectal biopsy 190
  relapse prevention 77
  relapse rate after allogeneic BMT 161
  scleroderma 187, 189, 195
  sickle cell anaemia BMT 44
  skin manifestations 186–7, 189, *190*
  staging *185*, *186*
  thalassaemia BMT 40, *43*
  thalassaemia donors 39
graft-versus-host disease (GvHD) prophylaxis 145–6, *147*, 148–50
  acute myeloid leukaemia (AML) 64
  anti-cytokine agents 149–50
  antibody therapy 149
  cyclophosphamide 146
  cyclosporin 146, *147*, 148, 161
  FK-506 146
  MAbs 124
  methotrexate 145–6
  methotrexate/cyclosporin combination 148
  steroids 148
  trimetrexate 146
granulocyte colony-stimulating factor (G-CSF) 14, 16, 59, 70
granulocyte-macrophage colony-stimulating factor (GM-CSF) 14, 16, 70, 77

GM-CSF *cont*
  multiple myeloma 73
  granulomatous disease, chronic 59–60
gravity sedimentation 121
growth effects of BMT 195
growth factors 14
  Hodgkin's lymphoma 70
growth hormone supplementation 195
guanethidine *121*
guidewire, central venous catheters 133, *134*, 135
Guillain-Barré syndrome 198

H
haematological malignancies 19
haematoma 135
haematopoiesis correction 10
haematopoietic growth factors 77
haematopoietic progenitors 58
haematopoietic stem cells
  engraftment 19
  positive selection 126
  source of normal 58
haemolytic anaemia 58
Haemophilus influenzae 171, 182
haemopoietic chimaerism 20
haemosiderosis 39, 42
harvest procedure 102, *103*, 104–5
  equipment 102, *103*, *104*, 105
HbE/ß-thalassaemia 38
HbF 46
  synthesis 40
HbS 43
HbS/ß-thalassaemia 38
hepatitis B virus 39
hepatitis C virus 39
herpes simplex 173
  cerebral infection *182*
  infection 162, 197
hexamethylmelamine 81
Hickman lines 131
  catheter tip position 138
  pneumothorax *134*
  pulmonary thromboembolism 137
  siting *131*
  tunnelling *132*
hilar adenopathy *84*
hip dislocation *25*
hirsutism *148*
HIV positivity in thalassaemia 39
HLA-identical BMT 29
HLA-matched donors 144
  see also human leucocyte antigen (HLA)
Hodgkin's lymphoma 69–70
host-versus-graft resistance 149
Howell-Jolly bodies *46*
human leucocyte antigen (HLA) 9
  assay 11
  inheritance *12*
  system 11–12
Hunter's disease (MPS-II) 25
Hurler's disease (MPS-IH) 15, 19, 20, 21, 22–5
  brain scan 25
  corneal clouding 24
  facial features *23, 24*
  kyphoscoliosis 24
  skeletal symptoms 22
4-hydroperoxycyclophosphamide 122
hydroxyethyl starch (HES) solution 110, 114
5-hydroxytryptamine (5HT) antagonists 162
hydroxyurea 44

hyperthermia 121
hyperthyroidism 198
hypothyroidism 198

I
a_i-iduronidase 15
a-iduronidase 19
IgE sensitivity transfer 198
IgG MAbs 123, 125
iliac crest, bone marrow aspiration 104
immune function, recovery post-transplant 58
immunocytochemical staining 118
immunodeficiency disease, primary 55–60
immunodeficiency disorders
  bone marrow transplants 55
  conditioning 56–7
  congenital 55
  graft rejection 57
  GvHD 57–8, *197*
immunodeficiency, post-transplant 51
immunosuppression
  chemotherapy conditioning 161
  post-transplant 12
  pretransplant 40, 57
implantable devices 138
inappropriate antidiuretic hormone secretion (SIADH) 163
inborn errors of metabolism 19–33
  Fanconi anaemia 30–3
  lysosomal enzyme deficiency 20, *21*
  lysosomal storage disease 21, *22*
infection
  central venous catheters 135–6
  post-BMT 197
a-interferon 68
interleukin-1 (IL-1) deficiency 56
interleukin-2 91
interleukin-3 77
interleukin-6 77
internal jugular vein 132
intravenous infusion 9
m-iodobenzylguanidine 121
iron accumulation, transfused 38
iron overload
  chronic transfusion therapy 44
  thalassaemia BMT 40, 42
irradiation
  atom bomb survivors 9
  blood products 102
  fractionated 195
  marrow aplasia 9
irradiation, total body 40
  aplastic anaemia BMT graft failure 51
  benefits 155
  conditioning for chronic granulocytic leukaemia BMT 68
  conditioning for multiple myeloma BMT 72
  conditioning for primary immunodeficiency diseases BMT 57
  with cyclophosphamide 163
  dosage 159
  dose distribution *157*
  fertility effects 196
  fractionation regimes 158–9
  graft failure 149
  idiopathic pneumonitis 178
  lung shielding 159
  patient conditioning 155–6, *157*, 158–9
  pre-graft ablation 161
  preconditioning for sickle cell anaemia BMT 44
  premedication 158
  sanctuary sites 159

irradiation, total body *cont*
  single fraction 158
  target cells 155
  test dose 156, *157*
irradiation, total lymphoid 40
  aplastic anaemia BMT graft failure 51
  graft failure 149
isohaemagglutinins 60

J
jaundice, cholestatic 185, 188
joint changes, degenerative *25*

K
Kaplan-Meyer survival curves for aplastic anaemia BMT *50, 51, 52*
Klebsiella 171
Kupffer cells 20
kyphoscoliosis *24*

L
lactic dehydrogenase 72
late effects of BMT 193–9
Legionella 171
Leishmania 53
leukaemia 63–8
  acute lymphoblastic 15, 65–7
  acute myeloid 63–5, 122
  acute promyelocytic *63*
  blast cells *63*
  BMT curing 143
  chronic granulocytic leukaemia (CGL) 67–8
  chronic myeloid 15, 143, 178
  GvHD in relapse 143
  monocytic *63*
  recurrence 197
  relapse 10
  relapse with T-cell depletion 149
  sickle cell anaemia 44
  T-cell 124
leukaemic progenitor cell detection 118
leukocyte adhesion defect
  gene therapy 60
  partial 57
leukocyte glucocerebrosidase *28*
leukodystrophy, metachromatic *27*
leukoencephalopathy, progressive multifocal 184
Leydig cell function 196
lichenoid effects
  mucosal lesions 194, *195*
  oral mucosa 188
  papular eruption *186*, 187
  skin 189
lip biopsy 190
liquid nitrogen
  safe handling *113, 114*
  storage of bone marrow 112, *113*
Listeria monocytogenes meningitis 182
liver
  chronic GvHD 194
  GvHD manifestations 188
  histological features of GvHD 191
  storage material reduction 29
lumbar gibbus *23*
lymphoblastic lymphoma 71
lymphocyte anti-killer cell (LAK) purging 123
lymphoid stem cell defects 56
lymphomas 69–72
  recurrence 197
lysosomal enzyme deficiency 20

lysosomal enzyme deficiency *cont*
  animal models 20, *21*
lysosomal enzyme transfer 19, 20
lysosomal storage disease 21, *22*
  BMT 29
  skeletal deformities 29
  transplantation in early life 29

M
macrophage replacement 20
maculopapular rash, erythematous 186, 187
major histocompatibility complex (MHC) 11–12
  antigens 144
malignant cells, purging 115, 116
Maroteaux-Lamy syndrome (MPS VI) *27*
marrow infusion, venous access 129
matched unrelated donor (MUD) BMT 14
  chronic granulocytic leukaemia (CGL) 68
Mathé, George 10
melanoma chemotherapy plus autologous BMT 90–91, *92*
melphalan 40
  breast cancer therapy *84*
  chemotherapy conditioning 106, 163
  conditioning for multiple myeloma BMT 72, 73
  fertility effects 196
  melanoma therapy 90
  ovarian carcinoma therapy 85, 86
  pre-graft ablation 161
renal function 198
  solid tumours of childhood 96
meningitis 181
  aseptic *184*
  bacterial *183*
  Listeria monocytogenes 182
2-mercaptoethane sulphonate sodium (MESNA) 163
6-mercaptopurine 66
Merocyanine 450 121
methotrexate 11, 13
  acute lymphoblastic leukaemia maintenance therapy 66
  breast cancer therapy 80
  familial haemophagocytic lymphohistiocytosis 57
  GvHD in aplastic anaemia BMT 52
  GvHD prophylaxis 44, 64, 145–6
  idiopathic pneumonitis 178
β_2-microglobulin 73
microspheres, monodispersed magnetic *124*, 125–6
mitoxantrone 86
mixed lymphocyte culture (MLC) 9
monoclonal antibodies (MAb)
  pretransplant immunosuppression 57
  purging techniques 123–7
  solid-phase matrix attachment 125
monocyte-macrophage system congenital disorders 55, *56*
monocytic leukaemia *63*
Morquio's disease (MPS-IV) *26*
  sickle cell anaemia 44
mucopolysaccharidosis I 20, 21
mucopolysaccharidosis II *25*
mucopolysaccharidosis III 21, 26
mucopolysaccharidosis IV *26*
mucopolysaccharidosis VI *27*
Mucor cerebral infection *181*
mucositis 162, 163
  oral 188
  oropharyngeal 171
multiple myeloma 72–3
  conditioning therapy 72
  survival 72
myasthenia gravis 198
Mycoplasma pneumonia 171

myelo-ablation
  pretransplant for primary immunodeficiency diseases 56
  thalassaemia 40
myelodysplastic syndromes 64

N
National Blood Transfusion Service 14
natural killer (NK) cells 145
needle biopsy 191
neoplastic cell cytotoxic conditioning 161
nephrotoxic agents 198
neuroblastoma 97
neuroblastoma cells
  identification *118*, 121
  IgG MAbs 125–6
neurological deficit 43
neurological disorders 198
neutropenia
  bacterial sepsis 197
  cerebral infections 181
nitrosoureas 161
Nocardia cerebral infection 182, *183*
non-Hodgkin's lymphoma 69, 70–71, 71–2
  aggressive 71
  survival 71
  thalassaemia BMT 40
non-IgG isotype 73
non-tunnelled lines 130

O
oesophageal stricture 33
OKT3 149
oligonucleotides 118, *119*
  antisense 121
ophthalmic complications of BMT 196
ostemoyelitis, clavicle 135
osteonecrosis 198
osteopetrosis 55, 56
  skeletal abnormalities 58
osteoporosis 198
ovarian cancer
  chemotherapy plus autologous BMT *83*, 85–6
  combination chemotherapy 80
oxymethalone 32

P
pancytopenia *28*, 30
  after BMT 129
  aplastic anaemia 49, 51
papovirus-JC infection 184
parainfluenza virus 174
patient conditioning 155–65
  chemotherapy 161–5
  total body irradiation 155-6, *157*, 158–9
penicillin 197
pentoxiphylline 80, 150
peripheral blood stem cell (PBSC) transplant
  chronic granulocytic leukaemia (CGL) 68
  Hodgkin's lymphoma 70
  multiple myeloma 73
peripheral blood stem cells (PBSC)
  cryopreservation 114
  reinfusion 106
phaeochromocytoma cells 121
Philadelphia chromosome 65, 67
phlebotomy 42
photoactive agent selective uptake 121
photofrin 121
PIXY-321 77
plasma depletion of bone marrow 110

plasmapheresis in bone marrow processing 110
platinum compounds 164
pluripotent progenitor cell selection techniques 128
pluripotent stem cells 13, 16
  absent 56
  disease 64
Pneumocystis carinii 171
  pneumonia 176–7, 197
pneumonitis
  idiopathic 177–8
  parainfluenza 174
  respiratory syncitial virus 173–4
pneumonitis, interstitial 162, 163, 196
  aplastic anaemia BMT 51, 52
  cytomegalovirus 171
polymerase chain reaction (PCR) 118, *119*
polyneuropathy 198
Pompe's disease *28*
pregnancy 196
Pseudomonas 171
puberty 196
  thalassaemia 38, 43
pulmonary artery *137*
pulmonary complications 168–78
  embolus 170
  haemorrhage 170
  infections 170–78
  long-term 178
  oedema 170
pulmonary embolus 170
pulmonary fibrosis *177*, *178*
pulmonary haemorrhage 170
pulmonary infection
  bacterial 170–71
  fungal 174–6
  idiopathic pneumonitis 177-8
  viral 171–4
pulmonary oedema 170
pulmonary thromboembolism 137
purine nucleoside phosphorylase (PNP) deficiency 59
  gene therapy 60
pyrimethamine 183

R
radiotherapy unit modification 155–6
rectal biopsy 190
red cell depletion 109–10
red cell production, inherited defects 37–40, *41*, 42–6
  thalassaemia 37–40, *41*, 42–3
red cells, filtered 38
renal function 198
respiratory function effects of BMT 196
respiratory syncitial virus (RSV) 173–4
reticular dysgenesis 56
ribavirin 174
ricin 123–4
Ricinus communis 123
right atrial catheters 130, 135

S
San Filippo's disease (MPS-III) 26–7
scleroderma 187, 189, 195
Seldinger technique 132
Senegal haplotype 46
sepsis, central venous catheters 130
Serratia 171
severe combined immunodeficiency disease (SCID) 11, 15, 19
  BMT outcome 59
  bone marrow transplants 55
  GvHD 57–8

SCID *cont*
  IL-1 deficiency 56
sexual dysfunction 42–3
sicca syndrome 196
sickle cell anaemia 43–6
  BMT 44–6
  conditioning 44
  life expectancy 44
skin
  chronic GvHD 194
  GvHD manifestations 185, 186–7
  histological features of GvHD 189, *190*
  lichenoid features 189
small non-cleaved cell lymphoma (SNCCL) 71
solid tumours 77–82, *83–4*, 85–6, *87*, 88–91, 93, *94*, 95–7
  chemotherapy plus autologous BMT 82–97
  of childhood 96–7
  dose escalation of drugs 79–80
  dose-response effect 77–8, 80–81
  recurrence 197
  see also brain tumours; breast cancer; germ cell tumours; melanoma; ovarian cancer
spleen
  sickle cell anaemia BMT *45*
  storage material reduction 29
splenectomy *28*, 29
splenomegaly *28*
Staphylococcus 171
  coagulase-negative 135
stem cells
  clonogenic assay 112, *113*
  cryopreservation 110, *111*, 112, *113*, 114, *115*
  cryopreservation quality control 114
  engraftment 56
  growth factor 77
  liquid nitrogen storage 112
  recovery 109
  transplants 14
Sternberg-Reed binucleated giant cells 69
sternum, bone marrow aspiration 104–5
steroids 148
streptavidin columns 127
Streptococcus 171
Streptococcus pneumoniae cerebral infection 182, *183*
streptokinase 136
stroke 43, 44
Strongyloides stercoralis 184
subclavian vein occlusion 137
subclavian venepuncture 130
  pleural injury 134
sulphadiazine 183
superior vena caval perforation 137
syngeneic BMT
  GvHD 144–5
  relapse 161
  T-cell depletion 115
  for GvHD attenuation 68
  GvHD prevention 148–9
  leukaemia survival 143

T
T-cell function, post-transplant 58
T-cell leukaemia purging 124
T-helper cells 12
teniposide 96
testicular carcinoma 86, *87–8*, 89–90
thalassaemia 37–40, *41*, 42-3
  BMT 38–9
  complications of BMT 40, *41*, 42–3
  cytomegalovirus (CMV) 39
  donors 39–40

thalassaemia *cont*
  hepatitis 39
  heterozygous donors 40
  HIV positivity 39
  inheritance 40
  preparative regime for BMT 40
  prognosis 37
  rejection of graft 40
ß-thalassaemia major 15
thalassaemia major
  liver biopsy *38*
  pre-graft ablation 161
  skull *37*
  survival *37*
thiotepa
  brain tumour therapy 93, *94*, 95
  breast cancer therapy 80, *83*
  chemotherapy conditioning 164
  melanoma therapy 90
  ovarian carcinoma therapy 85, 86
Thomas, E Donnall 9, 10–11
thrombosis
  central venous catheters 136–7
  implantable devices 138
  large-vessel 136–7
  preceding extravasation 138
  superior vena caval obstruction 132
thrombus formation
  catheter removal 135
  non-tunnelled lines 130
  right atrial 137
thumbs, Fanconi anaemia 31
thyroid stimulating hormone (TSH) 198
thyroid-releasing hormone (TRH) 198
thyroiditis, autoimmune 198
tissue typing 11–12
tongue hypertrophy *32*
Toxoplasma 52
  cerebral infection 182, *183*
transaminase 188
trimethoprim 177
trimetrexate 146, 148
Trypanosoma 52, *53*
tumour cells
  chemical separation methods 122
  immunological separation methods 123–8
  physical separation methods *120*, 121
  removal from bone marrow 117–18, *119*, 120
tunelled lines 130–31
twitcher mice 20, *21*

U
umbilical cord blood 58
upper airway obstruction *27*
urokinase 136

V
V-abl viral oncogene 67
vanishing bile duct syndrome 191
veno-occlusive disease, hepatic 162, 163
venous access 129–38
  central venous catheters 130–38
  implantable devices 138
  inadequate 129
  purposes 129
ventricular dilatation *25*
vinblastine 81, 85
VP-16 122

W
Wiskott-Aldrich syndrome 55, 56, 59

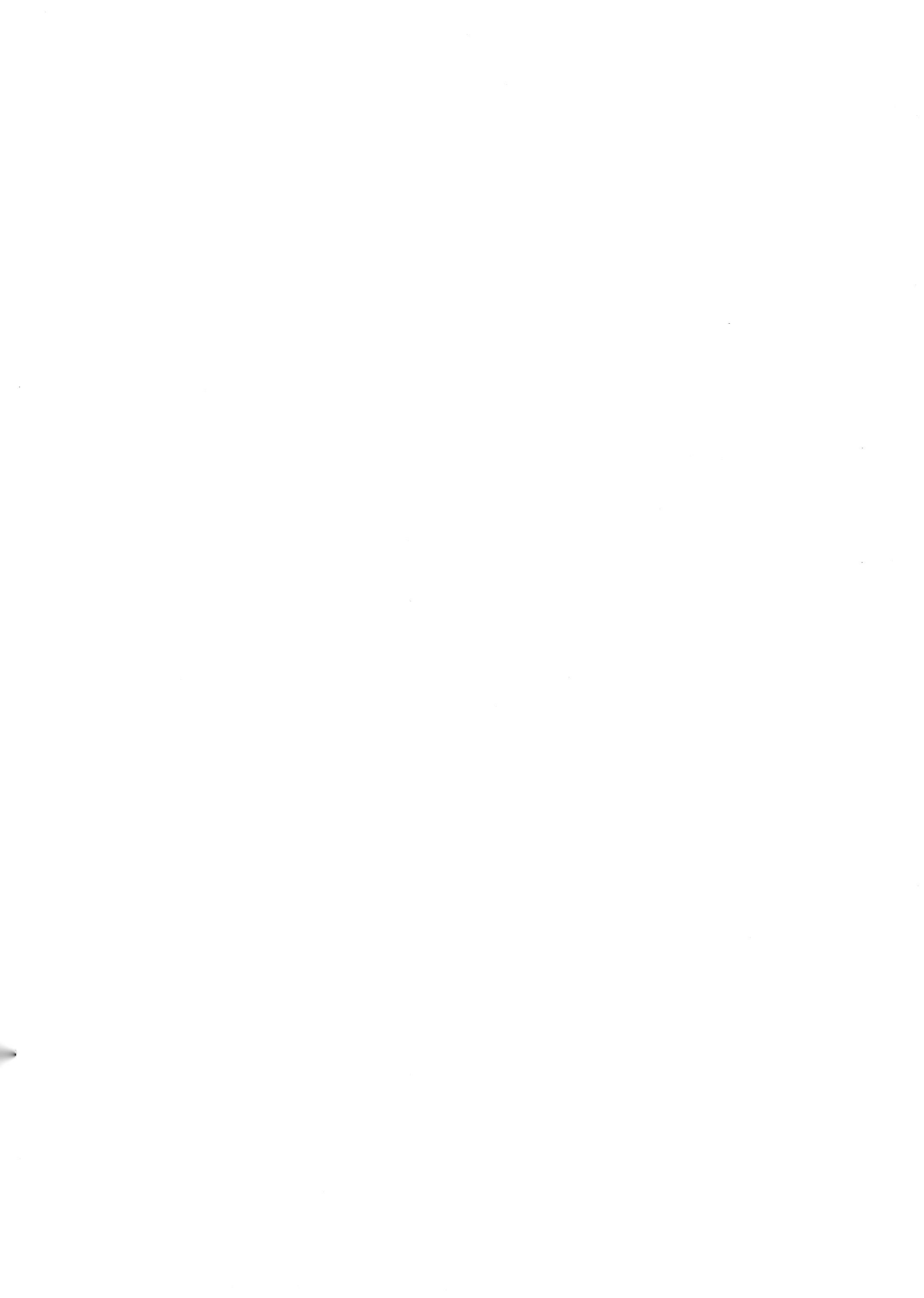